# Psychotherapy Is Worth It

## A Comprehensive Review of Its Cost-Effectiveness

*Edited by*

# Susan G. Lazar, M.D.

**The Committee on Psychotherapy
Group for the Advancement of Psychiatry**

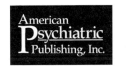

American **Psychiatric** Publishing, Inc.

Washington, DC
London, England

If you would like to buy between 25 and 99 copies of this or any other APPI title, you are eligible for a 20% discount; please contact APPI Customer Service at appi@psych.org or 800-368-5777. If you wish to buy 100 or more copies of the same title, please e-mail us at bulksales@psych.org for a price quote.

Copyright © 2010 American Psychiatric Publishing, Inc.
ALL RIGHTS RESERVED

Manufactured in the United States of America on acid-free paper
14  13  12  11  10    5  4  3  2  1
First Edition

Typeset in Adobe's Janson and Shannon.

American Psychiatric Publishing, Inc.
1000 Wilson Boulevard
Arlington, VA 22209-3901
www.appi.org

**Library of Congress Cataloging-in-Publication Data**
Psychotherapy is worth it : a comprehensive review of its cost-effectiveness / edited by Susan G. Lazar. — 1st ed.
    p. ; cm.
  Includes bibliographical references and index.
  ISBN 978-0-87318-215-7 (pbk. : alk. paper)
  1. Mental illness—Treatment. 2. Cost effectiveness. I. Lazar, Susan G., 1944–
II. American Psychiatric Publishing.
  [DNLM: 1. Mental Disorders—therapy. 2. Psychotherapy—economics.
3. Cost-Benefit Analysis. 4. Treatment Outcome. WM 420 P974355 2010]
  RC475.P736 2010
  616.89—dc22

                                                            2009052593

**British Library Cataloguing in Publication Data**
A CIP record is available from the British Library.

# Contents

Contributors . . . . . . . . . . . . . . . . . . . . . . . . . . . . .v

Acknowledgments . . . . . . . . . . . . . . . . . . . . . . . .vii

**1** Introduction . . . . . . . . . . . . . . . . . . . . . . . . . . 1
*Susan G. Lazar, M.D.*
*William H. Sledge, M.D.*
*Gerald Adler, M.D.*

**2** Psychotherapeutic and Psychosocial Interventions
in Schizophrenia: Clinical Outcomes and
Cost-Effectiveness . . . . . . . . . . . . . . . . . . . . . . . 31
*Lawrence H. Rockland, M.D.*

**3** Psychotherapy in the Treatment of Borderline
Personality Disorder. . . . . . . . . . . . . . . . . . . . . . 61
*Robert J. Waldinger, M.D.*

**4** Psychotherapy in the Treatment of Posttraumatic
Stress Disorder . . . . . . . . . . . . . . . . . . . . . . . . . 87
*Susan G. Lazar, M.D.*
*William Offenkrantz, M.D.*

**5** Psychotherapy in the Treatment of Anxiety
Disorders . . . . . . . . . . . . . . . . . . . . . . . . . . . 103
*Allan Rosenblatt, M.D.*

**6** Psychotherapy in the Treatment of Depression. . . 135
*Susan G. Lazar, M.D.*

**7** Psychotherapy and Psychosocial Interventions
in the Treatment of Substance Abuse . . . . . . . . 175
*William H. Sledge, M.D.*
*James Hutchinson, M.D.*

**8** Psychotherapy for Patients With Medical
Conditions . . . . . . . . . . . . . . . . . . . . . . . . . . 227
*William H. Sledge, M.D.*
*Joel Gold, M.D.*

**9** Psychotherapy for Children and Adolescents . . . . 267
*Jules Bemporad, M.D.*

**10** The Place of Long-Term and Intensive
Psychotherapy . . . . . . . . . . . . . . . . . . . . . . . 289
*Allan Rosenblatt, M.D.*

**11** Epilogue . . . . . . . . . . . . . . . . . . . . . . . . . . 311
*William H. Sledge, M.D.*
*Susan G. Lazar, M.D.*
*Robert J. Waldinger, M.D.*

Subject Index . . . . . . . . . . . . . . . . . . . . . . . . 315

Index of Treatment Studies . . . . . . . . . . . . . . . 341

# Contributors

**Susan G. Lazar, M.D., Volume Editor**
Past Chair, Committee on Psychotherapy, Group for the Advancement of Psychiatry; Clinical Professor of Psychiatry, Georgetown University School of Medicine, George Washington University School of Medicine, and Uniformed Services University of the Health Sciences; Supervising and Training Analyst, Washington Psychoanalytic Institute

## The Committee on Psychotherapy
## Group for the Advancement of Psychiatry

**William H. Sledge, M.D.**
Chair, Committee on Psychotherapy, Group for the Advancement of Psychiatry
Deputy Chair for Clinical Affairs and Program Development and George D. and Esther S. Gross Professor of Psychiatry, Yale University School Of Medicine, New Haven, Connecticut

**Gerald Adler, M.D.**
Training and Supervising Analyst, Boston Psychoanalytic Society and Institute, Boston, Massachusetts

**Jules Bemporad, M.D.**
Clinical Professor of Psychiatry, New York Medical College, Valhalla, New York

**Joel Gold, M.D.**
Clinical Assistant Professor of Psychiatry, New York University School of Medicine, New York, New York

**James Hutchinson, M.D.**
Teaching Analyst, Baltimore Washington Institute of Psychoanalysis, Washington, D.C.

**Susan G. Lazar, M.D.**
Past Chair, Committee on Psychotherapy, Group for the Advancement of Psychiatry; Clinical Professor of Psychiatry, Georgetown University School of Medicine, George Washington University School of Medicine, and Uniformed Services University of the Health Sciences; Supervising and Training Analyst, Washington Psychoanalytic Institute

**William Offenkrantz, M.D.**
Training and Supervising Analyst, Southwest Psychoanalytic Institute, Tucson

**Lawrence H. Rockland, M.D.**
Associate Professor of Clinical Psychiatry Emeritus, Weill Cornell College of Medicine, New York, New York

**Allan Rosenblatt, M.D. (deceased)**
Supervising and Training Analyst, San Diego Psychoanalytic Institute; Clinical Professor, Department of Psychiatry, University of California, San Diego Medical School, La Jolla, California

**Robert J. Waldinger, M.D.**
Associate Professor of Psychiatry, Harvard Medical School; Director, The Laboratory of Adult Development, Brigham and Women's Hospital, Boston, Massachusetts

*The following authors have no competing interests to report:*

Gerald Adler, M.D.
Jules Bemporad, M.D.
Joel Gold, M.D.
James Hutchinson, M.D.
Susan G. Lazar, M.D.
William Offenkrantz, M.D.
Lawrence H. Rockland, M.D.
William H. Sledge, M.D.
Robert J. Waldinger, M.D.

# Acknowledgments

The Editor is especially grateful for the unflagging support of co-author and current Chair of the Committee on Psychotherapy, Group for the Advancement of Psychiatry and Yale University School of Medicine George D. and Esther S. Gross Professor of Psychiatry, William H. Sledge, M.D.; for the help from his assistants Angelina Wing and Christine Holmberg; and the support of the George D. and Esther S. Gross Professorship Endowment.

The Editor could not have completed this volume without the invaluable help of her assistant, Susan P. Priester.

The Committee on Psychotherapy, Group for the Advancement of Psychiatry also wishes to acknowledge a grant for the support of this volume from the American Psychoanalytic Foundation.

# 1 | Introduction

Susan G. Lazar, M.D.
William H. Sledge, M.D.
Gerald Adler, M.D.

## Mental Illness and Psychotherapy: Background to Considerations of Cost-Effectiveness

This volume investigating the cost-effectiveness of psychotherapy examines many aspects of psychotherapeutic interventions for the major psychiatric diagnoses. Many variables affect the decision to provide psychotherapy. Often psychotherapy's efficacy and its ameliorative effect on patients' distress, functioning, family life, and work capacity are not well appreciated. This volume explores the costs of providing psychotherapy in relationship to the impact of psychotherapy both on health and on the costs of psychiatric illness and related conditions. Its intended audience includes psychotherapists, psychiatric benefits providers, policy makers, and others interested in the efficacy and impact on costs of providing psychotherapeutic treatments.

### Epidemiology of Mental Illness

According to the World Health Organization (2008), mental illness is the leading cause of global disability and the most important cause of disability, as represented by years lived with disability (YLDs), in adults ages 15 and over, accounting for one-third of YLDs in all regions. Substance abuse is the second leading cause of global disability. Neuropsychiatric disorders,

1

which include mental illness and substance use disorders, are more significant contributors to disease burden worldwide than are other noncommunicable diseases such as heart disease and cancer. Mood disorders including depression are a leading cause of disability for men and women, anxiety is an important cause in women, and alcohol and drug use disorders are disproportionately high in men. Schizophrenia and related psychotic disorders are the fourth leading cause of all disability in developed countries and the ninth leading cause of disability in people ages 19–44 worldwide.

The burden of mental illness in the United States and the enormous associated costs to society as a whole constitute a chronic, insufficiently recognized crisis in the health of the nation. Over a lifetime, 50% of the population will suffer from at least one psychiatric disorder (Kessler et al. 1994, 2005a), and every year in the United States, nearly 30% of the adult population over the age of 18 has a diagnosable psychiatric disorder. In a given year, of all patients with anxiety, mood, impulse control, and substance abuse disorders, only 41.1% receive treatment, 22.8% from a general medical provider, 16% from a nonpsychiatrist mental health provider, and only 12.3% from a psychiatrist. Of the patients treated, only 32.7% received minimally adequate treatment, with the likelihood of receiving minimally adequate care being highest in the mental health service sector and lowest in the general medical sector, which treats the majority of these mentally ill patients. In fact, most people with mental disorders in the United States remain untreated or poorly treated (Wang et al. 2005a, 2005b). However, despite the greater likelihood of receiving adequate care from the mental health service sector, an assessment of shifts in the pattern of mental health provider profile from that measured in the National Comorbidity Survey (1990–1992) compared with that measured in the more recent National Comorbidity Survey Replication (2001–2003) reveals that the general medical only profile has experienced the largest proportional increase (153%) between the two surveys and is now the most common provider of mental health services. The psychiatry profile increased 29%, as did the general medical in combination with other mental health specialty profile, which increased 72% (Wang et al. 2006).

In 1985 the cost of mental illness was $273 billion per year (Rice et al. 1990), including treatment costs, law enforcement costs, reduced productivity, and mortality. According to a different and less inclusive accounting, a 1999 report of the Surgeon General estimated the cost in 1996 of the direct treatment of mental disorders in the United States at $99 billion and the indirect costs at $79 billion, mostly from lost productivity secondary to illness and lesser amounts in lost productivity due to premature death or incarceration and for the time of individuals providing family care (U.S. Department of Health and Human Services 1999). Overall mental illness costs account for approximately 7% of total health care expenditures in the United States. In addition, the indirect costs of mental illness are substantially higher than the direct costs and account for 2% of U.S. gross domestic product (Hu 2006).

## Anxiety Disorders

The most prevalent psychiatric illness is the group of anxiety disorders, which affect 18.1% of adult Americans every year (Kessler et al. 2005b, 2006) and 28.8% of the population at some time during their lifetime (Kessler et al. 2005a). In addition, 22% of all children and adolescents have an anxiety disorder (Kashani and Orvaschel 1990).

The annual cost of anxiety disorders in 1990 was $42.3 billion or $1,542 per patient. The total includes $23 billion (54% of the total) in nonpsychiatric medical care costs, $13.3 billion (31%) in psychiatric treatment costs, $4.1 billion (10%) in indirect workplace costs, $1.2 billion (3%) in mortality costs, and $0.8 billion (2%) in prescription drug costs. Of the $256 in workplace costs per worker with anxiety, 88% is due to lost productivity at work as opposed to absenteeism (Greenberg et al. 1999).

## Affective Disorders

Affective disorders affect 19.3% of the U.S. population at some point in their lives, with major depression being the most common diagnosis affecting 17.1% of adults (Kessler et al. 1994) or 16.6% in the more recent National Comorbidity Survey Replication (Kessler et al. 2005a). Mood disorders also affect children and adolescents, with up to 2.5% of children and up to 8.3% of adolescents suffering from depression (Birmaher et al. 1996). In fact, suicide is the second leading cause of death in adolescent males (Centers for Disease Control 1986). Depression has a serious negative impact on a patient's functioning and well-being that is comparable to or worse than that of eight other serious chronic medical conditions, including back complaints, hypertension, diabetes, advanced coronary artery disease, angina, arthritis, pulmonary disease, and gastrointestinal disease (Wells et al. 1992).

The annual cost of depression in 1990 was $43.7 billion (Greenberg et al. 1993). In a 10-year update of this study (Greenberg et al. 2003), it was found that while the treatment rate of depression increased by over 50%, its economic burden rose only 7% from $77.4 billion in 1990 (inflation adjusted dollars) to $83.1 billion in 2001. Of the total, $26.1 billion (31%) were direct medical costs, $5.4 billion (7%) were suicide-related mortality costs, and $51.5 billion (62%) were losses in the workplace.

## Trauma and Abuse

Childhood trauma and abuse are important causes of psychiatric illness in the United States, leading to dissociative disorders and borderline personality disorders affecting 5% and 1.8% of the population, respectively (Swartz et al. 1990). The 12-month prevalence of posttraumatic stress disorder (PTSD) in American adults over the age of 18 is 3.5% (Kessler et al. 2005b) with a lifetime prevalence of 6.8% (Kessler et al. 2005a). One-third of all Vietnam war veterans have suffered from PTSD, and this group has twice as much divorce, homelessness, and substance abuse as those without PTSD. Over one-third of those with PTSD committed six or more acts of violence during 1 year, and nearly half are arrested or jailed at least once. Vietnam veterans with PTSD are five times as likely to be unemployed and three times as likely to have four or more chronic health problems as Vietnam veterans without PTSD (Kulka et al. 1988 ). For returning Iraq and Afghanistan war veterans, 14% screen positive for PTSD and 14% for major depression, and only about half of these have sought help from a physician or a mental health provider for their mental health problem in the past year (Tanielian and Jaycox 2008). Nearly 40% (Breslau et al. 1991) of inner-city residents experience severe trauma and nearly one-fourth of these develop PTSD. One-third of American females experience sexual abuse of incest, date rape, or other molestation (Russell 1984). One-fifth of rape victims attempt suicide (Kilpatrick et al. 1985). Criminally victimized women visit physicians twice as often as nonvictimized women, with two and a half times the medical costs (Koss 1991). Sexually abused children have high rates of anxiety, fear, sexually transmitted disease, suicide attempts, and borderline personality disorder (Briere and Runtz 1988; Friederich 1988; Herman et al. 1989; Schetky 1990).

## Other Diagnostic Groups

Of other diagnostic groups, 14.6% of the population suffers at some point during their lifetime from a substance abuse disorder abusing alcohol (18.6.%) or drugs (10.9%) (Kessler et al. 2005a). Antisocial personality disorder affects 3.5% of the population and schizophrenia affects 1% (Kessler et al. 1994).

The average prevalence of a psychiatric diagnosis among American workers is 18.2%. Psychiatric illness in the workforce accounts for significant work loss days (6 per month per 100 workers) and work cutback days (31 per month per 100 workers). The 3.7% of the workforce with more than one psychiatric disorder accounts for 49 work loss days and 346 work cutback days per month per 100 workers. Workers with only one diagnosis (14.5%) have 11 work loss days and 66 work cutback days per 100 workers.

These work losses compare starkly with the 81.8% of American workers with no psychiatric diagnosis who experience 2 work loss days and 11 work cutback days per month per 100 workers. It is clear that work impairment is a serious adverse consequence of psychiatric illness (Kessler and Frank 1997). In the National Comorbidity Survey Replication, an estimated 53.4% of American adults reported one or more of the mental or physical conditions assessed in the survey. These respondents reported an average of 32.1 more disability days in the past year than matched controls, with mental conditions accounting for more than half as many disability days as all physical conditions (Merikangas et al. 2007). Other findings from the National Comorbidity Survey Replication demonstrated that in 2002 American workers with serious mental illness in the preceding 12 months had earnings that averaged $16,306 less than other matched control respondents for a societal-level total of $193.2 billion (Kessler et al. 2008). Examining all American workers with mental illness, Marcotte and Wilcox-Gok (2001) estimated that mental illness decreases annual income by an amount between $3,500 and $6,000.

## Concepts of Mental Illness

The concept of mental illness is complex and involves an interplay of environmental, cultural, and biological factors. In addition, the definitions of mental illness can change over time and depend partly on a culture's view of what behavior is considered deviant. For example, hallucinations in some cultures are parts of religious experiences that are integrated into the basic structure of that culture rather than a possible manifestation of psychosis. A more current example of a cultural reappraisal of behavior that has been considered pathological is the debate over the past 25 years about homosexuality as a mental disorder or as a normal behavioral variant. During that period, the diagnosis of homosexuality as psychopathology was dropped from the *Diagnostic and Statistical Manual of Mental Disorders* prepared by the American Psychiatric Association. Discussions about homosexuality also illustrate changing perspectives of causation, moving from a certainty about environmental factors to a greater emphasis on a possible biological role as well as interactions between biology and environment.

Medical illness, in contrast to mental illness, can usually be more easily defined as a distinct syndrome, even though specifics are refined as more knowledge is accumulated. As an example, the importance of hypertension and its relationship to heart disease have been known for many years. New knowledge about medical illnesses leads to greater understanding of mechanisms of disease and treatment. For instance, the blood pressure level previously seen as normal has been lowered in recent years, but the basic understanding of hypertension and heart disease has remained intact. And while hereditary and environmental factors contributing to a predisposition to illness are more understood, cultural factors of stigma are largely irrelevant, in contrast to attitudes about mental illness.

Also important to this discussion is the way people minimize or deny the interconnection of the psyche and the soma in distinguishing between "mental illness" and "physical illness." In today's climate, with a biological emphasis, there is often a splitting off of emotional factors that interact with the biological. This biological approach also places some psychiatric illness into the physical illness category. In addition, within this framework, those mental illnesses with significant biological components are often treated with drugs alone, at times accompanied by the expectation that most psychopharmacologic treatments will be brief and inexpensive. Mental illness not seen as biological will often receive no treatment. However, evidence is growing that demonstrates the relevance of emotional factors and the use of psychotherapeutic interventions with illnesses clearly viewed as only or largely physical. For example, the work of Spiegel et al. (1989) and Lemieux et al. (2006) with women with metastatic breast cancer demonstrates the effectiveness of group psychotherapy in improving these patients' symptoms. Such studies illustrate the need for research on the impact of emotion and trauma, as well as the effect of psychotherapy on the immune system. Relatedly, Fawzy (1993) demonstrated the beneficial impact of a brief group therapy intervention for malignant melanoma patients who responded with improved natural killer cell levels and decreased mortality. In addition, Ornish (1990) showed that coronary heart disease can be reversed by a program that utilizes a combined approach, including extended group psychotherapy as well as exercise and diet.

Even though it is hard to clarify the multiple factors that lead to mental illness, there exist important attempts to develop pragmatic categories for clinicians and researchers. The most widely used current classification of mental illness consists of disorders defined in the *Diagnostic and Statistical Manual of Mental Disorders*, revised on a regular basis by a committee of the American Psychiatric Association, and presently in its fourth major revision (American Psychiatric Association 2000). DSM-IV-TR divides mental disorders into two axes: Axis I consists of all mental disorders with the exception of personality disorders and mental retardation. It thus includes such disorders as schizophrenia and other psychotic disorders, mood disorders, anxiety disorders, and eating disorders. Axis II defines categories of personality disorders (i.e., constellations of personality characteristics that are beyond the range of those considered within normal boundaries) and also includes mental retardation. DSM-IV-TR provides a way of collecting statistical data and sufficiently clear definitions for research purposes. Although the committees defining the different disorders do field trials to validate the clarity and use-fulness of these categories, the categories are also the work of clinicians and researchers influenced by their training and knowledge, the traditions of their training programs, and the influence of their cultural experiences. The evolution in these diagnostic categories of mental disorders is also determined by the advancing research knowledge in such areas as biology, early child-hood development, the impact of abuse and traumatic stress, and the results of biological and psychological treatment of mental disorders.

## Misconceptions, Stigma, and Prejudice With Respect to Psychiatric Patients

Western society often maintains a stoical work ethic that holds that people should be in control of their feelings, or even disregard them. Mental ill-ness, in this framework, demonstrates a failure of control. In addition to patients with severe mental illness, those patients with milder depressive disorders, character pathology, or reactions to a current stressor, such as the loss of a loved one, can readily be labeled as "the worried well" and seen as weak-willed and self-indulgent.

A frequent concern about these patients is the belief that their overuse of mental health services will deplete health care funds by the endless use of psychotherapy. These prejudices about mental illness contribute to insur-ance practices that seek greater limitations for inpatient and outpatient mental health services than for other medical treatment.

Inadequacy of psychiatric services including psychotherapy coverage in health care insurance systems is well known and has a long and complex his-tory. Its clearest current manifestation is the lack of parity (i.e., equally avail-able medical services for mental as well as physical illness) in U.S. medical insurance programs. The beginnings of these health care discrepancies re-late in some degree to basic attitudes about mental illness in U.S. society and those with mental illness. There is a relatively sharp contrast between society's perception of a physical illness in contrast to a mental illness. It is easy to view physical illness as inevitable, occurring as a person ages or as a tragic occurrence striking a person down in early life. Except perhaps for those illnesses caused by an individual's behavior that can be seen as self-destructive, such as the role of obesity in heart disease or poor diabetes con-trol, feelings of shame or guilt are ameliorated by sympathy for the patient who is stricken. The sick role is accompanied by an institutionalized "for-giveness" of a patient's usual social role obligations, as well as by the expec-tation that the patient has not been able to control the condition and will seek competent medical help. In contrast, mental illness in a family often arouses intense shame and guilt in connection to the anticipated perception of weakness in the ill person as well as in family members. Contributing to these feelings is an ethic in the industrialized Western world that values self-sufficiency and self-control without evidence of shameful weakness. Mental illness can readily be viewed as a failure to function in the self-contained mature way that is expected. To have a mental illness implies that one has an insufficient will to function maturely or has even willfully given up.

The social stigma attached to the mentally ill can also spread to those who treat them. Because therapists usually meet with their patients alone in an atmosphere of protective confidentiality, the resulting aura of mystery makes it easy for both caregivers and patients to be the targets of society's fears. Moreover, these fears are fueled by the awareness that therapists tend to be interested in "unconscious processes." Fears of dark, unknown forces can be related to biblical and historical beliefs in possession by demons (Group for the Advancement of Psychiatry 1978). The religious component of the stigma therefore includes associations to sin, guilt, punishment, and possible divine retribution for some transgression. It is therefore not unusual for responses both to the mentally ill and to their therapists to be tinged with denigration, sarcasm, disgust, anxiety, and avoidance.

## Psychotherapy

Just as mental illness is relatively unrecognized and too often undertreated, so is the importance of psychotherapy as a treatment unrecognized as a low-cost, effective lever to decrease many kinds of costs caused by mental illness. The effectiveness of psychotherapy has been established for many conditions. In addition, there is a growing body of evidence that providing psychotherapy is cost-effective, reducing disability, morbidity, mortality, and at times leading to a reduction of medical and surgical services (Lazar and Gabbard 1997). Older studies indicating a cost-offset effect include those by Duehrssen and Jorswiek (1965), Follette and Cummings (1970), and Jones and Vischi (1979). A meta-analysis examining the outcomes of a group of 58 studies of medical cost offset after outpatient psychotherapy demonstrates that 85% of the studies found a decline in subsequent medical charges ranging from 10% to 33% (Mumford et al. 1984). A study of a medical plan in Columbia, Maryland, also found significant decreases in medical utilization after outpatient psychiatric care in both adults and children, with individual therapy showing more dramatic cost offset than group therapy (Kessler et al. 1982). And as subsequent chapters will show, newer studies of psychotherapy for specific diagnostic groups of patients generally demonstrate both its effectiveness and cost-effectiveness.

Compounding third-party payers' and the public's bias against psychiatric illnesses is the fact that *psychotherapy* can be an ambiguous word to the general population. The term *psychotherapy* can be used to define a spectrum that includes a whole range of treatments from psychoanalysis and intensive psychoanalytic psychotherapy to weekly supportive psychotherapy and monthly meetings with chronically psychotic individuals to help them comply with medical and social programs. There are several theoretical approaches to psychotherapy, chief among them cognitive-behavioral and psychodynamic. In addition, many clinicians often integrate varying aspects of these different orientations. In the absence of adequate education, it is therefore not surprising that the general population would have little knowledge about the broad range of psychotherapy treatment options, about who can benefit from them, and about what psychotherapeutic interventions are appropriate for a specific patient. These uncertainties may add fuel to prejudice that attributes a lack of self-control, self-indulgence, and malingering to the wide and disparate psychiatric patient population. In this volume, we define psychotherapy broadly as the treatment of one or more patients through the use of psychological processes, primarily mediated through talking. This treatment includes a therapeutic relationship and the use of a trained therapist. Thus, psychotherapy can include individual, family, and group treatment from a variety of theoretical orientations (McGrath and Lowson 1986).

Measuring exactly what is psychotherapy is also an important problem. The delivery of psychotherapy has also only recently become more or less standardized with the development of a few relatively specific and behaviorally oriented "manualized" approaches. Psychotherapy manuals offer a way to specify indications, goals, and specific techniques of psychotherapy in order to give a more standardized approach. This approach was born out of the necessity to develop reliable, objective, and measurable ways of providing psychotherapy in a standardized manner for research purposes. In addition to furthering research goals of measuring the impact of psychotherapy, these approaches have assisted in the clinical training of psychotherapy. However, the manualized approach has been criticized for its "cookbook" quality and for the fact that it can never truly substitute for the expertise of an experienced, dedicated clinician.

As we have described, a psychiatric population that is viewed as weak and self-indulgent may be expected not only to seek psychotherapy services needlessly but to never want to end them. These views have colored the concerns of both insurers and the general population, despite significant research that demonstrates that available psychotherapy services do not lead to overuse or abuse by a large population. More research about the effect of different treatments in various health care environments is required to address a number of issues.

## Psychotherapists

When we turn to the treatment of mental illness, we are also faced with a decision about the most appropriate caregiver, because there are mental health care providers with different backgrounds and professional training. Among mental health professionals, we can define four major categories, including psychiatrists, psychologists, social workers, and nurses, any of whom may serve as a primary caregiver to a given patient. Clinicians who work as psychotherapists can also be defined by their emphasis on a psychodynamic approach (from psychoanalysis) or a cognitive-behavioral orientation.

All licensed mental health professionals have an undergraduate college degree as well as specialty graduate training. Psychiatrists are physicians who have completed medical school and have had four additional graduate years of training in psychiatry, neurology, and medicine. In addition to varying amounts of psychotherapy training, they are the provider group with the medical knowledge to make differential diagnoses between psychological and medical illness, to understand their interaction, and to prescribe psychopharmacological medications in addition to conducting psychotherapy. Psychiatrists can also take a two-part examination offered by the American Board of Psychiatry and Neurology to become board certified. Many well-trained psychologists have doctoral-level graduate degrees, have had a clinical internship, and often have a postdoctoral year. They have had varying amounts of training in psychotherapy and in psychological testing. Social workers have had 2 years of graduate training, including some psychotherapy experience, and 1 year of supervised clinical work postgraduation. Nurses may have pursued postgraduate specialty training in psychotherapy, and some acquire prescriptive authority through advanced practice certification. All of the four groups of providers must pass state licensure requirements for their particular profession to practice independently. All four groups of mental health professionals include a spectrum of providers with varying degrees of training, skill, and experience conducting psychotherapy.

However, because of their emphasis on containing costs, many managed care programs employ mental health workers with no graduate training to function as psychotherapists, arousing considerable concern about the adequacy of the treatment provided. In addition, with respect to the spectrum of providers of psychotherapy, Mojtabai and Olfson (2008) examined a survey of practice patterns from 1996 to 2005 of office-based psychiatry practices in the United States that shows that psychiatrists are providing increasingly more pharmacotherapy and increasingly less psychotherapy. These trends appear to be associated with changes in patterns of reimbursement for psychotherapy, the rise of managed care, and the growth in the prescription of medications, allowed only for psychiatric physicians and some nurse practitioners. Furthermore, in this era of managed care and health maintenance organizations (HMOs), short-term treatment and biological approaches to the treatment of mental illness are stressed. While these approaches can provide adequate treatment for certain patients, those who require a more intensive course of psychotherapy, either alone or in conjunction with psychotropic medication, may be at risk.

# Considerations of Cost, Cost-Effectiveness, and Insurance Coverage for Psychotherapy

## Costs

One difficulty in establishing a broad and coherent policy to address the support of psychotherapy has been the measurement of the various dimensions in psychotherapy. For instance, only recently has there been a growing consensus about the clinical outcomes, including not only symptomatic relief but also the need to consider and measure the capacity for greater social and vocational performance and quality of life. In addition, the whole dimension of cost has only recently come to be an important feature in the measure of outcome of psychotherapy.

### Dimensions of Costs

Cost is a complex idea. In reference to medical treatments, cost represents the value of the effort to bring about a particular treatment with a certain result. Cost is the value of the resources being withdrawn from society to bring about a particular treatment. Cost-effective analyses are a tool for determining the relationship between the value of an effort to carry out an intervention and the value of the intervention's ultimate impact. Costs are to be distinguished from charges that are simply a manager's efforts to recoup costs based on considerations of cost, market, and regulatory compliance (Finkler 1982). The methodology for estimating total costs (of an intervention, program, etc.) is generally based on determining the unit cost of services and multiplying it by the amount of such services consumed (Gold 1996; Weisbrod 1983; Weisbrod et al. 1980; Wolff 1998). However, there are methodological choices that vastly and differently influence how these costs are determined. One major issue is the perspective of the study that determines the breadth of what is being examined. Different perspectives include: 1) only the resources furnished by the provider (the *management* perspective), 2) all the explicit resource costs associated with production of the services (the *accountant* perspective), or 3) all explicit and implicit resource costs that would address opportunity costs such as those for resources that are both donated or already owned (the *economist* or *societal* perspective). For example, the management perspective of costs of developing a psychotherapy service in a public sector outpatient clinic would include, among other things, the number, type, and hours of the psychotherapists assigned to or hired for such a service; the amount of electricity and other utilities they consumed; and the cost of their malpractice insurance. The accountant would add the cost of the management of those services, as well as various other overhead expenses allocated to this function indirectly but directly incurred by the institution for doing business as an institution, such as the need to provide parking for all the workers, a security force, and so on. The economist would also consider the opportunity costs of using the resources (such as real estate, equipment, personnel) differently (even if they were "donated" without direct cost to the institution), as well as other hidden costs, such as the fact that the supervision of the staff was provided free to the institution and in exchange for a faculty appointment by another institution (Wolff 1998; Wolff et al. 1997).

In addition, production characteristics are also important in the methodology of determining unit costs. When an agency produces many different services, there are costs not directly attributable to the service in question but that are necessary to the agency's capacity to provide service. These include explicit as well as implicit off-budget agency costs such as, for example, the time and effort of management to lobby the legislature for increased mental health services. Furthermore, different programs within an agency may use different production strategies to produce similar treatments (Wolff 1998; Wolff et al. 1997). For instance, long-term psychotherapy provided by social workers may have a different cost structure from long-term psychotherapy provided by psychiatrists.

The final issue concerning the measurement of unit costs concerns the precise definition of the service unit. Service units can be defined in terms of output criteria that measure the services received by clients, whereas input criteria measure the number of hours of staff effort. For example, if a therapist sees five patients during an hour-long group session, the group session can be counted as five client visits and five group hours or as one group hour depending on whether one chooses to measure in terms of output or input (Wolff 1998).

Furthermore, there are multiple types of costs in addition to production costs. In mental health studies it is customary to address maintenance costs for food, shelter, and other necessities for patients involved because some of the interventions (inpatient settings, some partial hospital programs) provide these services. Law enforcement costs are another type of cost that are relevant in considering the possible cost shifting when the criminal justice system is used as a substitute for the psychiatric system. Other well-known costs are the considerable cost shifting between psychiatric and other health care costs, the "family burden" that addresses the resources allocated by a patient's family to provide care, and "mortality costs" that represent an effort to express in monetary terms the value of a person's life (Weisbrod 1983; Weisbrod et al. 1980).

# Cost-Effectiveness

With the increasing emphasis of the cost dimensions of the provision of health care and the sensitivity to market and economic forces of modern-day health care, analyses of cost and effectiveness of psychiatric and other health care interventions are becoming increasingly more complex and sophisticated. What follows below is a brief introduction and overview of some of the issues in considering economic analyses such as cost-effectiveness or cost-benefit analysis.

Cost-benefit and cost-effectiveness analyses are similar ways to express the value of an intervention in relation to that of the effort to bring it about. Cost-benefit analyses seek to represent all dimensions of the cost-benefit equation in monetary values, whereas cost-effectiveness analyses do not necessarily require the expression of every outcome in monetary terms. Cost-effectiveness analyses are preferred in most health service approaches because of the difficulty in expressing the outcome variables of symptoms, quality of life, and mortality experience in monetary terms.

Nonetheless, a comprehensive cost-effectiveness analysis does attempt to take careful account of the economic benefits of a particular intervention in assessing net economic costs. Just as costs have multiple dimensions, so do benefits. As Weisbrod (1983; Weisbrod et al. 1980) noted, these benefits include increased earnings of the individual affected, changes in labor market behavior that address the ability and willingness of the individual to seek employment, and improvement in decision making about the use of expensive services, improved role functioning in terms of family and economic behavior, and improved physical and mental health. It is enormously difficult to measure these benefits economically and to express them in monetary terms.

"Cost-effective" does not mean "cheap." Cost-effectiveness refers to the value returned per dollar spent as opposed to cost reduction, which refers to dollars saved. Cost-effectiveness also refers to a measure of efficiency that can at times be improved by spending more and at times by spending less. Thus, a treatment may be more cost-effective than an alternative by virtue of being more effective for the same or lesser cost or by virtue of being equally or even less effective for a lesser cost. A treatment that is both more effective and more expensive can also be more cost-effective than an alternative if the increased effectiveness is judged to be greater than the increased cost. Thus, efficiency is not achieved simply by cost cutting because a treatment's effectiveness must also be taken into account. Focusing solely on cost reduction may actually result in increased inefficiency (Clark 1996).

Effectiveness, therefore, refers to the effect of an intervention in terms of bringing about desired outcomes. Efficiency is the ratio of the cost to benefits; for instance, in a cost-benefit analysis, an efficiency ratio of less than 1 means that the intervention actually makes money.

In more recent years, considerations of costs and cost-effectiveness have become increasingly sophisticated. A systematic cost-effectiveness analysis, for example, can be calculated using incremental cost-effectiveness ratios in which the costs and effects of an intervention can be expressed as a ratio of its incremental cost to its incremental effect for comparison with the incremental cost/effectiveness ratio of another intervention. Researchers now often also use more refined concepts such as cost-utility analysis, which examines the costs and effectiveness of therapies in terms of the *quality-adjusted life year*, which is a unit of effectiveness that expresses the impact of various therapeutic approaches on both the quantity and quality of life. Quality of life is measured in utilities or values of varying health states. Lower ratios for cost-utility analysis are more favorable, the most favorable being cost saving in a case where a therapy is both more effective and less costly than an alternative. The gold standard of cost-utility analysis is to report from a societal perspective that values all costs and effects in order to determine the best allocation of societal resources (Gold 1996; Pirraglia et al. 2004; Siegel et al. 1996; Weinstein et al. 1996). A measure of "disease burden"—the *disability-adjusted life year*, or DALY—is a quantitative measure of years lost from a healthy life by disability or premature death (Murray and Lopez 1996). The disability component of the DALY is *years lived with disability* (YLDs), and a researcher using this measurement is interested in the YLDs averted by the intervention being studied. The cost of an intervention being investigated divided by the number of YLDs averted is another way of comparing the cost-effectiveness of one treatment regimen with another (Issakidis et al. 2004).

In some of the studies reviewed, cost-effectiveness implies effectiveness plus some relative cost savings in comparison with other treatment approaches. In other studies, cost-effective interventions do not actually save money but provide a superior measure of effectiveness per dollar spent (e.g., cost-effective does not mean cheap or even necessarily money saving in this kind of example). In such an instance the concept of threshold becomes germane in that it indicates the cost limits of societal willingness to pay for an effective treatment; in other words, the acceptable costs that policy makers, benefit managers, and stakeholders are willing to pay per health value gained.

## Cost-Effectiveness Studies of Patient Groups With a Mixture of Diagnoses

A survey of the literature on the economic impact of psychotherapy published between 1984 and 1994 used the standard of cost-effectiveness (Gabbard et al. 1997). This review of 18 studies, 10 with random assignment and 8 without random assignment, found that 80% of the former and 100% of the latter suggested that psychotherapy reduces total costs. This review found that psychotherapy appears to be cost-effective, especially for patients with severe disorders, including schizophrenia, bipolar affective disorder, and borderline personality disorder, in that it leads to improved work functioning and decreased use of hospitalization.

Ideally, when considering cost-effectiveness, one should also consider the other indirect costs such as the lost work of disabled homemakers and the lost lives and productivity of patients who commit suicide. The last mentioned study, Gabbard et al. (1997), applied the standard of cost-effectiveness in its review of the relevant literature as a more appropriate standard by which to measure any medical treatment. In fact, the need to demonstrate cost savings in medical and surgical services, or cost offset, by virtue of providing psychotherapy, can be construed as a double standard for psychotherapy versus other kinds of medical treatment. For example, it would be hard to envision a requirement to demonstrate cost offset in other kinds of costs before providing medically indicated surgical and medical services. These are more likely to be accepted as necessary and valuable in and of themselves.

One study demonstrating substantial cost offset is a Bell South pilot project from 1991 to 1993 and also hints at the complex relationship between medical services utilization and costs and psychiatric services utilization and costs. Three thousand Bell South workers and their families were given psychiatric benefits, including two psychotherapy visits per week or a total of 52 visits a year, a lowered copayment for psychotherapy visits, partial psychiatric hospitalization services, and an employee assistance program (EAP). There were significant subsequent decreases in psychiatric inpatient stays (by 30%) as well as in both outpatient and inpatient medical and surgical services (by 78% and 87%, respectively). Total health care expenses per company member declined from $17 to $8 per month even though outpatient psychiatric services increased by 33% and partial psychiatric hospitalization increased by 45% (Saeman 1994).

Two other studies demonstrate cost-effectiveness by virtue of a reduction in lost workdays. Klarreich et al. (1998) found that providing rational-emotive psychotherapy through an EAP of one large company led to a decrease in absenteeism from 10 to 3 days per year per employee, equal to a decrease of $1,054 in the annual cost of absenteeism per employee. For each dollar spent on psychotherapy, the corporation saved $2.74. In a British study (Mynors-Wallis et al. 1997) with a randomized controlled design, problem-solving therapy by a trained nurse was provided for 70 primary care patients with concomitant psychiatric illness and the outcome was compared with the usual treatment delivered by a general practitioner. There was no difference in clinical outcome as measured by four structured clinical assessment measures. However, the patients who received the psychotherapy had fewer subsequent lost workdays that more than offset the cost of providing the therapy.

Equivocal results were found in a review article of all controlled trials completed before July 2005 comparing counseling in primary care with other treatments for patients with psychological and psychosocial problems considered suitable for counseling (Bower and Rowland 2006). Fifteen separate publications describing eight trials were included. The objectives of the review were 1) to identify all randomized controlled trials (RCTs) of counseling in primary care, 2) to assess clinical effectiveness of counseling in primary care by reviewing these RCTs, and 3) to assess cost-effectiveness by reviewing economic analyses of RCTs of counseling in primary care. (In this study, the definition of counseling is consistent with the definition of psychotherapy used in selecting studies for this volume.) The authors found that counseling provided modest improvement in short-term outcome compared with usual care but provided no additional advantages in the long term. Patients were generally more satisfied with counseling than patients were with usual care. Although some types of health care utilization may have been reduced, counseling did not appear to reduce overall health care costs. It was suggested that while counseling was significantly more effective in reducing psychological symptoms in the short term, longer initial treatment, maintenance treatments, booster sessions, or interventions aimed at improving social circumstances may bring about more long-term improvement.

A study by Chiesa et al. (2002) used three treatment approaches for a variety of personality disorders. The first group received a 1-year inpatient stay that included individual and group psychotherapy and no treatment after discharge. The second group received 6 months of inpatient treatment with individual and group psychotherapy followed by 18 months of twice-weekly group psychotherapy. The third group received general psychiatric care (treatment as usual, or TAU) of community services and no psychotherapy. The first two groups experienced both significant improvement and a significant decrease in total service costs (greater in the second group). Patients in the third group experienced neither improvement nor lowered total service costs. A significant association between symptomatic improvement and reduction in costs at follow-up was found in the first two groups of patients but not in the third general psychiatric care group. The significant associations between cost reductions and clinical outcome indicate that the first two treatment programs, which included psychotherapy, were more effective in reducing health care costs and were more cost-effective than treatment based on general psychiatric management without psychotherapy.

In a second publication from the same study, Beecham et al. (2006) reported additional conclusions from the data reported in Chiesa et al. (2002). Because patients with personality disorder place large burdens on health and social care resources, make more extensive use of psychiatric services than patients without personality disorder, and have higher prevalence rates (36%–67% of psychiatric hospital populations vs. 10%–13% of the adult population), it becomes important to demonstrate that effective treatment may reduce service use and service costs over time. Of the three treatment groups, the second group, the step-down treatment program, yielded the greatest psychosocial benefits. The cost and outcome results suggested that patients in the first two groups had better outcomes than those in the general psychiatric care group, but the first two treatment programs were also much more expensive. Again, the patients in the second, step-down group improved most overall. The shorter inpatient step-down treatment followed by community-based psychotherapeutic support was felt to be the most cost-effective approach for these patients.

## Insurance Coverage for Psychotherapy

### Some Effects of Insurance Coverage

A survey of German patients who had concluded a course of psychodynamic psychotherapy demonstrated that greater improvement was associated with a longer duration of treatment. In addition, compared with pretreatment levels, use of all medications, days in the hospital, physician visits, and lost work days all declined significantly after treatment (Dossmann et al. 1997). This German study tends to support the findings of a survey of 4,000 readers of *Consumer Reports* that also found a correlation of treatment duration with the degree of improvement. In addition, those patients whose treatment had been artificially limited in length or intensity by insurance and managed care plans reported worse outcomes ("Mental Health: Does Therapy Help?" 1995).

Several other large-scale actuarial studies of mixed populations do not tend to support concerns about the potential for abuse of generous benefits for the provision of psychotherapy. One such study of Australian and New Zealand mental health care delivery systems showed a 44% lower cost per capita in Australia, where there is much more readily available outpatient psychotherapy and insurance coverage than in New Zealand, which has a hospital-based system and little outpatient treatment (Andrews 1989). In the United States, a study of the CHAMPUS system (the insurance program for military dependents and retirees) demonstrated that instituting utilization review of inpatient care plus a great expansion of outpatient psychotherapy between 1989 and 1992 led to tremendous savings in hospital costs of $4 for every extra $1 spent on outpatient treatment (Zients 1993).

With respect to psychoanalysis, in Ontario, Canada, where psychoanalysis has been fully covered, the length of psychoanalytic treatment is no different from that of patients in New York City, where virtually no insurance covers psychoanalysis at a comparable level (Doidge et al. 1994). This study also demonstrated the high prevalence of trauma and early loss in the history of patients who require the long-term, in-depth treatment course of psychoanalysis and also reported that 82% of patients in psychoanalysis in Ontario had failed to improve with briefer and less intensive treatments. While there were no data about the efficacy of psychoanalysis for these patients, there are data about the much greater efficacy of psychoanalytic treatments for seriously disturbed latency-age children under the age of 11 (Target and Fonagy 1994). In this retrospective chart review of child patients seen at the Anna Freud Centre, more than half of the more seriously disturbed children in this age group failed to improve with once to three-times-weekly psychotherapy, whereas over 80% improved with a frequency of treatment of four to five times per week.

A broad survey of the utilization of outpatient psychotherapy in the United States in 1987 demonstrated that 3% of the population has been in outpatient therapy, with the poor and near-poor using long-term treatment in proportion to their numbers in the general population (Olfson and Pincus 1994a, 1994b). This finding, in particular, tends to disconfirm one common stereotype about psychotherapy: that it is an unnecessary self-indulgence used by the more affluent. The authors also found the same percentage of out-of-pocket expenditures among both long-term and short-term therapy users. While patients in long-term psychotherapy (over 20 sessions) are 16% of therapy patients and account for 63% of psychotherapy costs, sicker people consume more services in most other chronic medical conditions as well. In addition, long-term therapy patients were documented to be more distressed, in poorer general health, had higher general medical costs and more functional impairment, were more likely to need psychotropic medication, and were more likely to have a psychiatric hospitalization than short-term therapy patients (Olfson and Pincus 1994a, 1994b). These findings tend to suggest that patients in extended psychotherapy are in treatment because of their need, not, as has been suggested, to take unnecessary advantage of an overly generous insurance benefit. In fact, one study found that expenditures for mental health care exclusive of substance abuse had been about 8.5% of total health care costs over the prior 20 years (Hay Huggins 1990), with outpatient costs about 1.6% of total health care costs (Krizay 1990). In addition, despite widespread fear that readily available outpatient psychotherapy would be overused, a RAND study demonstrated that when weekly outpatient psychotherapy is fully covered, only 4.3% of the insured population uses it and the average length of treatment is 11 sessions (Manning et al. 1986). The RAND study, however, did not find a cost-offset effect, probably because there were very few hospitalizations in the population studied. Cost savings subsequent to psychotherapy are generally due to reduced hospital costs.

In an update of their 1994 study, Olfson et al. (2002) found no significant change in the overall rate of use of psychotherapy between 1987 (3.2 per 100 persons) and 1997 (3.6 per 100 persons). However, the number of visits per patient was significantly lower than 10 years prior, and there was a marked decline in the proportion of patients who received longer term psychotherapy, defined as more than 20 visits. This proportion of patients declined from 15.7% in 1987 to 10.3% in 1997. It was also found that a much larger percentage of psychotherapy patients (61.5%) were also receiving medication (especially antidepressants) than in 1987 (31.5%). Approximately one-third of psychotherapy patients received only one or two sessions. The authors concluded that much of the psychotherapy in the United States is shallow and of limited benefit. Despite the lack of change in the rate of use of psychotherapy, the decline in the number of psychotherapy visits suggests a decreasing emphasis on a psychotherapeutic approach.

## Patterns of Insurance Coverage for Psychotherapy

Even before the current era of managed mental health care benefits when few patients are allowed the psychotherapy benefits they actually need, it was common practice for insurance companies to limit coverage for psychotherapy with higher copayments, stricter yearly limits, and lower lifetime limits than for other medical care. These discriminatory practices were considered justified by insurers because of the widespread assumption that psychotherapy benefits are vulnerable to abuse by those not in need and will therefore unnecessarily inflate health care expenditures in a way not shared by other medical benefits. In reality, recent studies have documented that higher copayments for mental health services do in fact reduce both initial access to and treatment intensity of mental health visits, but this reduction of care affects patients at all levels of clinical need (Landerman et al. 1994;

Simon et al. 1996). In other words, very ill psychiatric patients are equally affected by discriminatory copayments and are put at an arbitrarily increased risk of going without appropriate care due to the imposition of a financial disincentive meant to screen out a hypothetical group of patients who would capriciously abuse covered mental health services. Despite this history of insurance discrimination, studies document the need for and cost-effectiveness of psychotherapy benefits in several patient populations.

It is also instructive to note some data about insurance company practices. In 1990, commercial insurance companies spent 37.2 cents of every premium dollar on administrative costs and profits, almost 18 times more than that taken by Medicare (2.1 cents) and over 41 times more than that taken by the Canadian health system (0.9 cents) out of each premium dollar. Administrative expenses and profits took an even greater piece of the premium dollar (68.2 cents) for subscribers who could not obtain group coverage (Citizens Fund 1992). With the advent of managed care, profit-driven clinical decisions became even more the norm, with psychiatric treatment and psychotherapy in particular becoming vulnerable targets for benefit managers, leaving increasing numbers of psychiatric patients without access to appropriate care. These insurance and HMO practices persisted and worsened despite evidence for the very low additional expense of providing parity for all appropriate treatments for mental illness (Sturm 1997).

The concern over rising health care costs has led insurance companies to pressure providers to reduce costs by reducing inpatient care ostensibly by providing more (less expensive) outpatient care. However, an examination of claims from 3.9 million privately insured individuals from 1993 to 1995 showed that inpatient costs fell 30.4% in addition to a decline in outpatient care costs of 13.6% for patients also using inpatient services and 14.6% for patients receiving only outpatient care. The authors concluded that managed care has not caused a shift in the pattern of care but has caused an overall reduction of care for psychiatric patients (Leslie and Rosenheck 1999).

A 1999 report of the Surgeon General showed a widening gap in insurance coverage between mental health and other health services (U.S. Department of Health and Human Services 1999). Increasingly, plans have had multiple limits on their benefits and an increased use of managed care such that behavioral health care costs decreased, both absolutely and as a proportion of employers' total medical plan costs. Day limits on inpatient psychiatric care have been drastically cut, and the proportion of plans with outpatient visit limits rose between 1988 and 1997 from 26% to 48%, driving down the value of behavioral health care benefits from 6.1% to 3.1% of the total health benefit value (National Association of Psychiatric Health Systems and Association of Behavioral Group Practices 1999). The Surgeon General report also found that in the decade between 1986 and 1996, mental health care grew more slowly than health care spending in general, quite possibly from the greater reliance of mental health services on managed care cost-containment methods, the shifting of expenses to the public sector, increased reliance on non-mental health public human services, and increased barriers to service access. The findings included the refusal of some private insurers to cover mental illness treatment at all. Others imposed separate and lower annual and lifetime limits on mental health care with higher deductibles and copayments, exposing covered individuals to higher out-of-pocket expenses and potentially catastrophic financial losses and/or transfer to the public sector when the costs of care exceeded coverage limits. The report found that mental health coverage is singled out for special cost-sharing arrangements compared with other health services, that excessively restrictive managed care cost-containment strategies risk undertreatment, and that current incentives both within and outside managed care do not encourage an emphasis on quality of care (U.S. Department of Health and Human Services 1999).

## Parity

The idea of parity of insurance coverage for mental health benefits (i.e., at the same level as other medical benefits) has been hotly debated, with opponents arguing that parity mental health coverage is far too expensive to provide. A RAND study (Sturm 1997) examined assumptions about the high price of mental health parity expressed in the policy debates surrounding the Mental Health Parity Act of 1996. Twenty-four plans with 140,000 enrollees under United Behavioral Health with very generous benefits and no limits on coverage of all employees were selected for the study; the latter two criteria were used to avoid the impact of adverse selection from high users selecting more generous plans over time. These 24 plans were selected to simulate conditions of mandated mental health parity in a situation of managed care. The study demonstrated that although access to mental health specialty care increased to 7% of enrollees (compared with 5% of enrollees found in the free care condition in the earlier RAND Health Insurance Experiment), there was a relative shift to outpatient care, reduced hospitalization rates, and reduced payments per service. Children were the main beneficiaries of the expanded availability of benefits that were estimated to cost only an additional $1 per enrollee per year. The assumptions underlying concerns about the high costs of parity for mental health benefits were shown to be incorrect, based on outdated data, and dramatically overstated by a factor of four to eight.

One study found that parity increased costs by a few percentage points at most, reduced out-of-pocket costs for patients, and should be completely affordable on a national level ("Evaluation of Parity" 2005). And in October

2008, the Paul Wellstone and Pete Domenici Mental Health and Addiction Equity Act mandating equal insurance coverage for mental health treatment as for medical and surgical care was passed by Congress and signed into law. The mandate includes insurance plans that already cover mental health benefits in group plans covering 50 or more, will not take precedence over stronger state laws, and should take effect in 2010.

# Conclusion

While there are perhaps still too few large-scale studies addressing the cost-effectiveness of psychotherapy for specific diagnostic groups of patients, we can arrive at some important impressions from the studies that we do have. Those that exist do confirm that for many conditions, psychotherapy works, is cost-effective, can at times provide a significant cost offset in other medical and hospital expenses, and is not overused or abused by those not truly in need. Also, it is important to understand that a treatment that is cost-effective is not cheap, may not save money in other treatment costs, but does provide effective medical help at a cost acceptable to society, both in comparison with other effective treatments for the same condition and in comparison with medical treatments for other classes of medical disorder. Subsequent chapters in this volume will discuss in detail the evidence for the cost-effectiveness of psychotherapy for a variety of psychiatric conditions by exploring the use of psychotherapy with specific illnesses and conditions from the point of view of its cost-effectiveness.

# This Volume

Readers will note that this volume is a multiauthored work. Multiauthored acts of scholarship can sometimes be a challenge for users, as the tone, style, and perspective will be inconsistent across chapters. We have attempted to diminish this natural tendency by careful editing, but it is virtually impossible to eliminate the differences in voice and perspective even if we wanted to do so. Furthermore, a deeper familiarization with this volume will reveal that it is more like an encyclopedia than it is a text telling a story, although there are many substories within it. We have attempted to organize the chapters into groupings that allow for more ready and quick targeted access to material appropriate to the reader's interest. We have used tables to organize and present the material. Because of the variation of studies and their quality, by different subtopics of these disease-oriented chapters, one might find the tables useful. We have conceived the tables as a way of quickly summarizing the material that addresses either cost-effectiveness explicitly or provides quite compelling background material for cost-effectiveness study. These tables are typically organized by subcategories, and within the subcategories, the citations are chronologically listed.

Most of the chapters examining the literature on the cost-effectiveness for specific diagnoses were searched using the terms "psychotherapy + (specific diagnosis) + costs" for the years 1984 through 2007 (1984 was chosen as the starting point because it was the year of the Mumford, Schlesinger, et al. 1984 report on cost offsets provided by psychotherapy). We also included a number of studies cited with dates after 2007 if they were considered especially germane to a specific topic. In some instances, additional search terms to those mentioned above were used to provide other background information as required per topic. The chapters investigating psychotherapy for patients with medical illness, for children and adolescents, and on the role of long-term and intensive psychotherapy were done with different search criteria because of the nature of the available literature. The details of these literature searches are provided in each chapter. Most of the literature searches examined English language only publications except for the chapter on intensive psychotherapy, which reviews some German language publications.

Chapter 2, addressing the use of psychotherapy for a specific diagnosis, examines the issue of the clinical cost-effectiveness of psychotherapeutic approaches, especially that of family interventions and social skills training, as they are applied to the treatment of schizophrenia. It concludes that any treatment approach that reduces relapse will be cost-effective.

Chapter 3 reviews the psychotherapy of borderline personality disorder and explores recent empirical research and its implications for clinical effectiveness and cost offset. It notes that the available studies meeting the criteria for inclusion and review indicate that outpatient psychiatric services, including group and individual psychotherapy, in borderline patients reduce the use of psychiatric inpatient services, the utilization of outpatient medical services, absenteeism at work, and self-destructive episodes.

Chapter 4 examines the literature on the psychotherapeutic treatment of patients with PTSD and finds that victims of trauma, victims of sexual and physical abuse, and combat veterans are all highly vulnerable to the development of PTSD, a highly costly illness. While there are few cost-effectiveness studies, the efficacy of multiple psychotherapeutic approaches in reducing pain and disability can be presumed to indicate their cost-effectiveness.

Chapter 5 addresses what is known in terms of cost-effectiveness in the psychotherapy of anxiety disorders. It notes that anxiety disorders, the most common of all mental health problems, account for 31% of total mental health costs. It reviews studies of panic disorder, obsessive-compulsive disorder, phobic disorder, and general anxiety disorder.

Chapter 6 examines the cost-effectiveness of psychotherapy for depression, noting that unipolar depression is a major cause of disability in the world. It examines data on treatments for depression and concludes that inadequate treatment and complete lack of recognition and treatment of depression rather than direct treatment costs have resulted in the enormous costliness of depression.

Chapter 7, on the cost-effectiveness of psychosocial interventions for substance abuse, notes that despite the ambivalence surrounding treatment of substance abuse and the difficulties in achieving abstinence among those addicted, brief interventions by medical professionals can improve success rates. It also indicates that more intensive treatments involving multiple modalities can be effective.

Chapter 8 addresses psychotherapy in the medically ill. A review of the literature notes support for the concept that treating the psychological as well as the physical ailments of medical patients provides an approach that is often both medically more effective and financially sound.

Chapter 9, examining psychotherapy for children, notes that while cost-effectiveness studies with children and adolescents are generally not available, efficacy studies of psychological treatment have demonstrated effectiveness. The implications of these findings for public policy are discussed.

A final chapter, not focused on a specific diagnosis, is organized differently from the others. This chapter examines the place of more intensive and extended psychotherapy than is usually available to patients, covered by medical insurance, or included in recent research designed to study specific diagnostic groups.

These works provide an almost comprehensive review by disease entity demonstrating the cost-effectiveness of psychotherapy.

# References

American Psychiatric Association: Diagnostic and Statistical Manual of Mental Disorders, 4th Edition, Text Revision. Washington, DC, American Psychiatric Association, 2000

Andrews G: Private and public psychiatry: a comparison of two health care systems. Am J Psychiatry 146:881–886, 1989

Beecham J, Sleed M, Knapp M, et al: The costs and effectiveness of two psychosocial treatment programmes for personality disorder: a controlled study. Eur Psychiatry 21:102–109, 2006

Birmaher B, Ryan ND, Williams DC, et al: Childhood and adolescent depression: a review of the past ten years, Part I. J Am Acad Child Adolesc Psychiatry 35:1427–1439, 1996

Bower P, Rowland N: Effectiveness and cost effectiveness of counselling in primary care. Cochrane Database Syst Rev 3:CD001025, 2006

Breslau N, Davis GC, Andreski P, et al: Traumatic events and postraumatic stress disorder in an urban population of young adults. Arch Gen Psychiatry 48:216–222, 1991

Briere J, Runtz M: Post sexual abuse trauma, in Lasting Effects of Child Sexual Abuse. Edited by Wyatt GE, Powell GJ. Newbury Park, CA, Sage, 1988, pp 85–99

Centers for Disease Control: Suicide Surveillance, 1970–1980. Atlanta, GA, U.S. Department of Health and Human Services Public Health Services, 1986

Chiesa M, Fonagy P, Holmes J, et al: Health service use costs by personality disorder following specialist and nonspecialist treatment: a comparative study. J Pers Disord 16:160–173, 2002

Citizens Fund: Premiums Without Benefits: The Decade-Long Growth in Commercial Health Insurance Industry Waste and Inefficiency. Washington, DC, Citizens Fund, April 1992

Clark R: Searching for cost-effective mental health care. Harv Rev Psychiatry 4:45–48, 1996

Doidge N, Simon B, Gillies L, et al: Characteristics of psychoanalytic patients under a nationalized health plan. Am J Psychiatry 151:586–590, 1994

Dossmann R, Kutter P, Heinzel R, et al: The long-term benefits of intensive psychotherapy: a view from Germany. Psychoanalytic Inquiry 17 (suppl):74–86, 1997

Duehrssen A, Jorswiek E: [An empirical and statistical inquiry into the therapeutic potential of psychoanalytic treatment.] Nervenarzt 36:166–169, 1965

Evaluation of parity in the Federal Employees Health Benefits (FEHB) program: final report. Psychiatric News, September 16, 2005, p 1

Fawzy F, Fawzy N, Hyun C: Malignant melanoma: effects of an early structured psychiatric intervention, coping and affective state on recurrence and survival 6 years later. Arch Gen Psychiatry 50:681–689, 1993

Finkler SA: The distinction between costs and charges. Ann Intern Med 96:102–109, 1982

Follette WT, Cummings NA: Psychiatric services and medical utilization in a prepaid health plan setting.Med Care 8:419–428, 1970

Friedrich WN: Behavior problems in sexually abused children, in Lasting Effects of Child Sexual Abuse. Edited by Wyatt GE, Powell GJ. Newbury Park, CA, Sage, 1988, pp 171–192

Gabbard GO, Lazar SG, Hornberger J, et al: The economic impact of psychotherapy: a review. Am J Psychiatry 154:147–155, 1997

Gold M: Panel on cost-effectiveness in health and medicine. Med Care 34 (suppl 12):DS197–DS199, 1996

Greenberg P, Stiglin LE, Finkelstein SN, et al: The economic burden of depression in 1990. J Clinical Psychiatry 54:405–418, 1993

Greenberg P, Sisitsky T, Kessler R, et al: The economic burden of anxiety disorders in the 1990s. J Clin Psychiatry 60:427–435, 1999

Greenberg P, Kessler R, Birnbaum H, et al: The economic burden of depression in the United States: how did it change between 1990 and 2000? J Clin Psychiatry 64:1465–1475, 2003

Group for the Advancement of Psychiatry, Committee on Therapy: Psychotherapy and Its Financial Feasibility Within the National Health Care System (GAP Report Vol X, Publ No 100). New York, Group for the Advancement of Psychiatry, Mental Health Materials Center, 1978

Hay Huggins: Report to the American Psychoanalytic Association, 1990

Herman JL, Perry JC, van der Kolk BA: Childhood trauma in borderline personality disorder. Am J Psychiatry 146:490–495, 1989

Hu T: An international review of the national cost estimates of mental illness, 1990–2003. J Ment Health Policy Econ 9:3–13, 2006

Issakidis C, Sanderson K, Corry J, et al: Modelling the population cost-effectiveness of current and evidence-based optimal treatment for anxiety disorders. Psychol Med 34:19–35, 2004

Jones KR, Vischi TR: Impact of alcohol, drug abuse and mental health treatment on medical care utilization. Med Care 17 (suppl 2):1–82, 1979

Kashani JH, Orvaschel H: A community study of anxiety in children and adolescents. Am J Psychiatry 147:313–318, 1990

Kessler F, Frank R: The impact of psychiatric disorders on work loss days. Psychol Med 27:861–873, 1997

Kessler LG, Steinwachs DM, Hankin JR: Episodes of psychiatric care and the medical utilization. Med Care 20:1209–1221, 1982

Kessler RC, McGonagle KA, Zhao S, et al: Lifetime and 12-month prevalence of DSM-III-R psychiatric disorders in the United States: results from the National Comorbidity Survey. Arch Gen Psychiatry 5:8–19, 1994

Kessler RC, Berglund P, Demler O, et al: Lifetime prevalence and age-of-onset distributions of DSM-IV disorders in the National Comorbidity Survey replication. Arch Gen Psychiatry 62:593–602, 2005a

Kessler RC, Chiu WT, Demler O, et al: Prevalence, severity, and comorbidity of 12-month DSM-IV in the National Comorbidity Survey replication. Arch Gen Psychiatry 62: 617–627, 2005b

Kessler RC, Chiu WT, Jin R, et al: The epidemiology of panic attacks, panic disorder, and agoraphobia in the National Comorbidity Survey replication. Arch Gen Psychiatry 63:415–424, 2006

Kessler RC, Heeringa S, Lakoma M, et al: Individual and societal effects of mental disorders on earnings in the United States: results from the National Comorbidity Survey replication: Am J Psychiatry 165:703–711, 2008

Kilpatrick DG, Best CL, Veronen LJ, et al: Mental health correlates of criminal victimization: a random community survey. J Consult Clin Psychol 53:866–873, 1985

Klarreich S, DiGiuseppe R, DiMattia D: Cost-effectiveness of an employee assistance program with rational-emotive therapy. Professional Psychology: Research and Practice 18:140–144, 1987

Koss MP, Koss PG, Woodruff WJ: Deleterious effects of criminal victimization on women's health and utilization. Arch Intern Med 151:342–347, 1991

Krizay J: Open Minds. April 1990

Kulka AR, Schlenger WE, Fairbank JA, et al: Contractual Report of Findings from the Vietnam Veterans Readjustment Study. Research Triangle Park, NC, Research Triangle Institute, 1988

Landerman L, Burns B, Swartz M, et al: The relationship between insurance coverage and psychiatric disorder in predicting use of mental health services. Am J Psychiatry 151:1785–1790, 1994

Lazar SG, Gabbard GO: The cost-effectiveness of psychotherapy. J Psychother Pract Res 6:307–314, 1997

Lemieux J, Topp A, Chappell H, et al: Economic analysis of psychosocial group therapy in women with metastatic breast cancer. Breast Cancer Res Treat 100:183–190, 2006

Leslie D, Rosenheck R: Shifting to outpatient care? Mental health care use and cost under private insurance. Am J Psychiatry 156:1250–1257, 1999

Manning WG Jr, Wells KB, Duan N, et al: How cost sharing affects the use of ambulatory mental health services. JAMA 256:1930–1934, 1986

Marcotte D, Wilcox-Gok V: Estimating the employment and earnings costs of mental illness: recent developments in the United States. Soc Sci Med 53:21–27, 2001

McGrath G, Lowson K: Assessing the benefits of psychotherapy: the economic approach. Br J Psychiatry 150:65–71, 1986

Mental health: does therapy help? Consumer Reports, November 1995, pp 734–739

Merikangas KR, Ames M, Cui L, et al: The impact of comorbidity of mental and physical conditions on role disability in the US adult household population. Arch Gen Psychiatry 64:1180–1188, 2007

Mojtabai R, Olfson M: National trends in psychotherapy by office-based psychiatrists. Arch Gen Psychiatry 65:962–970, 2008

Mumford E, Schlesinger HJ, Glass GV, et al: A new look at evidence about reduced cost of medical utilization following mental health treatment. Am J Psychiatry 141:1145–1158, 1984

Murray C, Lopez A: The Global Burden of Disease: A Comprehensive Assessment of Mortality and Disability from Diseases, Injuries, and Risk Factors in 1990 and projected to 2020. Cambridge, MA, Harvard School of Public Health on behalf of the World Health Organization and the World Bank, 1996

Mynors-Wallis L, Davies I, Gray A, et al: A randomised controlled trial and cost analysis of problem-solving treatment for emotional disorders given by community nurses in primary care. Br J Psychiatry 170:113–119, 1997

National Association of Psychiatric Health Systems and Association of Behavioral Group Practices: Health care plan design and cost trends—1988 through 1998, Arlington, VA, HayGroup, 1999

Olfson M, Pincus H: Outpatient psychotherapy in the United States, I: volume, costs and user characteristics. Am J Psychiatry 151:1281–1288, 1994a

Olfson M, Pincus H: Outpatient psychotherapy in the United States, II: patterns of utilization. Am J Psychiatry 151:1289–1294, 1994b

Olfson M, Marcus S, Druss B, et al: National trends in the use of outpatient psychotherapy. Am J Psychiatry 159:1914–1920, 2002

Ornish D, Brown SE, Scherwitz LZ, et al: Can lifestyle changes reverse coronary heart disease? The Lifestyle Heart Trial. Lancet 336(8708):129–133, 1990

Pirraglia PA, Rosen AB, Hermann RC, et al: Cost-utility analysis studies of depression management: a systematic review. Am J Psychiatry 161:2155–2162, 2004

Rice D, Kelman S, Miller L, et al: The economic costs of alcohol and drug abuse and mental illness (DHHS Publ No ADM-90-1694). Rockville, MD, Alcohol, Drug Abuse, and Mental Health Administration, 1990

Russell D: Sexual Exploitation: Rape, Child Sexual Abuse and Sexual Harassment. Beverly Hills, CA, Sage, 1984

Saeman H: Integrated care model works, says Bell South. National Psychologist 3:12–13, 1994

Schetky DH: A review of the literature of the long-term effects of childhood sexual abuse, in Incest-Related Syndromes of Adult Psychopathology. Edited by Kluft RP. Washington, DC, American Psychiatric Press, 1990, pp 35–54

Siegel JE, Weinstein MC, Russell LB, et al: Recommendations for reporting cost-effectiveness analyses. JAMA 276:1339–1341, 1996

Simon G, Grothaus L, Durham M, et al: Impact of visit copayments on outpatient mental health utilization by members of a health maintenance organization. Am J Psychiatry 153:331–338, 1996

Spiegel D, Kraemer H, Gottheil E: Effective psychosocial treatment on survival of patients with metastatic breast cancer. Lancet 2:888–891, 1989

Sturm R: How expensive is unlimited mental health care coverage under managed care? JAMA 78:1533–1537, 1997

Swartz M, Blazer D, George L, et al: Estimating the prevalence of borderline personality disorder in the community. J Pers Disord 4:257–272, 1990

Tanielian T, Jaycox LH (eds): Invisible Wounds of War: Psychological and Cognitive Injuries, Their Consequences, and Services to Assist Recovery. Santa Monica, CA, RAND Center for Military Health Policy Research, 2008

Target M, Fonagy P: Efficacy of psychoanalysis for children with emotional disorders. J Am Acad Child Adolesc Psychiatry 33:361–371, 1994

U.S. Department of Health and Human Services: Mental Health: A Report of the Surgeon General. Rockville, MD, U.S. Department of Health and Human Services, Substance Abuse and Mental Health Services Administration, Center for Mental Health Services, National Institutes of Health, National Institute of Mental Health, 1999

Wang PS, Berglund P, Olfson M, et al: Failure and delay in initial treatment contact after first onset of mental disorders in the National Comorbidity Survey replication. Arch Gen Psychiatry 62:603–613, 2005a

Wang PS, Lane M, Olfson M, et al: Twelve-month use of mental health services in the United States. Arch Gen Psychiatry 62:629–640, 2005b

Wang PS, Demler O, Olfson M, et al: Changing profiles of service sectors used for mental health care in the United States. Am J Psychiatry 163:1187–1198, 2006

Weinstein MC, Siegel JE, Gold MR, et al: Recommendations of the panel on cost-effectiveness in health and medicine. JAMA 276:1253–1258, 1996

Wells KB, Burnam MA, Rogers W, et al: The course of depression in adult outpatients. Results from the Medical Outcomes Study. Arch Gen Psychiatry 49:788–794, 1992

Weisbrod BA: A guide to benefit-cost analyses, as seen through controlled experiments in treating the mentally ill. Journal of Health, Politics and the Law 7:808–845, 1983

Weisbrod BA, Test MA, Stein LI: Alternative to mental hospital treatment, II: economic benefit-cost analysis. Arch Gen Psychiatry 37:400–405, 1980

Wolff N: Measuring costs: what is counted and who is accountable? Disease Management and Clinical Outcomes 1(4):114–128, 1998

Wolff N, Helminiak TW, Tebes J: Getting the cost right in cost-effectiveness analyses. Am J Psychiatry 154:736–743, 1997

World Health Organization: Global Burden of Disease: 2004 Update. Geneva, World Health Organization, 2008

Zients A: A Presentation to the White House Mental Health Working Group, White House Task Force for National Health Care Reform, April 23, 1993

# 2 | Psychotherapeutic and Psychosocial Interventions in Schizophrenia

## Clinical Outcomes and Cost-Effectiveness

Lawrence H. Rockland, M.D.

According to an examination of 188 studies of the prevalence of schizophrenia published between 1965 and 2002, the median value of the lifetime prevalence of schizophrenia worldwide is 4 per 1,000 persons (Saha et al. 2005). The severe psychological, social, and functional deficits associated with schizophrenia, and its chronicity, require that these patients and their families receive extensive medical and rehabilitation services. In addition, both patients and caretakers suffer significant losses of productivity.

Wyatt et al. (1995) estimated that for 1991, the cost of treating and caring for patients with schizophrenia, plus the productivity lost to the illness, was $65 billion. Of the $65 billion, $19 billion represented direct treatment-related expenses, whereas indirect costs, the illness-associated lost productivity of wage earners and homemakers, added an additional $46 billion. In 2002 the U.S. total excess societal costs associated with patients with schizophrenia were $62.7 billion, including $22.7 billion in excess direct health care costs, $7.6 billion in direct non-health care costs, and $32.4 billion in total excess costs of productivity loss, this last figure representing 52% of all schizophrenia-related costs. The authors of this later study reviewed the earlier studies and concluded that atypical antipsychotics had reduced the risk of relapse and had thus changed treatment patterns, resource utilization, and the cost profile of schizophrenic patients (Wu et al. 2005). Thus schizophrenia constitutes a major public health problem, medically and financially, because of 1) its prevalence, severity, and chronicity, and 2) the enormous costs associated with the effects of the illness and its treatment.

Schizophrenia is a disease, or group of diseases, of the mind and of the brain characterized by strange perceptual experiences, odd thinking, poor control of feelings, inappropriate behaviors, and severe social and vocational dysfunction. It is a chronic relapsing illness, and even well-established and effective treatments do not carry with them any promise of a cure. Thus far, no treatment produces durable results that persist indefinitely after the treatment is stopped.

The DSM-IV-TR (American Psychiatric Association 2000) diagnostic criteria for schizophrenia provide a more current and detailed description. Criteria for the diagnosis are:

A.  Symptoms (two or more are required)
    1.  Delusions
    2.  Hallucinations
    3.  Disorganization of speech
    4.  Disorganized or catatonic behavior
    5.  Negative symptoms (e.g., anhedonia, affective flattening, avolition)
B.  Social or occupational dysfunction—impairment in one or more major areas of function.
C.  Duration—signs of the illness last for 6 months or more, including the 1 month that meets Criteria A.
D.  Schizoaffective disorder, mood disorder with psychotic features, substance abuse, and generalized medical illness have all been ruled out.

Once the diagnosis of schizophrenia is established, the illness is subdivided into five subtypes:

1.  Paranoid
2.  Disorganized
3.  Catatonic
4.  Undifferentiated
5.  Residual

Increasing evidence has implicated brain pathology, particularly in the frontal and limbic areas. Psychopharmacologic agents are usually effective against positive symptoms such as hallucinations and delusions, and they thereby reduce relapse rates. But they are much less effective treating cognitive and social deficits, whether from developmental defects, chronic disuse, or secondary to the illness itself. Therefore, an effective treatment plan for schizophrenic patients should include both pharmacologic and psychosocial interventions, skillfully integrated and individually tailored to the patient's strengths and deficits (Hogarty 2002).

Prior to 20 years ago, there was little reason for enthusiasm about any psychotherapeutic or psychosocial treatment for patients with schizophrenia. Charismatic psychoanalytic writers, for example, Fromm-Reichmann (1950) and Searles (1965), published elegant accounts of intensive psychotherapies of individual schizophrenic patients, but the generally negative results of the large *N* studies (Gunderson et al. 1984; May 1968) led to widespread disillusionment with the usefulness of psychodynamic therapies for these patients, and this pessimism spread to all psychological interventions.

However, since the 1980s, newer psychosocial treatments, particularly family interventions (FIs) and social skills training (SST), have produced impressively positive results, leading to a more optimistic view of psychological treatments for schizophrenic patients. Family interventions generally begin with education about the nature of schizophrenic illness. This is followed by the main tasks of the intervention, attempting to improve family problem solving and management of conflict and stress, and more effective family communication. The identification of stressors and symptoms associated with patient relapse is usually also included. Social skills training uses the principles of learning theory to improve the interpersonal skills and work competency of the patient. Its goals are improvements in the patient's social function, work-related capacity, and quality of life.

This chapter reviews the schizophrenia literature from 1984 to 2007, focusing largely on the results of well-designed outcome studies of FIs and SST and on cost-effectiveness data where available.

# Search Methodology

The studies that are the focus of this chapter were gathered from two literature searches. The first searched MEDLINE, 1984–1994, for papers on the cost-effectiveness of psychotherapy applied to patients with a wide variety of psychiatric diagnoses; they are summarized in "The Economic Impact of Psychotherapy: A Review" by Gabbard et al. (1997). That search yielded six studies related to schizophrenia, and they provided a very useful nucleus for this paper.

The second literature search used MEDLINE and PsycLIT, 1984–2007, utilizing the key words "schizophrenia" + "costs or economics" + "therapy, or psychotherapy, or psychoeducation, or patient education." That search yielded 16 additional studies.

These studies are listed by subcategories in the review table at the end of this chapter, and within the subcategories, the studies are listed chronologically.

# Literature

Of the 22 studies yielded by the literature searches, 17 addressed FIs and 2 addressed SST. Five of the FI papers included cost-effectiveness data; neither of the SST studies did. The treatments were all behaviorally oriented, and all patients were treated with antipsychotic drugs. However, there was very variable attention to drug compliance issues from study to study. Two studies were not clinical trials but estimates of the cost-effectiveness of adding effective treatments for a number of disorders, including schizophrenia. Another study examined the cost-effectiveness of seven different clinical interventions, including psychotherapy, for schizophrenic patients in Spain.

## Clinical Effectiveness

In virtually all 13 studies through 1998 charted in the review table at the end of this chapter, the Experimental treatment (E) was superior to the Control treatment (C). Control treatments comprised a wide variety of treatments-as-usual. This finding held whether the treatments were delivered simultaneously (Falloon et al. 1987) or at different times (Rund et al. 1994); whether the subjects were outpatients (Leff et al. 1989, 1990), inpatients (Glick et al. 1990, 1993; Haas et al. 1988), or both (Eckman et al. 1992); whether treatments were prolonged and infrequent (Hogarty et al. 1986, 1991) or brief and intense (Glick et al. 1990,1993; Haas et al. 1988); and whether outcome measures were obtained only during treatment (McFarlane et al. 1995a, 1995b) or continued after termination of treatment (Tarrier et al. 1989, 1991, 1994).

Three studies (Falloon et al. 1987; Leff et al. 1989; Spiegel and Wissler 1987) delivered the family intervention in the patient's home, one on the inpatient unit (Glick et al. 1990), and the remainder in an outpatient clinic. Duration of treatments varied widely, from eight sessions (Glick et al. 1990, 1993; Haas et al. 1988) to 24 months (Falloon et al. 1987). The collection of outcome measures was also very variable. As noted above, some investigators evaluated patients only during treatment (McFarlane et al. 1995a, 1995b), whereas others continued assessments for up to 24 months after treatment termination (Spiegel and Wissler 1987). One study (Hogarty et al. 1986,

1991) compared FI with SST and with combined FI and SST. The Leff et al. (1989) study contrasted FI delivered in the home with a relatives' group in the clinic.

Despite the wide variations in design, FIs were generally consistently effective in the studies prior to 1998. They decreased relapse rates by an average of 50% and had positive effects on the mental and physical health of the patient and his or her caretakers. For example, Zhang et al. (1994) found that male patients with schizophrenia given a family intervention after hospital discharge had a significantly lower rate of hospital readmission and, for those who were readmitted, significantly longer hospital-free periods than patients in the standard-care control group. Brooker et al. (1994) reported decreased frequency and severity of symptoms after family interventions for schizophrenia patients compared with patients in the waitlist control or delayed intervention groups.

Family interventions not only decreased relapse rates but also reduced the number and duration of in-hospital stays and the dose of antipsychotic drug required. The results demonstrated the efficacy of FIs for patients with schizophrenia and strongly supported the critical role of family expressed emotion (EE) on the course of the patient's illness.

Expressed emotion (Koenigsberg and Handley 1986) refers to the attitudes of family caretakers toward the identified patient. It is measured by rating the extent to which caretakers express critical, hostile, or overinvolved attitudes toward the patient while discussing his or her illness with the interviewer. The assumption is that caretaker attitudes in the interview reflect enduring traits and chronic interaction patterns with the patient. A number of studies (Brown et al. 1972; Vaughn et al. 1982) have provided convincing support for the predictive value of EE. For example, patients in high EE families relapsed more frequently. More recent studies reviewed here demonstrate that FIs can reduce family EE and decrease the risk of relapse. Presumably, the reduced patient relapse rates resulted from decreased EE in the family.

The EE concept has also been applied to other psychopathology such as depression (Hooley et al. 1986) and to physical illnesses such as diabetes mellitus (Koenigsberg et al. 1993). In the latter study, levels of family EE predicted the success of blood sugar control in the diabetic children, an impressive example of the interaction between psychological and biological issues.

The positive effects of FIs decrease progressively after treatment ends and long-term family treatment appears to be necessary. However, even if relapse is not prevented but only delayed by FIs (i.e., illness-free periods are lengthened), significant medical and economic advantages accrue. Incidentally, an exception to the short-lived effects of FIs is the Tarrier et al. (1994)

study, in which a 9-month FI was associated with decreased relapse rates up to 8 years later.

Although cost-effectiveness remained an important concern after 1998 (Mosher 1999), interest and studies shifted to more theoretical questions, for example: How do family interventions work? What is the minimal effective family intervention? Costs were not calculated, but it is clear that all studies had cost-effectiveness implications. Simultaneously, the consistently positive outcomes prior to 1998 became much more variable after 1998.

Zhang et al. (1998) compared conventional aftercare (C) with conventional services plus group therapy (14 lectures and five discussion groups) (E). The authors found the usual positive effects for the E group on relapse rates, work activities, family burden, caretaker health, and family knowledge and skills.

By contrast, the Treatment Strategies in Schizophrenia Study (Schooler et al. 1997) found no significant differences in outcome between behavioral family therapy (BFT) (E) and a supportive family intervention (C); both produced essentially equivalent positive effects on patient outcome. BFT did not lead to greater improvement in family communication and problem solving, and in those families that improved, positive changes were not associated with better patient outcomes. The authors concluded that intensive BFT interventions may not be cost-effective.

Montero et al. (2001) compared similar experimental and control conditions, namely relatives' group (C) and BFT group (E), and found mixed results. Relapse rates were similar in both groups, but in areas such as social function and neuroleptic dose required, the results favored BFT.

Schooler et al.'s negative results were expanded and supported by Bellack et al. (2000) and Mueser et al. (2001). Mueser et al. compared supportive family management (SFM) (C) with applied family management (AFM) (E). The latter added a year of BFT after the SFM that both E and C groups received. The experimental condition improved "family atmosphere" but did not improve patient social function, family behavioral patterns, or patient outcomes.

Similarly, Bellack et al. using the same design concluded that AFM (E) did not produce superior patient outcomes to SFM (C). Further, improvements in family communication and problem solving were not associated with decreased relapse rates or other positive changes in the patient's clinical condition.

By contrast, Berglund et al. (2003), using a design very similar to that of Schooler, Mueser, and Bellack but with inpatients, found very positive results for the E condition. Family burden was decreased and accompanied by more positive attitudes toward patient care. In addition, relapse rates and neuroleptic doses strongly favored the E condition.

In the two SST papers, both experimental treatments were superior to controls. Liberman et al. (1986) demonstrated that patients treated with SST (E) manifested better social functioning, decreased relapse rates, and reduced days in hospital over a 2-year follow-up than did patients in the control group, who were treated with stress reduction techniques. Eckman et al. (1992) found that patients could learn self-management skills even in the presence of severe psychopathology and that these skills persisted without significant deterioration over a 12-month follow-up. (The persisting benefits of SST in this study are inconsistent with Hogarty et al.'s [1991] findings, in which patients lost the positive effects of SST late in the 2nd year of treatment.)

The effects of combined FI and SST appear to be additive. After 12 months of treatment, Hogarty et al. (1986, 1991) found the following relapse rates: controls (individual supportive therapy) 40%, FIs 20%, SST 20%, and combined FI and SST 0%.

Noting that both FIs and SSTs lost their effectiveness in the 2nd year posttreatment, Hogarty et al. (1995, 1997a, 1997b; Hogarty 2002) designed personal therapy, an individual psychological treatment that takes account of the patient's neuropsychological impairments and current level of function. Affective dysregulation is central to Hogarty's view of schizophrenia, and a key aspect of the treatment is teaching the patient better strategies for the control of escalating affects.

Personal therapy produced widespread improvements in social and vocational adjustment that persisted, and increased, in the 2nd and 3rd years posttreatment. By contrast, the positive effects of the control treatments, individual supportive and family interventions, peaked at about 12 months posttreatment and then faded. Personal therapy decreased relapse rates in patients living with their families but increased relapse in patients living independently; the reasons are unclear.

Starting from a much broader and more cost-centered focus, two interesting studies from 2005 estimate directly the impact on costs obtainable by increased implementation of effective interventions for several diagnostic groups of psychiatric patients. Chisholm (2005) provided an overview of the mental health component of the World Health Organization's CHOICE project, the goal of which is to generate cost-effectiveness evidence for a large number of interventions for various illnesses in a range of geographical and epidemiological settings around the world. Expected costs and effects of effective pharmacological and psychosocial interventions were modeled for four disorders: schizophrenia, bipolar disorder, depression, and panic disorder. A number of conclusions emerged with respect to the treatment of schizophrenia. The impact of pharmacological treatment for schizophrenia with either older or newer antipsychotic drugs is modest, not reducing the incidence or duration of the disease but providing approximately a 25% improvement in day-to-day functioning over no treatment. The improvement is closer to 45% when psychosocial treatment is also given. In fact, the addition of psychosocial treatment to pharmacotherapy is projected to have a far greater benefit than switching from older to newer antipsychotic agents. (A similar trend is noted for bipolar disorder.) Psychosocial treatment for schizophrenia (and bipolar treatment), with its relatively modest additional costs, yields significant health gains and is more cost-effective than pharmacotherapy alone. Vos et al. (2005) also estimated the impact on improved health and costs of using the most effective treatment strategies for Australian patients with depression schizophrenia, attention-deficit/hyperactivity disorder, and anxiety disorder. For schizophrenia, they concluded that more efficient drug intervention would save $68 million (Australian dollars) that would more than cover an estimated $36 million (Australian dollars) annual cost of providing family psychotherapy interventions to eligible schizophrenic patients, which would lead to an estimated 12% improvement in their health status.

Gutierrez-Recacha et al. (2006) examined the cost-effectiveness of seven different clinical interventions for schizophrenic patients in Spain: 1) current situation (treatment patterns used in Spain in the year 2000), referring to a variety of both older and newer antipsychotic psychotropic agents; 2) older antipsychotics alone; 3) new antipsychotics alone (risperidone); 4) older antipsychotics plus psychosocial treatment; 5) new antipsychotics plus psychosocial treatment; 6) older antipsychotics plus case management and psychosocial treatment; and 7) new antipsychotics plus case management and psychosocial treatment. Results included that the addition of a psychosocial treatment (family psychotherapy, SST, cognitive-behavioral therapy) to pharmacotherapy increased both the efficacy and the cost-effectiveness of clinical interventions for schizophrenia. While risperidone was slightly more effective than haloperidol, the addition of psychosocial treatment considerably increased the health gain achieved. Concurrent psychosocial treatment along with antipsychotic medication improved the cost-effectiveness of treatment for schizophrenia as a result of better compliance and because the additional costs of psychosocial treatment were largely offset by reduced hospital admissions. The advantages derived from the addition of psychosocial treatments were far greater than those derived from switching from older to newer antipsychotics. Intervention with generic risperidone plus psychosocial treatment plus case management was the most cost-effective treatment option.

## Cost-Effectiveness

Effective therapeutic interventions reduce costs in two major ways: 1) by decreasing relapse and the need for in-hospital treatment (direct costs), and 2) by maximizing function and productivity (indirect costs).

Most FIs appear to decrease patient relapse rates and also to improve general family health, well-being, and function. Social skills training improves social and vocational abilities, with the clear implication of improved function and increased productivity. Cost-effectiveness data are available for FIs but not for SST.

In the FI studies that included cost data, the general pattern was that the more effective treatments under study (E) increased outpatient costs, but the increase was far outweighed by the savings from reduced relapse rates and decreased hospital days. Therefore, overall total costs were markedly decreased. For example, in Falloon et al.'s (1987; Liberman et al. 1987) study, behavioral family management cost $13,000 more per patient than the control treatment, but in-hospital costs per patient were $41,000 less. Thus, total cost per patient for the FI (E) group was $28,000 less than for the controls. The same pattern of costs was found in the Tarrier et al. (1989, 1991, 1994) study; total costs were 37% less for the FI group than for the control group. Similarly, in the Rund et al. (1994) study, whole group total costs were $720,000 less for the FI cohort than for the controls.

The Lehtinen (1993) study was unusual in that while mean total costs were 50% less for the FI group (E) than for the control group, the outpatient costs for the experimental FI group were also less than for the control group.

McFarlane et al.'s (1995a, 1995b) study had a different focus. It compared two different family interventions: multiple family groups (MFGs) and single family therapy (SFT). Compared with SFT, MFGs were not only more effective but also less expensive. Patients had lower relapse rates in MFGs than in SFT, and MFGs required only half the number of professional staff. McFarlane et al. calculated cost-benefit ratios of 1:34 for MFGs and 1:17 for SFTs, both compared with no family treatment.

# Clinical Vignette

The following vignette illustrates some of the techniques used in FIs and SST and how they are applied to the treatment of a young man with schizophrenia.

Ben W. was a 37-year-old unmarried man, diagnosed as paranoid schizophrenic, when he was brought for hospitalization by his parents. The parents were in their late 60s and felt increasingly unable to care for Ben at home. He had stopped his antipsychotic medication 6 months previously, had quit his volunteer job, and had become increasingly isolated and then more aggressive and violent. The precipitant for the hospitalization was that Ben punched his father in the face, loosening several teeth. In addition, the parents were worried about Ben's future as they became older and less capable of caring for him.

Ben had previously been on the antipsychotic drug haloperidol, and this was restarted in the hospital. The unit social worker met with Ben's parents to educate them about Ben's illness and to support their self-esteem and morale. She stressed the organic aspects of schizophrenia, decreasing the parents' guilt and helping them to focus more effectively on planning for Ben's future. After 1 week on haloperidol with modest clinical improvement, Ben was discharged from the hospital.

He did not continue to respond positively to the haloperidol and developed severe akathisia, characterized by very uncomfortable feelings of restlessness. The akathisia did not respond to the usual agents and the haloperidol was changed to perphenazine, another antipsychotic agent; intractable akathisia developed again. The newer antipsychotic agent clozapine was suggested, but now Ben was refusing all medications.

The outpatient therapist continued the family meetings, expanded them to include Ben, and also met with Ben alone on a weekly basis. The family meetings focused on: 1) educating the family about the nature and treatment of schizophrenia, and 2) practical strategies for dealing more effectively with family conflicts and stresses.

The parents gradually became less critical, more objective, and less intensely involved with Ben. For example, they began to feel less responsible for Ben's inactivity and therefore less critical; when Ben became hostile they learned to distance temporarily instead of arguing with him.

The atmosphere of the family meetings began to change. The parents became able to discuss current stressors more objectively and to think more realistically about Ben's future. From his side, Ben gradually became less guarded and less suspicious; he began to discuss his options for the future more rationally. He felt that side effects made standard antipsychotic agents intolerable, but became increasingly curious about clozapine, asking what made it different from other drugs, what were its side effects, and so on.

Ben agreed to try clozapine and fortunately responded well to it. After a month on the drug, he actively and willingly participated in moving to a halfway house and a day program. He began a vocational rehabilitation program in which he learned techniques for communicating more clearly and for dealing more effectively with coworkers and bosses. Ben functioned well at the halfway house and gradually progressed back to his former volunteer job.

# Conclusion

The first issue to be addressed is the discrepancy between the almost consistently positive studies through 1998 and the mixed outcomes of the literature after 1998. In addition, during the 1997–2007 period, even when investigators used very similar designs and similar or identical experimental and control conditions, the results were inconsistent and even contradictory (e.g., Berglund et al. 2003; Mueser et al. 2001).

It is difficult to understand this variable mix of outcomes. There were differences in patient populations (outpatients only in Mueser et al. 2001; inpatients only in Berglund et al. 2003). Skills in delivering both E and C treatments or in the effectiveness of the C treatment probably varied. Recall, for example, that Schooler et al. (1997) did not conclude that the BFT (E) treatment was ineffective. Rather, there were no significant differences between the E and C conditions, probably because the C condition was so effective. The inpatient/outpatient discrepancy between Mueser et al.'s and Berglund et al.'s studies may be a crucial factor. Berglund et al.'s findings could suggest that FIs are most effective when there is a crisis and the patients are hospitalized.

Schooler, Mueser, and Bellack are all very experienced and sophisticated investigators, particularly in the area of schizophrenia and its nonbiologic treatments. Therefore, the similar results from all three of their studies must carry a lot of weight.

The discrepant up-to-1998 and post-1998 results are also puzzling. The pre-1998 studies used a wide variety of FIs, differing in length, techniques, place delivered, and so on; the only common element was the goal of decreasing family EE. By contrast, by 1998 the most accepted FI was BFT, which was utilized by almost all investigators. One could speculate that BFT, although well regarded and widely utilized, was not the ideal FI to produce the desired changes; that is, the decreased family EE leads to less relapse, less inpatient days, lower levels of antipsychotic drugs, and so on.

As noted earlier, there was very variable and inconsistent attention to medication compliance. This major clinical variable was not a major focus of attention in any of the studies, pre- or post-1998. Further, one can assume that pre-1998, the drugs used were primarily first-generation antipsychotics; after 1998 there was widespread use of second-generation drugs. One could speculate that the more effective second-generation antipsychotics, delivered to both E and C groups, were sufficiently more potent than the psychosocial interventions to overwhelm the differences between the E and C conditions.

What can be said at this time about the effectiveness of FIs and SST for schizophrenic patients?

1. Family interventions produce mainly positive effects, but perhaps BFT is not the ideal FI. When effective, FIs reduce relapse rates and inpatient days, improve family problem solving and atmosphere, and lead to better mental and physical health of the patient and his or her caretakers. This is particularly true when the FI is delivered for a sufficiently

long period of time. Decreased family EE is, in all probability, the critical mechanism that produces the other positive changes.

2. The durability of FIs is limited, and positive effects tend to fade progressively after treatment ends.

3. Patients with schizophrenia can learn and retain social and vocational skills, even while acutely ill. Positive changes appear to be more durable than those of FIs, but probably also have less effect on relapse rates. One can imply their cost-effectiveness because of the very high costs of impaired function in these patients; however, confirmatory data are lacking.

4. The lack of durability of psychosocial interventions, particularly FIs, does not negate their value. Delayed relapse (i.e., longer illness-free periods) has significant positive consequences, both health and cost related.

5. Hogarty's personal therapy, an individual treatment that focuses on the patients' neuropsychological deficits, level of function, and maladaptive handling of intense affects, may well be the psychosocial intervention with the most promise, at least for some patients. Its effects are durable and increase in the 2–3 years after termination. Why it appears to be effective for patients living with their families but ineffective or even destructive for those living independently remains a serious and puzzling drawback.

The impression from all of these studies is that any effective treatment for schizophrenia, psychosocial or biologic, that reduces relapse rates and days in hospital will be cost-effective. Treatments that significantly improve social and vocational function (i.e., SST) will, in all probability, also be cost-effective. Further, the more clinically powerful the intervention, the more likely it is to be cost-effective.

The same cost-effectiveness questions directed to psychosocial interventions have also been raised about the newer second-generation antipsychotic agents. The atypical serotonin/dopamine antagonists (e.g., risperidone and olanzapine) tend to be clinically superior to the older antipsychotics but also much more expensive by a factor of 30 to 40 times. These drugs frequently help patients whose positive symptoms were not responsive to first-generation agents, they are more effective for negative symptoms, and they tend to have less problematic side-effect profiles. Despite their greatly increased costs, when they keep patients out of the hospital, decrease visits to emergency rooms, and make rehabilitation efforts more successful, the total costs of the illness are decreased. Several studies have demonstrated the cost-effectiveness of clozapine and risperidone utilizing this approach (Aronson 1987; Meltzer et al. 1993; Rosenheck et al. 1993).

With respect to psychosocial treatments, estimates on the cost impact obtainable by the increased use of effective treatment interventions do suggest their cost-effectiveness for schizophrenia (Chisholm 2005; Vos et al. 2005). And these estimates seem to be borne out by the study of Spanish patients with schizophrenia demonstrating that family psychotherapy, SST, and cognitive-behavioral therapy do contribute both to efficacy and to cost-effectiveness and magnify the effectiveness of psychopharmacological treatment (Gutierrez-Recacha et al. 2006).

# References

American Psychiatric Association: Diagnostic and Statistical Manual of Mental Disorders, 4th Edition, Text Revision. Washington, DC, American Psychiatric Association, 2000

Aronson SM: Cost-effectiveness and quality of life in psychosis: the pharmacoeconomics of risperidone. Clin Ther 19:139–147; discussion 126–137, 1997

Bellack AS, Haas GL, Schooler NR, et al: Effects of behavioural family management on family communication and patient outcomes in schizophrenia. Br J Psychiatry 177:434–439, 2000

Berglund N, Vahlne JO, Edman A: Family intervention in schizophrenia: impact on family burden and attitude. Soc Psychiatry Psychiatr Epidemiol 38:116–121, 2003

Brooker C, Falloon I, Butterworth A, et al: The outcome of training community psychiatric nurses to deliver psychosocial intervention. Br J Psychiatry 165:222–230, 1994

Brown GW, Birley JL, Wing JK: Influence of family life on the course of schizophrenic disorders: a replication. Br J Psychiatry 121:241–258, 1972

Chisholm D: Choosing cost-effective interventions in psychiatry: results from the CHOICE programme of the World Health Organization. World Psychiatry 4:37–44, 2005

Eckman TA, Wirshing WC, Marder SR, et al: Technique for training schizophrenic patients in illness self-management: a controlled trial. Am J Psychiatry 149:1549–1555, 1992

Falloon IR, McGill CW, Boyd JL, et al: Family management in the prevention of morbidity of schizophrenia: social outcome of a two-year longitudinal study. Psychol Med 17:59–66, 1987

Fromm-Reichmann F: Principles of Intensive Psychotherapy. Chicago, IL, University of Chicago Press, 1950

Gabbard GO, Lazar SG, Hornberger J, et al: The economic impact of psychotherapy: a review. Am J Psychiatry 154:147–155, 1997

Glick ID, Spencer JH Jr, Clarkin JF, et al: A randomized clinical trial of inpatient family intervention, IV: Follow-up results for subjects with schizophrenia. Schizophr Res 3:187–200, 1990

Glick ID, Clarkin JF, Haas GL, et al: Clinical significance of inpatient family intervention: conclusions from a clinical trial. Hosp Community Psychiatry 44:869–873, 1993

Gunderson JG, Frank AF, Katz HM, et al: Effects of psychotherapy in schizophrenia, II: comparative outcome of two forms of treatment. Schizophr Bull 10:564–598, 1984

Gutierrez-Recacha P, Chisholm D, Haro JM, et al: Cost-effectiveness of different clinical interventions for reducing the burden of schizophrenia in Spain. Acta Psychiatr Scand Suppl 432:29–38, 2006

Haas GL, Glick ID, Clarkin JF, et al: Inpatient family intervention: a randomized clinical trial, II: results at hospital discharge. Arch Gen Psychiatry 45:217–224, 1988

Hogarty GE: Personal Therapy for Schizophrenia and Related Disorders. New York, Guilford, 2002

Hogarty GE, Anderson CM, Reiss DJ, et al: Family psychoeducation, social skills training, and maintenance chemotherapy in the aftercare treatment of schizophrenia, I: one-year effects of a controlled study on relapse and expressed emotion. Arch Gen Psychiatry 43:633–642, 1986

Hogarty GE, Anderson CM, Reiss DJ, et al: Family psychoeducation, social skills training, and maintenance chemotherapy in the aftercare treatment of schizophrenia, II: two-year effects of a controlled study on relapse and adjustment. Environmental-Personal Indicators in the Course of Schizophrenia (EPICS) Research Group. Arch Gen Psychiatry 48:340–347, 1991

Hogarty GE, Kornblith SJ, Greenwald D, et al: Personal therapy: a disorder-relevant psychotherapy for schizophrenia. Schizophr Bull 21:379–393, 1995

Hogarty GE, Greenwald D, Ulrich RF, et al: Three-year trials of personal therapy among schizophrenic patients living with or independent of family, I: Description of study and effects on relapse rates. Am J Psychiatry 154:1504–1513, 1997a

Hogarty GE, Greenwald D, Ulrich RF, et al: Three-year trials of personal therapy among schizophrenic patients living with or independent of family, II: Effects on adjustment of patients. Am J Psychiatry 154:1514–1524, 1997b

Hooley JM, Orley J, Teasdale JD: Levels of expressed emotion and relapse in depressed patients. Br J Psychiatry 148:642–647, 1986

Koenigsberg HW, Handley R: Expressed emotion: from predictive index to clinical construct. Am J Psychiatry 143:1361–1373, 1986

Koenigsberg HW, Klausner E, Pelino D, et al: Expressed emotion and glucose control in insulin-dependent diabetes mellitus. Am J Psychiatry 150:1114–1115, 1993

Leff J, Berkowitz R, Shavit N, et al: A trial of family therapy v. a relatives group for schizophrenia. Br J Psychiatry 154:58–66, 1989

Leff J, Berkowitz R, Shavit N, et al: A trial of family therapy versus a relatives' group for schizophrenia: two-year follow-up. Br J Psychiatry 157:571–577, 1990

Lehtinen K: Need-adapted treatment of schizophrenia: a five-year follow-up study from the Turku project. Acta Psychiatr Scand 87:96–101, 1993

Liberman RP, Mueser KT, Wallace CJ: Social skills training for schizophrenic individuals at risk for relapse. Am J Psychiatry 143:523–526, 1986

Liberman RP, Cardin V, McGill CW, et al: Behavioral family management of schizophrenia: clinical outcome and costs. Psychiatric Annals 17:610–619, 1987

May P: Treatment of Schizophrenia: A Comparative Study of Five Treatment Methods. New York, Science House, 1968

McFarlane WR, Link B, Dushay R, et al: Psychoeducational multiple family groups: four-year relapse outcome in schizophrenia. Fam Process 34:127–144, 1995a

McFarlane WR, Lukens E, Link B, et al: Multiple-family groups and psychoeducation in the treatment of schizophrenia. Arch Gen Psychiatry 52:679–687, 1995b

Meltzer HY, Cola P, Way L, et al: Cost effectiveness of clozapine in neuroleptic-resistant schizophrenia. Am J Psychiatry 150:1630–1638, 1993

Montero I, Asencio A, Hernandez I, et al: Two strategies for family intervention in schizophrenia: a randomized trial in a Mediterranean environment. Schizophr Bull 27:661–670, 2001

Mosher LR: Soteria and other alternatives to acute psychiatric hospitalization: a personal and professional review. J Nerv Ment Dis 187:142–149, 1999

Mueser KT, Sengupta A, Schooler NR, et al: Family treatment and medication dosage reduction in schizophrenia: effects on patient social functioning, family attitudes, and burden. J Consult Clin Psychol 69:3–12, 2001

Rosenheck R, Massari L, Frisman L: Who should receive high-cost mental health treatment and for how long? Schizophr Bull 19:843–852, 1993

Rund BR, Moe L, Sollien T, et al: The Psychosis Project: outcome and cost-effectiveness of a psychoeducational treatment programme for schizophrenic adolescents. Acta Psychiatr Scand 89:211–218, 1994

Saha S, Chant D, Welham J, et al: A systematic review of the prevalence of schizophrenia. PLoS Med 2:E141, 2005

Schooler NR, Keith SJ, Severe JB, et al: Relapse and rehospitalization during maintenance treatment of schizophrenia: the effects of dose reduction and family treatment. Arch Gen Psychiatry 54:453–463, 1997

Searles H: Collected Papers on Schizophrenia and Related Subjects. London, Hogarth Press, 1965

Spiegel D, Wissler T: Using family consultation as psychiatric aftercare for schizophrenic patients. Hosp Community Psychiatry 38:1096–1099, 1987

Tarrier N, Barrowclough C, Vaughn C, et al: Community management of schizophrenia: a two-year follow-up of a behavioural intervention with families. Br J Psychiatry 154:625–628, 1989

Tarrier N, Lowson, Barrowclough C: Some aspects of family intervention in schizophrenia. Br J Psychiatry 159:481–484, 1991

Tarrier N, Barrowclough C, Porceddu K, et al: The Salford Family Intervention Project: relapse rates of schizophrenia at five and eight years. Br J Psychiatry 165:829–832, 1994

Vaughn CE, Snyder KS, Freeman W, et al: Family factors in schizophrenic relapse: a replication. Schizophr Bull 8:425–426, 1982

Vos T, Haby MM, Magnus A, et al: Assessing cost-effectiveness in mental health: helping policy-makers prioritize and plan health services. Aust N Z J Psychiatry 39:701–712, 2005

Wu EQ, Birnbaum HG, Shi L, et al: The economic burden of shcizophrenia in the United States in 2002. J Clin Psychiatry 66:1122–1129, 2005

Wyatt RJ, Henter I, Leary MC, et al: An economic evaluation of schizophrenia—1991. Soc Psychiatry Psychiatr Epidemiol 30:196–205, 1995

Zhang M, Wang M, Li J, et al: Randomised control trial of family interventions for 78 first-episode male schizophrenic patients. Br J Psychiatry 165:96–102, 1994

Zhang M, He Y, Gittelman M, et al: Group psychoeducation of relatives of schizophrenic patients: two-year experiences. Psychiatry Clin Neurosci 52 (suppl): S344–S347, 1998

## Summary of studies on psychotherapy of schizophrenia

| Article | Patients | Treatment | Outcome |
|---|---|---|---|
| **Family therapy** | | | |
| 1. Hogarty et al. 1986 | 103 patients with schizophrenia or schizoaffective disorder, residing in high expressed emotion (EE) households. | Random assignment to four treatment groups; assessment at 12 and 24 months of treatment: | At 12 months, no patient treated with FI plus SST relapsed. Each (FI and SST) decreased relapse rate by 50%. |
| 2. Hogarty et al. 1991 | | Treatment 1 (Experimental): family psychoeducation and management (family intervention, FI) | Treatment (Rx.) relapse rates 1: 20% 2: 20% 3: 0% 4: 40% |
| (both papers discuss same study) | | Treatment 2 (Experimental): social skills training (SST) | At 24 months, FI continued to be effective, but SST lost its effectiveness. |
| | | Treatment 3 (Experimental): combined FI and SST | Rx. relapse rates 1: 30% 2: 50% 3: 25% 4: 62% |
| | | Treatment 4 (Control): supportive therapy, individual | (see Treatment column) |

## Summary of studies on psychotherapy of schizophrenia *(continued)*

| Article | Patients | Treatment | Outcome |
|---|---|---|---|
| **Family therapy** *(continued)* | | | |
| 1. Falloon et al. 1987 | 39 patients with schizophrenia. | Random assignment to individual or family treatment: | A. Clinical<br>Home-based family treatment superior on all clinical measures: relapses, psychiatric symptoms, days in hospital, smaller doses of neuroleptic. |
| 2. Liberman et al. 1987 | Patients stabilized on neuroleptic and living with, or in daily contact with, high EE families. | Treatment 1 (Experimental): home based, behavioral family therapy, problem solving, and management.<br>Treatment 2 (Control): clinic based, problem oriented, supportive, individual therapy<br>Assessment at baseline, 9 months, 24 months of treatment. | B. Economic<br>Family treatment produced higher outpatient costs, much lower inpatient costs; lower total costs. (Mean cost per patient—$41,690 Rx.1 vs. $70,200 Rx.2.) |
| (both papers discuss same study) | | | |
| Spiegel and Wissler 1987 | 36 veterans with schizophrenia who lived with their families. | Patients randomly assigned to:<br>Treatment 1 (Experimental): problem solving, consultative home visits, plus treatment as usual (TAU)<br>Treatment 2 (Control): TAU<br><br>TAU = psychotherapy and medications as outpatient or day hospital, vocational guidance | 3 months<br>Rx.1 superior to Rx.2: fewer days in hospital, higher ratings on adjustment scales.<br>12 months<br>Trend to higher adjustment ratings, no difference in days in hospital. |

## Summary of studies on psychotherapy of schizophrenia *(continued)*

| Article | Patients | Treatment | Outcome |
|---|---|---|---|
| **Family therapy *(continued)*** | | | |
| 1. Glick et al. 1993<br><br>2. Haas et al. 1988<br><br>3. Glick et al. 1990<br><br>(all three papers discuss the same study) | 92 patients with schizophrenia, schizoaffective, or schizophreniform disorder; live with, or regular contact with, family. | Schizophrenia patients divided into good and poor premorbid patients on the basis of prehospitalization function and randomly assigned to:<br>Treatment 1 (Experimental): TAU, plus inpatient family intervention (IFI)<br>Treatment 2 (Control): TAU | A. Patients with schizophrenia with good premorbid course; for females, trend favoring IFI; for males, better outcome for control (TAU) treatment.<br><br>B. Patients with schizophrenia with poor premorbid course; IFI had significantly better outcomes for all patients, more marked in females.<br><br>C. For all families, more positive attitudes to female patients in IFI group.<br><br>In poor premorbid patients, IFI produced more positive family attitudes for all patients, regardless of gender. |

## Summary of studies on psychotherapy of schizophrenia *(continued)*

| Article | Patients | Treatment | Outcome |
|---|---|---|---|
| **Family therapy *(continued)*** | | | |
| 1. Leff et al. 1989<br><br>2. Leff et al. 1990<br><br>(both papers discuss same study) | 23 patients with schizophrenia and their families, ages 16–65, living in high contact (> 35 hr/week) with high EE families. | Patients maintained on neuroleptic, 18 of 23 on depot drug. Randomly assigned to family therapy (12) or relatives' group (11).<br><br>Patient randomly assigned to:<br>Treatment 1 (Experimental): education, plus family therapy in the home; patient included<br>Treatment 2 (Experimental): education, plus relatives' group at clinic; patient not included<br><br>Two treatments not equally accepted; 11 of 12 families accepted family therapy, 6 of 11 accepted relatives' group.<br>Treatments every 2 weeks, then at decreasing frequency for 9 months. | At 9 months:<br>Relapse rates 8% for family therapy patients, 36% for relatives' group patients. When relatives attended at least one group, relapse rate decreased to 17%. All differences not significant.<br><br>At 24 months:<br>Relapse rates 33% for family therapy, 36% for relatives' group; both psychosocial interventions produced lower relapse rates (40%), compared with no intervention (75%). |

## Summary of studies on psychotherapy of schizophrenia *(continued)*

| Article | Patients | Treatment | Outcome |
|---|---|---|---|
| **Family therapy** *(continued)* | | | |
| 1. Tarrier et al. 1989<br>2. Tarrier et al. 1991<br>3. Tarrier et al. 1994<br><br>(all three papers discuss the same study) | 73 patients with schizophrenia and their families were subdivided into high and low EE families. | Families divided into low and high EE; high EE families randomly received:<br>Treatment 1 (Experimental): behavioral family intervention for high EE families<br>Treatment 2 (Control): brief psychoeducation, plus TAU for high EE families<br><br>Treatment 2a (Control): brief psycho-education, plus TAU for low EE families<br>FI group with the goal of decreasing high EE. | A. Clinical<br>Behavioral family intervention with high EE families was more effective than TAU. Outcomes of FI in high EE families were similar to low EE families.<br><br>B. Costs<br>Rx.1 less costly than Rx.2 (total costs) Savings of £432 (27%) per patient, £17,112 (37%) for whole group. |

**Summary of studies on psychotherapy of schizophrenia** *(continued)*

| Article | Patients | Treatment | Outcome |
|---|---|---|---|
| **Family therapy** *(continued)* | | | |
| Lehtinen 1993 | 28 first-contact patients with schizophrenia treated 1983–1984 (Treatment 1 group). 56 first-contact patients with schizophrenia treated 1976–1977 (Treatment 2 group). | Nonrandom distribution; the two treatment groups were studied over different time periods: Treatment 1 (1983) (Experimental): family and network therapy; general systems approach Treatment 2 (1976) (Control): long-term dynamic psychotherapy, long hospital stays, and intensive milieu treatment | A. Clinical 5-year follow-up: Rx.1 patients had more positive clinical course than Rx.2 patients: a) Less psychotic symptoms b) Better social function c) Less days in hospital d) Less outpatient visits e) Less patients on disability<br><br>B. Economic Rx.1, decreased total costs. Mean Rx. cost/patient (ECU = European Currency Unit): Rx.1 = 30,000 ECU Rx.2 = 59,000 ECU |
| Brooker et al. 1994 | 48 patients with schizophrenia living, or sustained contact, with "relative or significant other." | Patients nonrandomly assigned 24 to each group: Treatment 1 (Experimental): weekly family psychoeducation, problem solving, and crisis intervention Treatment 2 (Control): wait list (treated later) | Rx.1 > Rx.2: Decreased positive symptoms Decreased negative symptoms Improved social function Decreased time in hospital (not significant) Improved general health and satisfaction in caretakers |

**Summary of studies on psychotherapy of schizophrenia *(continued)***

| Article | Patients | Treatment | Outcome |
|---|---|---|---|
| Family therapy *(continued)* | | | |
| Rund et al. 1994 | 24 young patients with schizophrenia (onset 13–18). | No random distribution; the two treatments were delivered at different times; 12 patients in each treatment group.<br>Treatment 1 (Experimental): psychoeducational problem solving, parent seminars, improving social networks<br>Treatment 2 (Control) (same hospital, earlier time): individual and milieu therapy; TAU for the time<br>Assessment at 24 months of treatment. | A. Clinical<br>Rx.1 more effective; patient function and EE of parents improved. Poor-prognosis patients benefited most.<br>Relapse rate:<br>Rx.1 more effective than Rx.2<br>Rx.1: 7 of 12 families changed from high to low EE<br>Rx.2: 0 of 12 families changed from high to low EE<br><br>B. Economic<br>Whole group direct costs (Norwegian krone, NOK):<br>17.4 million (Rx.1) vs. 22.8 million (Rx.2). (The 5 million NOK difference is about $720,000.) |

## Summary of studies on psychotherapy of schizophrenia *(continued)*

| Article | Patients | Treatment | Outcome |
|---|---|---|---|
| **Family therapy** *(continued)* | | | |
| Zhang et al. 1994 | 78 male patients with schizophrenia, first admission, living with family, treated with oral neuroleptics. | Patients randomly distributed to two treatments; patients evaluated Q 3 months for 18 months postdischarge from hospital. Treatment 1 (Experimental): FI Q 1–3 months, with focus on psychoeducation and management Treatment 2 (Control): as needed to outpatient department | Treatment 1 superior to Treatment 2: Rx.1 vs. Rx.2 A. Rehospitalization 6 vs. 21 B. Hospital free 245 days vs. 130 days C. Global Assessment Scale (GAS) scores: +6 –9 (Similar results for Brief Psychiatric Rating Scale and GAS scores.) |
| 1. McFarlane et al. 1995b 2. McFarlane et al. 1995a (both papers discuss same study) | 172 patients (18–45) with schizophrenia, schizoaffective, or schizophreniform disorder and their families. Inpatient at recruitment, living with family, or more than 10 hours of contact per week. | Random assignment to: Treatment 1 (Experimental): multiple family groups (MFGs) Treatment 2 (Control): single family therapy (SFT) | A. Clinical 1. Relapse—Rx.1 less relapses $P$=0.06 2. Hospitalization—equal rates 3. Positive and negative symptoms— Rx.1>Rx.2 ns 4. Employment—both groups improved over time, no difference B. Economic Both Rxs. cost-effective. Rx.1>Rx.2. Rx.1 used 50% of the staff of Rx.2. Rx.1 $3,875 per patient per year less expensive than Rx.2. Cost-benefit Rx.1 (MFG)=1:34 Cost-benefit Rx.2 (SFT)=1:17 |

**Summary of studies on psychotherapy of schizophrenia *(continued)***

| Article | Patients | Treatment | Outcome |
|---|---|---|---|
| *Family therapy (continued)* | | | |
| Schooler et al. 1997 | 313 male and female patients with schizophrenia or schizoaffective disorder. | Patients randomly assigned to one of three medication strategies using fluphenazine decanoate of 1) continuous moderate dose, 2) continuous low dose, or 3) targeted early intervention only when symptomatic. Subjects were then randomly assigned to one of two family treatment interventions: 1. Supportive family management (SFM) monthly group meetings 2. More intensive family management with monthly group meetings and home visits teaching communication and problem solving skills All treatments were given for 2 years. | Both continuous low dose and targeted treatment increased use of rescue medication and relapse; targeted treatment increased rehospitalization. Compliance was enhanced for all subjects although there were no differences between the two family treatment groups. |

## Summary of studies on psychotherapy of schizophrenia *(continued)*

| Article | Patients | Treatment | Outcome |
|---|---|---|---|
| **Family therapy** *(continued)* | | | |
| Zhang et al. 1998 | Relatives of schizophrenia patients:<br>1. 682 cases in experimental group<br>2. 366 cases in control group | Group psychotherapy including 14 lectures and 5 group discussions with conventional services. Control group received conventional services only. No significant differences in sociodemographic characteristics between the two groups. | Annual relapse rate in the experimental group was much lower than in control group and rate of regular work was higher in experimental group. At the end of the 2nd year, the relatives in the experimental group had less care burden, better mental and physical health status, and more knowledge of caring for schizophrenics than those in the control group. Experimental group dropout rate was only 18.4% during the 2-year treatment period. |
| Bellack et al. 2000 | 77 patients with schizophrenia and their families. | Random assignment to one of two family treatments:<br>1. Behavioral family intervention, applied family management (AFM), provided structured training in communication and problem-solving skills to reduce family conflict and increase nonhostile communication<br>2. Family support program, SFM, including monthly multiple family group meetings and case management as needed | No group differences in acquisition of communication skills for either patients or family. Change in communication was unrelated to patient outcomes. |

## Summary of studies on psychotherapy of schizophrenia *(continued)*

| Article | Patients | Treatment | Outcome |
|---|---|---|---|
| **Family therapy *(continued)*** | | | |
| Montero et al. 2001 | 41 patients with schizophrenia and their families. | Random assignment to two different FIs:<br>1. A relatives' group<br>2. A single family behavioral family therapy (BFT) | Relapse rate at 12 months was not significantly different for the two groups. The BFT group had better social adjustment, greater reduction on psychotic symptoms, and a lower dropout rate. |
| Mueser et al. 2001 | 528 patients with schizophrenia, schizoaffective, or schizophreniform disorder, with symptom relapse or psychiatric hospitalization in prior 3 months, currently outpatients. | Treatment 1 (Experimental)<br>AFM BFT × 1 year, plus Support Groups × 2 years<br>Treatment 2 (Control): SFM × 2 years<br>Treatment 3: three different fluphenazine enanthate doses: standard, low, and intermittent | 1. Rx.1 led to less patient rejection by relatives and less family friction.<br>2. Both Rx.1 and Rx.2 improved patient social function but did not differ from each other.<br>3. Family burden in both E and C conditions was unchanged.<br>4. Medication conditions had little effect, but patients on standard dose did best.<br>5. Medication conditions did not interact with FIs. |
| Berglund et al. 2003 | 31 families in which 1) one member was diagnosed as schizophrenic or schizoaffective disorder and 2) patients had regular contact with their families. | Treatment 1 (Experimental): BFT<br>Treatment 2 (Control): conventional family support<br>Both treatments started when the patient suffered a relapse and was psychiatrically hospitalized and terminated when the patient was discharged.<br>During treatments, all patients were in hospital. | 1. At discharge, Rx.1 > Rx.2 in measurements of family burden.<br>2. Rx.1 > Rx.2 in reducing neuroleptic dose.<br>3. Rx.1 > Rx.2 in relapse rates in the 1 year following discharge. This was highly significant ($P<0.001$).<br>4. Rx.1 > Rx.2 in improved family attitudes to patient. |

## Summary of studies on psychotherapy of schizophrenia (continued)

| Article | Patients | Treatment | Outcome |
|---|---|---|---|
| **Social skills training for individuals at risk for relapse** | | | |
| Liberman et al. 1986 | 48 male patients (ages 19–35) with schizophrenia, inpatients, stabilized on neuroleptic, at least two previous hospitalizations. | Randomly assigned to: Treatment 1 (Experimental) SST: 1. "Receiving"—perception of others' feelings 2. "Processing"—evaluating possible responses 3. "Sending"—communication to others, e.g., voice volume Treatment 2 (Control): "holistic" health treatment: 1. Stress reduction techniques 2. Increasing self-esteem | A. Psychopathology ratings decreased significantly in both groups, but Rx.1 > Rx.2: a. Better social adjustment ratings b. Decreased symptomatology c. Lower relapse rate d. Better course of illness e. Less rehospitalizations B. Families of Rx.1 patients showed decreased EE. |
| Eckman et al. 1992 | 41 male (mean age 40) patients with schizophrenia, moderately ill, no substance abuse; 25% had been married. | Random assignment to: Treatment 1 (Experimental): skills training in groups; medication and symptom self-management Treatment 2 (Control): supportive group therapy—insight, support, psycho-education (All patients also received case management, psychiatric, medical, and social services.) | Assessments at pretreatment baseline, treatment termination, and 6 and 12 months posttermination. A. Patients in both Rxs. improved over time. Differences favored skills training, but not significant. B. Patients treated with skills training learned and retained those skills, regardless of severity of psychopathology. C. More dropouts from Rx.2. |

## Summary of studies on psychotherapy of schizophrenia *(continued)*

| Article | Patients | Treatment | Outcome |
|---|---|---|---|
| **Studies estimating cost-effectiveness of different interventions for large patient populations** | | | |
| Chisholm 2005 | From the mental health component of World Health Organization CHOICE PROJECT, the costs and effects of pharmacological and psychological interventions were modeled for four disorders, including schizophrenia. | Generating cost-effectiveness evidence for effective pharmacological and psychosocial interventions for various illnesses, including schizophrenia, in a range of geographical and epidemiological settings around the world. | 1. Impact of psychotropic drugs for schizophrenia is modest, with a 25% improvement in functioning compared with no treatment, but no reduction in the incidence or duration of illness. <br> 2. Improvement in functioning approaches 45% when psychosocial treatment is also given. Adding psychosocial treatment to psychotropic medication provides far greater benefit than switching from older to newer antipsychotic medication. <br> 3. Psychosocial treatment, for a modest additional cost, provides greater benefit and is more cost-effective than pharmacotherapy alone. |
| Vos et al. 2005 | Estimates made on impact of expenditures and health status if recommended mental health treatments for schizophrenia were to be implemented in Australia. | 1. More efficient drug *intervention*; and <br> 2. Provision of family psychotherapy interventions | More efficient drug *interventions* would save $68 million (Australian), which would more than cover an estimated $36 million (Australian) annual cost of providing family psychotherapy interventions. The above changes would lead to an estimated 12% improvement in health status. |

## Summary of studies on psychotherapy of schizophrenia *(continued)*

| Article | Patients | Treatment | Outcome |
|---|---|---|---|
| **Studies estimating cost-effectiveness of different interventions for large patient populations** *(continued)* | | | |
| Gutierrez-Recacha et al. 2006 | Spanish patients with schizophrenia. | An estimate of the cost-effectiveness of seven different types of clinical interventions for schizophrenic patients in Spain: <br><br> 1. Current situation (treatment patterns used in Spain in 2000) referring to a variety of both older and newer antipsychotic psychotropic agents <br> 2. Older antipsychotics alone <br> 3. New antipsychotics alone (risperidone) <br> 4. Older antipsychotics plus psychosocial treatment <br> 5. New antipsychotics plus psychosocial treatments <br> 6. Older antipsychotics plus case management and psychosocial treatment <br> 7. New antipsychotics plus case management and psychosocial treatment | The relatively low added costs of adding psychosocial treatment would yield significant health gains making such a combined strategy for schizophrenia more cost-effective than medication alone. |

# 3

# Psychotherapy in the Treatment of Borderline Personality Disorder

Robert J. Waldinger, M.D.

This chapter reviews the research literature on psychotherapy of borderline personality disorder (BPD). A search was conducted of MEDLINE and PsycINFO from 1980 to 2007, and studies for this review were limited to those with more than 10 subjects, well-defined measures of outcome, and specific outcome variables (e.g., number of inpatient days used per patient per year) that had direct bearing on economic considerations involved in decision making about mental health care policy. The 10 published studies and one unpublished doctoral dissertation that met these criteria are reviewed and summarized in the table at the end of this chapter. The studies strongly suggest that providing outpatient group and/or individual psychotherapy for patients with borderline personality disorder reduces their use of psychiatric inpatient services and outpatient medical services, and reduces self-destructive episodes requiring emergency room care. Long-term follow-up of subjects in several of these studies (most often 1-year posttermination) shows that patients maintain the gains achieved by the end of a 1-year course of treatment.

# Defining the Problem

Borderline personality disorder is a crippling condition characterized by self-destructive behaviors (e.g., self-mutilation, substance abuse, high-risk sexual behaviors), chronic suicidality, and notoriously unstable and intense relationships. Crises are the hallmark of this disorder, so much so that BPD is often considered a disorder marked by stable instability. The very nature of the disorder—particularly the desperate, help-seeking quality of many borderline patients' relationships, makes these patients disproportionately high consumers of medical and mental health care. While the prevalence of BPD has been estimated at 1.8% of the general population in the United States (Swartz et al. 1990), borderline patients account for 19% of psychiatric inpatients and 11% of psychiatric outpatients (Widiger and Frances 1989). In primary care, the prevalence of BPD is high (6.4% or four times that in the general population), with patients experiencing a high rate of current suicidal ideation, anxiety and depressive disorders, and functional impairment. Nearly half of these patients are not recognized or diagnosed, and half report not receiving mental health treatment in the past year (Gross et al. 2002). Patients with BPD commonly seek help in psychiatric emergency rooms after suicide gestures and more serious attempts. Moreover, the rate of completed suicides among individuals with BPD is high: An estimated 7% to 10% of borderline patients ultimately kill themselves (McGlashan 1986; Paris et al. 1987; Stone et al. 1987). The following clinical vignette is typical of the complexity of BPD and the variety of demands that BPD places on social, medical, and mental health care systems.

## Clinical Vignette

Mrs. N is a 35-year-old married secretary and mother of two daughters, ages 12 and 15. She first sought psychiatric treatment at age 18 after a suicide attempt in her dormitory room 3 months into her freshman year of college. She moved back home with her parents at that time, and at age 19, married her high school boyfriend "to get away from home once and for all." She described an unhappy childhood notable for her mother's unavailability and unpredictability due to chronic alcoholism, and her father's violence and intermittent alcohol abuse. Mrs. N describes her husband as "my rock, an anchor when I'm tossed around by storms." She made occasional suicide gestures during her 20s, usually precipitated by arguments in which her husband threatened to leave her. These resulted in emergency room visits and one brief hospitalization.

When she was 32, her older daughter's menarche triggered Mrs. N's recollection of multiple episodes of sexual abuse (intercourse) by her father at age 12. Flashbacks of the abuse experiences precipitated an episode of serious self-laceration requiring emergency surgery and subsequent medical and psychiatric hospitalization. During the next 4 years, she was hospitalized seven times, was chronically absent from work, and was increasingly unable to share in household tasks and child-rearing activities. During the height of Mrs. N's illness, her younger daughter refused to go to school for 2 months and became depressed and suicidal. This daughter required intensive outpatient psychotherapy for 12 months, and a psychiatric hospitalization was narrowly averted. Mrs. N's older daughter began spending most of her time away from home. Mrs. N's husband initiated divorce proceedings and filed for custody of both children.

Mrs. N's story is sadly familiar to mental health professionals who treat patients with BPD. Suicide attempts, emergency room visits, medical complications, and frequent hospitalizations are common stigmas of the borderline syndrome. BPD exacts a heavy toll on others as well as on the individual suffering from the disorder. Failed relationships, unstable work histories, and poor or inconsistent parenting are common themes in the lives of individuals with BPD. The intergenerational transmission of inadequate parenting is one of the environmental routes by which the borderline syndrome may be passed on from parent to child (Masterson 1971). The costliness of BPD in individual, societal, and socioeconomic terms has prompted a search for treatments that can ameliorate the disorder and help patients achieve and maintain their best level of functioning.

Psychotherapy is the cornerstone of treatment for BPD. It is the most widely used treatment modality, and it is most widely believed to be of long-term benefit to borderline patients. Although pharmacotherapy has proved to be effective for managing some symptoms of BPD, it does not affect the core deficits in ego functioning that lie at the heart of the borderline syndrome (Waldinger and Frank 1989). Day hospital and inpatient treatment are costly, and feasible only as short-term measures for crisis intervention. This chapter examines existing research on the efficacy and cost offset of psychosocial treatments for BPD. This literature was reviewed several years ago by Gabbard et al. (1997), and what follows is informed by and based on their earlier work.

There is a rich literature on the psychotherapy of BPD (Buie and Adler 1982; Kernberg 1975; Waldinger 1987). Case reports indicate that borderline individuals are capable of making substantial improvements in mood, in occupational and social functioning, and in their ability to function without extensive use of costly mental health services (Abend et al. 1983; Waldinger and Gunderson 1987). However, the majority of treatments of borderline patients end in premature termination and/or failure (Waldinger and Gunderson 1984), leaving clinicians to question the representativeness of case reports that report favorable responses to psychotherapeutic treatments.

The natural development of research toward more rigorously designed outcome studies of treatments for BPD has been slow and fraught with difficulties (Aronson 1989). The obstacles to measuring the effects of psychotherapy on the course and outcome of BPD are formidable. Definition of the borderline syndrome has, until the advent of DSM-III, been poor, and even now definitions of BPD used by clinicians and researchers are fraught with ambiguity (Waldinger 1993). The current diagnostic standard is the set of criteria used in DSM-IV-TR (American Psychiatric Association 2000), and most researchers apply these criteria or earlier versions of them in recent research. These difficulties are by no means unique to the study of BPD but rather are paradigmatic of the challenges faced by psychotherapy outcome research in all areas of the field.

Psychotherapy outcome studies rely on patients to remain in treatment long enough for the intervention to have effects. Borderline patients drop out of treatment at particularly high rates (Perry et al. 1999). As many as 50% of patients can be expected to leave long-term treatment within the first 6 months (Waldinger and Gunderson 1984). Thus, high rates of dropouts and missing data plague most studies of long-term (greater than 6 months) treatment of BPD.

Definitions of psychotherapy vary widely. While the literature on the psychotherapy of BPD is vast, there have been few attempts to write down treatment protocols in manuals that can be used to train therapists to deliver a more or less uniform intervention. And once therapists are trained in a given technique, they must be monitored for adherence to this technique to combat the natural tendency to revert to more habitual ways of doing psychotherapy. Few investigators have monitored adherence among therapists. Several of the studies reviewed here (e.g., Linehan et al. 1991; Munroe-Blum and Marziali 1995) have made significant strides toward standardizing both the treatments and their delivery by psychotherapists.

Perhaps most daunting is the high cost of psychotherapy outcome research. Therapists, trainers, supervisors, and raters must all be paid for the large investment of time that such studies require. Not surprisingly, few outcome studies of long-term treatments have been funded by public or private agencies. Among existing studies, financial arrangements can confound observed differences between groups. For example, in Linehan et al.'s (1991) comparison of dialectical behavior therapy (DBT) with treatment-as-usual (TAU) in the local community, the DBT condition was paid for as part of the study, but patients in the TAU had to finance their own therapy.

Despite all of the above obstacles, studies of long-term psychotherapy of BPD have begun to demonstrate that borderline individuals make significant improvements in treatment, and these improvements are not only in quality of life but also in behaviors that have direct economic implications: most particularly, decreases in use of emergency rooms, psychiatric inpatient days, psychiatric day hospital days, outpatient visits to medical and surgical providers, and days absent from work.

Considerations of the costs and benefits of psychotherapy for BPD are complex. Generally, cost-effectiveness studies have emphasized cost issues more than questions of efficacy. Costs of any treatment must be assessed in terms of the actual costs of delivering the treatment as well as the costs of disability, lost productivity, and problems on the job. Modeled on the review by Gabbard et al. (1997), the following discussion uses a broader standard of cost-effectiveness: 1) reduction in medical/surgical outpatient visits and reduction in medical inpatient days, 2) reduction in psychiatric inpatient days, and 3) reduction in indirect expenses associated with work productivity.

As noted above, several studies stand apart from the bulk of research on psychotherapy of BPD, in that they are more rigorously designed, attempt to control important factors in the delivery of treatments, and/or use larger numbers of subjects than have other studies of psychotherapy outcome. These studies are discussed below and are summarized in the review table at the end of this chapter.

# Individual Psychotherapy

Individual psychotherapy is the most widely used psychotherapeutic modality in the treatment of BPD. Numerous theoretical orientations have guided such therapies. The most prevalent orientations currently used by mental health professionals to treat BPD in the United States are 1) psychodynamic therapy, which aims to help patients understand the childhood origins of many psychological symptoms and interpersonal problems; and 2) cognitive-behavioral therapy (CBT), which aims to uncover and change distorted cognitions about the self and others, as well as maladaptive behaviors. Both orientations are represented in studies of the outcome of individual psychotherapy for borderline patients.

Stevenson and Meares (1992) used individual psychodynamic psychotherapy in a study of 30 patients who met DSM-III criteria for BPD who were selected for persisting social dysfunction (e.g., absence of or severely dysfunctional social behavior, antisocial behavior). These patients were given twice-weekly psychodynamic psychotherapy for 12 months by closely supervised trainee therapists. The treatment was not manualized but was based on a psychology of the self and intensively supervised by experienced psychotherapists. This was a repeated measures design in which each patient was assessed before and after treatment. These patients improved significantly during the course of treatment. There was marked and statistically significant decline in the time these patients spent away from work: an av-

erage of 1.37 months per year in the 12 months following treatment, compared with 4.47 months per year in the year prior to treatment. As compared with the year prior to treatment, patients studied for 12 months after
treatment also improved significantly in the following areas that have major
economic consequences: 1) the number of visits to medical professionals
dropped to one-seventh of pretreatment rates; 2) the number of self-harm
incidents dropped to one-quarter of pretreatment rates; 3) the number of
hospital admissions decreased by 59%, and 4) the time patients spent on inpatient units decreased by half. Thirty percent of the cohort were no longer
diagnosable as borderline at the conclusion of the year-long treatment.
When these patients were followed up 5 years posttreatment, the improvements recorded at 1-year follow-up were largely maintained (Stevenson and
Meares 1995). Time away from work, drug use, medical visits, self-harm,
hospital admissions, and time spent as an inpatient remained significantly
reduced from pretreatment levels. Meares et al. (1999) then compared these
30 patients with a group of 30 BPD patients who remained on a clinic waiting list for psychotherapy for at least 12 months and received TAU (e.g.,
medication, supportive therapy, crisis intervention) but did not receive the
specific treatment described above. DSM symptom scores for the treatment
group were significantly reduced at follow-up, whereas scores for the control group were unchanged.

An economic analysis of the cost-effectiveness of treating this cohort of
30 patients was conducted by Stevenson and Meares (1992) in conjunction
with two health economics researchers (Hall et al. 2001). They used data on
inpatient stays, emergency room usage, ambulatory care, and diagnostic testing and medications to estimate the net costs of health service use during
the 12 months prior to the psychotherapy and the 12 months after comple-
tion of the therapy. Data were culled from hospital records and patient recall. For the 30 patients as a group, the cost of health services in the 12
months posttreatment was $670,000 less than it had been in the 12 months
prior to treatment, and most of this reduction was in use of inpatient care.
The psychotherapy cost $130,050 to administer, resulting in a net savings of
$546,509 or approximately $18,000 per patient. When the patients were divided into high users ($n=12$ who had used more than $10,000/year in services
prior to treatment) and low users ($n=18$ who had used less than $10,000/
year), savings were primarily in the high users group. For low users, the
costs of the psychotherapy were about the same as the savings in health service use. However, had other factors been considered, such as improvement
in general health outcomes, savings for the low users group may well have
been demonstrable.

Patient recall of health service use is not wholly reliable, and this is one
limitation of the study. In addition, other outcomes (e.g., absenteeism from

work, nonpsychiatric health care usage) were not considered in this study. Nevertheless, this is one of the first definitive and well-designed studies of the cost-effectiveness of psychotherapy for BPD. The results strongly suggest that a focused, intensive year-long psychotherapy can be of considerable benefit to borderline patients and result in substantial savings in health care costs.

Ryle and Golynkina (2000) studied the effectiveness of time-limited psychotherapy with BPD. They used cognitive analytic therapy (CAT), a treatment model developed by Ryle (1997) that emphasizes collaboration between therapist and patient in identifying the patient's varying self states and switches between them. These understandings are recorded in writing and in diagrams that become the shared tools of therapy, in which therapist and patient work to understand how to avoid negative interpersonal patterns and self-fragmentation. Twenty-seven patients at an inner-city London clinic who met DSM-IV (American Psychiatric Association 1994) criteria for BPD completed 24 sessions of CAT over 6 months. Pre- and posttreatment assessments demonstrated significant changes following CAT. Fourteen patients (52%) no longer met diagnostic criteria for BPD and were judged to require no further treatment. As a group, patients' levels of depression, as measured by the Beck Depression Inventory (Beck et al. 1961), were significantly diminished. Global psychological functioning, as indexed by the global severity index on the Hopkins Symptom Checklist–90–Revised (Derogatis 1983) was significantly improved, as was interpersonal functioning. Although economic factors were not explicitly addressed in this study, there is some indication that these patients used fewer health care resources following treatment. For example, 3 patients were hospitalized after overdoses in the year prior to treatment, but none were hospitalized during the 6 months after treatment ended. The absence of a control group and high attrition rate (33.3%) are significant limitations of this study.

Clarkin et al. (2001) studied 23 female patients who met DSM-IV criteria for BPD and were treated with a manualized transference-focused psychotherapy twice weekly for 12 months. Treaters were well trained, and adherence to the psychotherapy protocol was carefully monitored. In this group, compared with the year prior to treatment, the number of patients who made suicide attempts decreased significantly (from 53% to 18%), as did the medical risk and severity of medical condition following self-injurious behavior. Nineteen percent of patients dropped out of treatment during the study period. Comparing the year prior to treatment with the 12-month period of psychotherapy, the group had significantly fewer hospitalizations (a 67% reduction) as well as fewer inpatient days (an 89% reduction) during the year of treatment. The study sample was a relatively homogeneous group of severely disturbed borderline patients, none of whom abused psychoactive substances. The absence of a control group leaves open the question of the extent to which positive change might have occurred in this group without psychotherapy. However, the results strongly suggest that a twice-weekly treatment that focuses specifically on the relationship between patient and psychotherapist may be both clinically useful and cost-effective.

Other research has suggested that continuous long-term psychotherapy with the same therapist may be advantageous in terms of outcome and cost offset. In research for her doctoral dissertation, Hoke (1989) followed 58 borderline patients for up to 7 years. This was a nonrandomized, naturalistic study of TAU in the community. Half of this group ($n=29$) had intermittent or inconsistent psychotherapeutic treatments, whereas the other half had stable, consistent individual psychotherapy for at least 2 out of 7 years. The group of patients who had stable, long-term psychotherapy had better outcomes than the group with inconsistent psychotherapy in the following areas: fewer emergency room visits, fewer hospitalizations, less use of day treatment facilities, decreased impulsivity, and better mood. The partly retrospective nature of this work, the absence of standardized treatment conditions, and the lack of a control group all limit the generalizability of Hoke's findings. Nevertheless, the study provides a view of the natural course of BPD patients in the community with currently available standard treatments. Hoke's findings of limited but substantial improvement are consistent with those of the other investigators cited in this review.

These four studies vary widely in design and have significant limitations. Only the Stevenson and Meares (1992) study had a control group, and that group was not in active treatment. All four studies compared patient functioning pre- and posttreatment, but only Stevenson and Meares directly addressed cost-effectiveness issues. Although none offers conclusive evidence linking the therapy to functional outcomes, all four studies strongly suggest that individual psychotherapy with borderline patients results in significant gains in functioning that have economic implications. All point to a reduction in the use of costly health care services, particularly of psychiatric inpatient days. None of these studies test the efficacy of a particular approach (e.g., transference-focused therapy, CAT) against other approaches, leaving open the question of which treatment components bring about positive change.

Several more recent studies of psychotherapy for BPD yield more equivocal results. In one (Tyrer et al. 2004), 480 patients with a mixture of diagnoses were treated after an episode of self-harm in a multicenter randomized trial with a brief form of cognitive therapy, manual-assisted cognitive-behavior therapy (MACT), and followed up for over a year. Being 10% cheaper and cost-effective compared with TAU, MACT led to a 50% decrease in the frequency of self-harm episodes with the notable exception of BPD patients who had increased costs after MACT and were the most likely patients to have repeat self-harm episodes. This form of CBT was thus not found to be cost-effective for borderline patients, although Tyrer et al. noted that the absence of effect of MACT for more severe BPD was not surprising because it is a very much briefer treatment, using only a fraction of the resources of the more comprehensive program.

In another study, Palmer et al. (2006) reported on outcomes of the Borderline Personality Disorder Study of Cognitive Therapy (BOSCOT) multicenter randomized controlled trial of CBT (providing up to 27 with average of 16 sessions) plus TAU compared with TAU alone for 106 borderline patients. A cost-effectiveness analysis assessed the quality-adjusted life year of patients at baseline and at 6-monthly intervals over 2 years and also measured both health care utilization costs and related non-health care costs at the same intervals. Total costs per patient in the CBT cohort were lower than patients receiving usual care alone, but the CBT patients also had a lower quality of life. These differences were small and not statistically significant. Although the CBT patients had fewer suicidal acts, lowered anxiety, lessened dysfunctional beliefs, and less inpatient hospitalization costs than the TAU group (and thus slight evidence of a cost advantage for CBT), there did not appear to be a significant cost-effective advantage for CBT based on this study.

# Group Psychotherapy

Group psychotherapy has been used widely in the treatment of BPD patients. Groups have been used both in conjunction with individual psychotherapy and alone. However, there has been little empirical work on the efficacy of group therapy for BPD, and rarely do authors deal with issues related to cost-effectiveness. For example, Joyce et al. (1999) studied 40 borderline patients in an intensive 18-week group psychotherapy, and though they found improvement in psychological functioning over the course of treatment, the study had no control group and did not address specific behavioral outcomes that have economic implications.

Munroe-Blum and Marziali (1995) conducted a randomized, controlled trial of time-limited group psychotherapy compared with individual psychodynamic psychotherapy. The 110 subjects (81% female) who met criteria for BPD on the Diagnostic Interview for Borderlines (Gunderson et al. 1981) were randomly assigned to interpersonal group psychotherapy (IGP), a manualized group treatment of thirty 90-minute sessions over 12 months, or to individual dynamic psychotherapy (IDP). Dropouts at the point of randomization and missing data resulted in final cohorts of 22 subjects in

IGP and 26 subjects in IDP. Subjects were measured at the beginning and end of treatment and at 12 months posttermination using measures of behavioral dysfunction, social adjustment (Social Adjustment Scale), global severity index (Hopkins Symptom Checklist–90), and depression (Beck Depression Inventory). Both groups showed significant improvement on all four measures. In particular, subjects showed significant decreases in impulse control problems and in the use of mental health and social services during both the year of the study and the year following termination of treatment. There were no significant differences in outcome between the group therapy and individual therapy cohorts.

To date, Munroe-Blum and Marziali's (1995) work is the only randomized controlled trial of group treatment specifically for patients with BPD. It lends empirical weight to the more anecdotal findings of case-based research and corroborates clinical evidence that BPD patients in ongoing group psychotherapy rely less heavily on mental health and social services than those patients who do not have such treatment.

# Dialectical Behavior Therapy (Combined Individual and Group Psychotherapy)

Dialectical behavior therapy (Linehan 1987) is a manualized treatment that combines treatment strategies from behavioral, cognitive, and supportive therapies (Linehan 1993). Treatment consists of weekly individual psychotherapy sessions and weekly group psychotherapy sessions and is 1 year in duration. Therapists meet weekly in group supervision to discuss treatment problems and monitor adherence to the treatment protocol. Group therapy sessions teach interpersonal skills, skills for tolerating distress, and skills for regulating emotional arousal. Individual therapy sessions address behavioral goals according to a hierarchy, with parasuicidal behaviors addressed first, followed by behaviors that jeopardize the success of therapy (e.g., noncompliance), followed by behaviors outside treatment sessions that are distressing to the patient. The therapist actively teaches and reinforces adaptive behaviors and withholds reinforcement for maladaptive behaviors.

Linehan et al. (1991) conducted a randomized controlled trial of DBT versus TAU with 44 women who met criteria for BPD according to DSM-III and the Diagnostic Interview for Borderlines (Gunderson et al. 1981). The TAU group's treatment averaged approximately 20 mental health visits per year. Compared with TAU patients during the 12 months of treatment, DBT patients had significantly fewer psychiatric hospital days (8.46 per year compared with 38.86 for TAU) and fewer parasuicidal incidents that required medical treatment. The gains made by patients who had received DBT were largely maintained at 6-month and 1-year follow-up (Linehan et al. 1993); and at 12 months posttreatment, DBT patients continued to have significantly fewer days of psychiatric hospitalization and demonstrated better employment performance than their TAU counterparts. Factoring in the costs of the psychotherapies, Linehan et al. calculated the cost savings of providing DBT instead of TAU in the community to be on average $10,000 per patient per year. Much of this savings was due to decreased use of inpatient beds (Heard 1994). Linehan et al. noted that the 1-year course of DBT was more effective at bringing behavior under control than it was at increasing subjective well-being. This is consistent with the goals of DBT, which are to help patients control parasuicidal and other dysfunctional behaviors prior to engaging in serious work on alleviating the patients' sense of emotional desperation. Linehan et al. cautioned that this study supports the clinical observation that 1 year of treatment is not sufficient for this highly treatment-seeking population.

A second randomized controlled trial of DBT versus TAU was conducted with Veteran's Affairs outpatients (Koons et al. 1998). Twenty BPD patients were randomly assigned to receive TAU in the Veteran's Affairs or standard DBT. After 6 months of treatment, DBT patients showed a trend toward fewer hospital admissions and fewer inpatient days than those in the TAU group. The failure to meet criteria for statistical significance at the .05 alpha level was attributed to the small sample, as well as to the fact that base rates of hospitalization in both groups of patients prior to treatment were low.

As many as two-thirds of patients who meet criteria for BPD also meet criteria for a concurrent substance use disorder (Dulit et al. 1990). Linehan et al. have conducted two randomized controlled trials of DBT with borderline patients who had concurrent substance use disorders. In a study of 28 women with carefully diagnosed BPD (Linehan et al. 1999), the investigators used a form of DBT modified to address additional problems stemming from substance use. Patients were assigned randomly to DBT or TAU, and the two groups did not differ with respect to severity of psychopathology. Regular urinalyses were used to monitor substance use. Participants were assessed at 4, 6, 8, and 12 months from the beginning of treatment, as well as at 4 months posttreatment. DBT patients had significantly greater reductions in substance abuse throughout the year and at follow-up than TAU patients. However, no significant differences were found between the groups in the amount of medical or psychiatric hospitalization required during the year of treatment or at follow-up. It is unclear whether this negative finding was due to the greater severity of psychopathology in this study population as compared with previously studied groups, to the modification of the DBT protocol used for substance abusers, or to some other factor not evident in the analyses.

Taken together, these studies of DBT suggest that it is effective in reducing suicidal behavior and, with the exception of one study, in reducing the use of inpatient psychiatric care. Cost-offset data were presented only for the original study by Linehan et al., but the high cost of hospitalization compared with outpatient psychotherapy suggests that the inpatient care reductions noted in the other studies would likely result in economic savings. The evidence for the superiority of DBT over TAU in the community is preliminary and in need of further testing. In most studies, both treatment conditions reduce psychiatric symptoms and use of medical and psychiatric care from pretreatment levels. TAU is defined differently in each study, and treatment norms are likely to vary across communities (e.g., between outpatient private practice and Veteran's Affairs practices). So, for example, the TAU condition in Linehan et al.'s study of substance abusers provided on average smaller "doses" of time and attention than those provided in DBT, thereby calling into question whether the DBT modality was superior to TAU or whether the differences between groups could be attributed to differences in therapist time and attention. One analysis concluded that the naturalistic follow-up of patients treated with DBT provided uneven results and that the putative clinical improvement in suicidality in these patients is highly equivocal (Levy 2008). The "active ingredients" of DBT that are helpful, such as the combination of skills training and Zen principles, have yet to be elucidated (Koerner and Linehan 2000).

# Partial Hospitalization With Combined Individual and Group Psychoanalytic Psychotherapy

In a randomized controlled study of 38 patients with BPD (Bateman and Fonagy 1999), 19 patients were treated with the study intervention of partial hospitalization with individual and group psychoanalytic psychotherapy for up to 18 months and 19 were treated with the control of standard psychiatric care including regular psychiatric review with a senior psychiatrist, inpatient admission, and partial hospitalization as needed and outpatient and community follow-up aftercare with no formal psychotherapy. Compared with those treated with standard care, patients treated with the study intervention showed a statistically significant decrease in depressive symptoms, need for medication, suicidal and self-mutilatory acts, and inpatient days, and they had better social and interpersonal function beginning at 6 months until the end of treatment at 18 months. In a subsequent study of the health care costs (psychiatric care, pharmacological treatment, and emergency room care) for the 6 months before treatment, the 18 months of treatment, and for an 18-month follow-up period, no cost differences were found between the groups during pretreatment or treatment. The higher costs of care for patients treated with partial hospitalization were offset by less psychiatric inpatient care and reduced emergency room care for them during this period. During the 18-month treatment period, the annual costs were also significantly lower for both groups compared with their 6-month pretreatment costs. However, while the overall costs between the two groups were comparable during treatment, after discharge the average annual cost of health care for the partial hospitalization group was one-fifth of that for the general psychiatric care group. At follow-up, the mean annual cost savings associated with the study intervention were $12,000, thus recouping over 2 years the cost of the treatment and suggesting its cost-effectiveness for borderline patients (Bateman and Fonagy 2003). At 5-year follow-up after discharge from mentalization-based treatment, these patients, although evidencing some impaired social functioning, continued to have far superior clinical outcomes compared with TAU patients with respect to suicidality (23% vs. 74%), diagnostic status (13% still diagnosable with BPD compared with 87%), psychiatric outpatient service use (2 years vs. 3.5 years), use of medication (0.02 vs. 1.90 years using three or more medications), global function above 60 (45% vs. 10%), and vocational status (employed or in school 3.2 years vs. 1.2 years) (Bateman and Fonagy 2008).

# Problems To Be Addressed in Future Research

As noted in the introduction, research on the cost-effectiveness of psychotherapy with borderline patients is plagued by a number of methodological problems, some of which are common to all psychotherapy studies and some of which are more specific to the study of a group of individuals who, by definition, have highly unstable relationships with others. Each of the 11 studies reviewed here attempts to overcome one or more of these limitations. Considered together, they offer a view of where research needs to go in order to provide convincing corroboration of current findings.

## Defining and Standardizing the Treatment

Studies vary from completely nonstandardized treatments, as in the Hoke (1989) study, to carefully manualized treatment protocols such as those used by Linehan et al. (1991, 1999) and by Munroe-Blum and Marziali (1995).

Treatments need to be standardized in some way to assure that, to the extent possible, different therapists are delivering the same therapeutic agents. Manualization aids in this process, but by itself is not sufficient to assure homogeneous treatments. Careful supervision and systematic measurement of each therapist's adherence to the prescribed treatment protocol are essential elements in studies that propose to understand the particular elements of therapy that foster positive change.

## Treatment Duration

While Ryle and Golynkina's (2000) 6-month study of CAT, Tyrer et al.'s (2004) study of MACT (7 sessions of psychotherapy plus patient manual), Palmer et al.'s (2006) study of CBT (average of 16 sessions), and Koons et al.'s (1998) study of DBT for 6 months examined psychotherapy treatments of 6 months or less, the remainder of the studies reviewed in this chapter tested treatments that lasted at least 1 year. Longitudinal studies and clinical experience suggest that BPD is a chronic condition that is slow to change (see, e.g., Stone 1990). Howard et al. (1986) found supporting evidence in a meta-analysis of 15 psychotherapy outcome studies spanning 30 years of research. Using clinical chart ratings, they found that borderline patients take significantly longer to demonstrate improvement in psychotherapy than do anxious and depressed patients. While 50% of anxious and depressed patients improve in 8–13 sessions, borderline patients require 26–52 psychotherapy sessions to achieve similar levels of improvement. These findings suggest that borderline patients, while able to make significant gains in psychotherapy, may need longer term treatment than patients in other diagnostic groups. However, further research is needed to determine whether specific shorter term psychotherapies can be equally effective.

## Control Groups

Finding adequate comparison groups in psychotherapy outcome studies is difficult. Many studies (e.g., Clarkin et al. 2001; Ryle and Golynkina 2000) have no control groups but simply compare patient functioning before and after treatment. These studies leave open the question of whether patients might have improved whether they had been in treatment or not. Stevenson and Meares (1992) used the strategy of comparing a treated group with a group on a waiting list. However, leaving people who suffer from severely dysfunctional disorders without treatment for many months poses ethical problems that make such designs problematic. A more palatable strategy is the one used by Linehan et al. (1991, 1999), Koons et al. (1998), Bateman and Fonagy (1999), Tyrer et al. (2004), and Palmer et al. (2006), using TAU in the community as the comparison condition. However, this design compares a standardized treatment with one that is not standardized. In addition, the standardized treatment is often delivered by enthusiastic treaters who themselves receive more attention and support for their efforts than practitioners in the community. Thus, it is difficult to know whether differences found between a specific treatment and TAU stem from the treatments themselves or from the contexts in which those treatments are delivered. Nevertheless, for cost-effectiveness studies, such designs may offer a real-world comparison condition against which to test a particular type of treatment.

## Randomization

Random assignment of participants to one study condition or another helps assure comparability of the groups under consideration. However, borderline patients are notoriously difficult to engage in treatment, and when randomization leads to assignments that are incongruent with patient expectations, patients may be more likely to drop out (Bateman and Fonagy 2000). Thus, comparability of groups on major demographic and psychological variables must be examined regardless of whether patients are randomly assigned to different conditions or are given choice in the matter.

## Comorbid Disorders

A significant proportion of patients with BPD have concurrent mood, anxiety, or substance use disorders. When the symptoms of these other disorders (e.g., depressive symptoms) improve, patients' personality functioning often improves as well, and use of health care resources is reduced. It is therefore important to examine cost-effectiveness with relatively homogeneous groups of borderline patients, as was done in the study of BPD patients with substance use disorders (Linehan et al. 1999). At a minimum, comparison groups should be carefully assessed for comparability with respect to the presence of comorbid psychiatric disorders.

## Attention to Economic Variables

While the Linehan and Stevenson and Meares studies explicitly addressed the costs of health care utilization before and after treatment, both relied to some extent on patient recall of how much they used health care services during specific time periods (Hall et al. 2001; Heard 1994). Ideally, all information would be gleaned from health service records, which are more reliable. However, this is possible only where health records are consolidated within one system. Cost-effectiveness measures should be used at follow-up beyond 12 months to understand more about the duration of cost savings that result from psychotherapy. Use of inpatient hospital facilities remains the most widely cited indicator of cost-effectiveness of psychotherapy, because it is relatively easy to measure and accounts for a large proportion of health care costs among borderline patients. The Bateman and Fonagy (2003) study overcomes these limitations to some degree in that it extends beyond 12 months (with its 18-month posttreatment follow-up) and captures a wider scope of health expenditures (psychiatric care plus pharmacotherapy and emergency room visits) from case records as opposed to patient report. However, future cost-effectiveness studies should broaden the scope of assessments to include the cost of using other social services, the cost of job absenteeism, and the cost of nonpsychiatric medical treatments. Finally, there is some evidence in the studies by Hall et al. (2001) and others to suggest that the greatest cost savings in the use of psychiatric care during and after outpatient psychotherapy is among that subgroup of borderline patients who were particularly high users of health care resources prior to treatment. Studies that look at subgroups of BPD patients may help identify those individuals for whom an investment in long-term psychotherapy could result in the greatest savings in health services utilization. Bateman and Fonagy's (1999, 2003, 2008) findings lend support to the idea of a greater cost-effectiveness of longer treatment for borderline patients. The failure for borderline patients both of the brief psychotherapy in the MACT (Tyrer et al. 2004) and of the average of 16 sessions in the BOSCOT study (Palmer et al. 2006) may in fact underscore the point that briefer treatments do not address the serious needs of this patient population.

In their own systematic review and economic evaluation of six randomized controlled trials of different kinds of psychotherapy for BPD, Brazier et al. (2006) concluded that the overall efficacy of psychological therapies is not yet conclusive. They found the cost-effectiveness of partial hospitalization with psychotherapy to be "promising" and see a "potential" for the cost-effectiveness for DBT. They also concurred that MACT is not cost-effective for borderline patients.

# Conclusion

Although rigorous empirical research on the cost-effectiveness of psychotherapy for BPD has been scarce due to methodological and economic constraints, the studies described above all point to the substantial benefits of long-term (minimum 1 year) psychotherapeutic treatment. The studies by Linehan et al. (1991), Stevenson and Meares (1992), and Bateman and Fonagy (2003) demonstrate most directly that the costs of providing ongoing psychotherapy for borderline patients are more than offset by decreased utilization of other forms of mental health and medical care, even without considering the substantial improvements in productive work time that are another result of these treatments. Most of the other studies are more suggestive of cost-effectiveness, finding that compared with pretreatment levels, borderline patients exhibit fewer self-destructive behaviors and use fewer inpatient hospital days at the end of outpatient psychotherapeutic treatment. Only the Tyrer et al. (2004) and Palmer et al. (2006) studies found negative results for psychotherapy for borderline patients, possibly due to the brevity of the psychotherapy interventions studied.

Bateman and Fonagy (2000) identified several elements common to treatments that have been found to be moderately effective in empirical studies of borderline patients. These include several ingredients of treatments found to be effective in the studies reviewed in this chapter: 1) a clear treatment structure, 2) efforts to enhance patient compliance with treatment, 3) a clear focus for discussion in treatment sessions, 4) a theoretical orientation that is coherent to both therapist and patient, and 5) a long-term format. It is possible that the particular theoretical orientation (e.g., psychodynamic vs. cognitive) of psychotherapy is less important than that both patient and therapist have a clear common orientation that they believe to be potentially effective.

Further research is needed to refine our understanding of which elements of psychotherapies are the "active ingredients" that promote improved functioning and whether we can identify particular subgroups of borderline patients for whom long-term psychotherapy is most cost-effective. But the evidence at present suggests that there is a substantial cost to *not* providing psychotherapy for borderline patients, both in human and in economic terms (Gabbard et al. 1997).

# References

Abend S, Porder M, Willick M: Borderline Patients: Psychoanalytic Perspectives. New York, International Universities Press, 1983

American Psychiatric Association: Diagnostic and Statistical Manual of Mental Disorders, 4th Edition. Washington, DC, American Psychiatric Association, 1994

American Psychiatric Association: Diagnostic and Statistical Manual of Mental Disorders, 4th Edition, Text Revision. Washington, DC, American Psychiatric Association, 2000

Aronson TA: A critical review of psychotherapeutic treatments of the borderline personality. Historical trends and future directions. J Nerv Ment Dis 177:511–528, 1989

Bateman A, Fonagy P: Effectiveness of partial hospitalization in the treatment of borderline personality disorder: a randomized controlled trial. Am J Psychiatry 156:1563–1569, 1999

Bateman A, Fonagy P: Effectiveness of psychotherapeutic treatment of personality disorder. Br J Psychiatry 177:138–143, 2000

Bateman A, Fonagy P: Health service utilization costs for borderline personality disorder patients treated with psychoanalytically oriented partial hospitalization versus general psychiatric care. Am J Psychiatry 160:169–171, 2003

Bateman A, Fonagy P: 8-Year follow-up of patients treated for borderline personality disorder: mentalization-based treatment versus treatment as usual. Am J Psychiatry 165:631–638, 2008

Beck AT, Ward CH, Mendelson M, et al: An inventory for measuring depression. Arch Gen Psychiatry 4:561–571, 1961

Brazier J, Tumur I, Holmes M, et al: Psychological therapies including dialectical behaviour therapy for borderline personality disorder: a systematic review and preliminary economic evaluation. Health Technol Assess 10:iii, ix–xii, 2006

Buie DH, Adler G: Definitive treatment of the borderline personality. Int J Psychoanal Psychother 9:51–87, 1982

Clarkin JF, Foelsch PA, Levy KN, et al: The development of a psychodynamic treatment for patients with borderline personality disorder: a preliminary study of behavioral change. J Pers Disord 15:487–495, 2001

Derogatis L: SCL-90-R Administration, Scoring, and Procedures Manual-II for the Revised Version, 2nd Edition. Towson, MD, Clinical Psychometric Research, 1983

Dulit RA, Fyer MR, Haas GL, et al: Substance use in borderline personality disorder. Am J Psychiatry 147:1002–1007, 1990

Gabbard GO, Lazar SG, Hornberger J, et al: The economic impact of psychotherapy: a review. Am J Psychiatry 154:147–155, 1997

Gross R, Olfson M, Gameroff M, et al: Borderline personality disorder in primary care. Arch Intern Med 162: 53–60, 2002

Gunderson JG, Kolb JE, Austin V: The diagnostic interview for borderline patients. Am J Psychiatry 138:896–903, 1981

Hall J, Caleo S, Stevenson J, et al: An economic analysis of psychotherapy for borderline personality disorder patients. J Ment Health Policy Econ 4:3–8, 2001

Heard H: Behavior therapies for borderline patients. Paper presented at the 147th annual meeting of the American Psychiatric Association. Philadelphia, PA, May 21–26, 1994

Hoke L: Longitudinal patterns of behaviors in borderline personality disorder. Unpublished doctoral dissertation, Boston University, Boston, MA, 1989

Howard KI, Kopta SM, Krause MS, et al: The dose-effect relationship in psychotherapy. Am Psychol 41:159–164, 1986

Joyce AS, McCallum M, Piper WE: Borderline functioning, work, and outcome in intensive evening group treatment. Int J Group Psychother 49:343–368, 1999

Kernberg O: Borderline Conditions and Pathological Narcissism. Northvale, NJ, Jason Aronson, 1975

Koerner K, Linehan MM: Research on dialectical behavior therapy for patients with borderline personality disorder. Psychiatr Clin North Am 23:151–167, 2000

Koons C, Robins C, Bishop G: Efficacy of dialectical behavior therapy with borderline women veterans: a randomized controlled trial. Paper presented at the annual meeting of the Association for the Advancement of Behavior Therapy, Washington, DC, 1998

Levy K: Psychotherapies and lasting change. Am J Psychiatry 165:556–559, 2008

Linehan MM: Dialectical behavior therapy for borderline personality disorder. Theory and method. Bull Menninger Clin 51:261–276, 1987

Linehan MM: Skills Training Manual for Treating Borderline Personality Disorder. New York, Guilford, 1993

Linehan MM, Armstrong HE, Suarez A, et al: Cognitive-behavioral treatment of chronically parasuicidal borderline patients. Arch Gen Psychiatry 48:1060–1064, 1991

Linehan MM, Heard HL, Armstrong HE: Naturalistic follow-up of a behavioral treatment for chronically parasuicidal borderline patients. Arch Gen Psychiatry 50:971–974, 1993

Linehan MM, Schmidt H 3rd, Dimeff LA, et al: Dialectical behavior therapy for patients with borderline personality disorder and drug-dependence. Am J Addict 8:279–292, 1999

Masterson JF: Treatment of the adolescent with borderline syndrome. A problem in separation-individuation. Bull Menninger Clin 35:5–18, 1971

McGlashan TH: The Chestnut Lodge follow-up study. III. Long-term outcome of borderline personalities. Arch Gen Psychiatry 43:20–30, 1986

Meares R, Stevenson J, Comerford A: Psychotherapy with borderline patients: I. A comparison between treated and untreated cohorts. Aust N Z J Psychiatry 33:467–472; discussion 478–481, 1999

Munroe-Blum H, Marziali E: A controlled trial of short-term group treatment for borderline personality disorder. J Pers Disord 9:190–198, 1995

Palmer S, Davidson K, Tyrer P, et al: The cost-effectiveness of cognitive behavior therapy for borderline personality disorder: the results from the BOSCOT trial. J Pers Disord 20:466–481, 2006

Paris J, Brown R, Nowlis D: Long-term follow-up of borderline patients in a general hospital. Compr Psychiatry 28:530–535, 1987

Perry JC, Banon E, Ianni F: Effectiveness of psychotherapy for personality disorders. Am J Psychiatry 156:1312–1321, 1999

Ryle A: Cognitive Analytic Therapy and Borderline Personality Disorder: The Model and the Method. Chichester, England, Wiley, 1997

Ryle A, Golynkina K: Effectiveness of time-limited cognitive analytic therapy of borderline personality disorder: factors associated with outcome. Br J Med Psychol 73 (part 2):197–210, 2000

Stevenson J, Meares R: An outcome study of psychotherapy for patients with borderline personality disorder. Am J Psychiatry 149:358–362, 1992

Stevenson J, Meares R: Borderline patients at five-year follow up. Paper presented at the Annual Congress of the Royal Australia and New Zealand College of Psychiatrists, Cairns, Australia, 1995

Stone MH: The Fate of Borderline Patients: Successful Outcome and Psychiatric Practice. New York, Guilford, 1990

Stone MH, Stone DK, Hurt SW: Natural history of borderline patients treated by intensive hospitalization. Psychiatr Clin North Am 10:185–206, 1987

Swartz M, Blazer D, George L, et al: Estimating the prevalence of borderline personality disorder in the community. J Pers Disord 4:257–272, 1990

Tyrer P, Tom B, Byford S, et al: Differential effects of manual assisted cognitive behavior therapy in the treatment of recurrent deliberate self-harm and personality disturbance: the POPMACT study. J Pers Disord 18:102–116, 2004

Waldinger RJ: Intensive psychodynamic therapy with borderline patients: an overview. Am J Psychiatry 144:267–274, 1987

Waldinger RJ: The role of psychodynamic concepts in the diagnosis of borderline personality disorder. Harv Rev Psychiatry 1:158–167, 1993

Waldinger RJ, Frank AF: Transference and the vicissitudes of medication use by borderline patients. Psychiatry 52:416–427, 1989

Waldinger RJ, Gunderson JG: Completed psychotherapies with borderline patients. Am J Psychother 38:190–202, 1984

Waldinger RJ, Gunderson JG: Effective Psychotherapy With Borderline Patients: Case Studies. New York, MacMillan, 1987

Widiger T, Frances A: Epidemiology, diagnosis, and comorbidity of borderline personality disorders, in Review of Psychiatry, Vol. 8. Edited by Tasman A, Hales R, Frances A. Washington, DC, American Psychiatric Press, 1989, pp 8–24

## Summary of studies on psychotherapy of borderline personality disorder

| Article | Patients | Treatment | Outcome |
|---|---|---|---|
| **Individual psychotherapy** | | | |
| Hoke 1989 | 58 patients with borderline traits or borderline personality disorder (BPD). Half had stable psychotherapy for 2 or more years, half had inconsistent or unstable psychotherapy. | 29 patients had intermittent or inconsistent psychotherapy and 29 had stable individual psychotherapy for at least 2 out of 7 years. Semi-retrospective follow-along design; subjects interviewed every 4–6 months for up to 7 years to assess change in impulsivity, mood, use of mental health services, global functioning. | Stable psychotherapy group had fewer emergency room (ER) visits, fewer hospitalizations, less use of day treatment facilities, decreased impulsivity, and better mood by end of 7-year follow-up period. |
| 1. Stevenson and Meares 1992<br><br>2. Meares et al. 1999<br><br>3. Hall et al. 2001 | 30 severely dysfunctional BPD patients referred from community. | Outpatient individual psychodynamic psychotherapy 2x/week for 12 months, follow-up 12 months after termination. Patients served as own controls (pre- vs. posttreatment), along with a wait-list comparison group. | Significant reduction in impulsivity, anger, suicidal behavior; medical visits cut to one-seventh of pretreatment rates; work absenteeism, hospital admissions, and inpatient days decreased significantly after treatment; significant decrease in BPD symptoms compared with waiting-list group; substantial savings in health care usage comparing 12 months pre- and posttreatment. |

## Summary of studies on psychotherapy of borderline personality disorder *(continued)*

| Article | Patients | Treatment | Outcome |
|---|---|---|---|
| *Individual psychotherapy (continued)* | | | |
| Ryle and Golynkina 2000 | 27 patients with BPD, mean age 34 years, from public hospital outpatient department. | Cognitive-analytic therapy, a 6-month, 24-session outpatient treatment protocol. Naturalistic design, no comparison group, patients served as own controls. Follow-up at 6 and 18 months post-treatment. | 14 patients no longer met diagnostic criteria for BPD and judged to require no further treatment. Significant decreases in measures of depression, psychiatric distress, interpersonal difficulties, and social and occupational functioning. |
| Clarkin et al. 2001 | 23 female patients with BPD and at least two incidents of self-injurious behavior in the last 5 years, no substance abuse, mean age 32.7 years. | Outpatient psychotherapy two times per week for 12 months, using manualized transference-focused psychotherapy. Patients served as own controls (pre- vs. posttreatment). No separate control group. | Comparing 12 months prior to treatment with 12 months of treatment: decreased self-destructive acts, decreased number and severity of suicide attempts, decreased medical and psychiatric hospitalizations and number of hospital days. 17 of 23 patients completed treatment. |
| Tyrer et al. 2004 | 480 patients with a mixture of diagnoses after an episode of self-harm in a multicenter randomized trial | Patients randomly assigned to either treatment-as-usual (TAU) or manual-assisted cognitive-behavioral therapy, a brief form of cognitive therapy; and follow-up for over a year. | MACT was 10% cheaper and cost-effective compared with TAU and led to 50% decrease in frequency of self-harm episodes, except for BPD patients who had increased costs after MACT and were most likely to repeat self-harm. MACT is not cost-effective for borderline patients possibly because of being a very brief treatment. |

## Summary of studies on psychotherapy of borderline personality disorder *(continued)*

| Article | Patients | Treatment | Outcome |
| --- | --- | --- | --- |
| **Individual psychotherapy** *(continued)* | | | |
| Palmer et al. 2006 | 106 borderline patients. | Multicenter randomized controlled trial of cognitive-behavior therapy (CBT) (providing up to 27 sessions, average of 16) plus TAU compared with TAU alone. | Assessment of quality-adjusted life year of patients at baseline and 6 monthly intervals over 2 years, measurement of health care utilization costs and related non-health care costs at same intervals. Total costs per patient in CBT cohort lower than for patients receiving usual care alone, but CBT patients also had lower quality of life—differences small, not statistically significant. CBT patients had fewer suicidal acts, lowered anxiety, lessened dysfunctional beliefs, lower inpatient hospitalization costs than TAU group (slight evidence of cost advantage for CBT) but no significant cost-effective advantage for CBT. |

**Summary of studies on psychotherapy of borderline personality disorder *(continued)***

| Article | Patients | Treatment | Outcome |
|---|---|---|---|
| **Group psychotherapy** | | | |
| Munroe-Blum and Marziali 1995 | 110 patients with BPD ages 18–52 years. | Interpersonal group psychotherapy (IGP), a 12-month, 30-session treatment protocol vs. individual dynamic psychotherapy (IDP). Patients randomly assigned to IDP or IGP, final analyses after dropouts and missing data were on 22 IGP and 26 IDP subjects. | Both treatment groups experienced significant decline in impulsivity and in use of mental health and social services at 12- and 24-month follow-up. No significant differences on outcome variables between groups. |
| **Dialectical behavior therapy (DBT)** | | | |
| Linehan et al. 1991 | 44 patients with BPD, ages 18–45 years, at least two parasuicide incidents in previous 5 years. | Patients randomly assigned to DBT, weekly individual, and group therapy for 1 year, or TAU in community, usually individual psychotherapy. | During 1 year of treatment: TAU patients had more medically treated parasuicide episodes (1.76 vs. 0.64) and more psychiatric inpatient days (38.86 vs. 8.46) than DBT patients. These differences held at 1-year follow-up. |
| Koons et al. 1998 | 20 female patients with BPD but not parasuicide. | Patients randomly assigned either to DBT weekly individual and group therapy or to TAU in community, usually individual psychotherapy. | DBT patients showed trend toward reduced psychiatric hospitalization compared with TAU and greater improvement in depression. |

## Summary of studies on psychotherapy of borderline personality disorder *(continued)*

| Article | Patients | Treatment | Outcome |
|---|---|---|---|
| **Dialectical behavior therapy (DBT)** *(continued)* | | | |
| Linehan et al. 1999 | 28 female patients with BPD and substance use disorder. | Patients randomly assigned to DBT, weekly individual and group therapy modified for substance abusers for 1 year, or TAU in community, usually individual psychotherapy. | DBT patients showed significantly greater decreases in substance abuse, global adjustment, and social functioning during and after treatment compared with TAU patients. No significant differences between the two groups in rates of parasuicide and hospitalization (both decreased over pretreatment levels). |
| **Individual and group psychoanalytic psychotherapy** | | | |
| 1. Bateman and Fonagy 1999 | 38 patients with BPD. | Psychoanalytic psychotherapy; individual and group in a partially hospitalized setting for up to 18 months vs. the control treatment of standard psychiatric care patients assigned in a randomized controlled design. | |
| 2. Bateman and Fonagy 2003 | | | Health care utilization costs were compared for the two groups of patients before treatment, during treatment, and at 18-month follow-up. Costs were the same for both groups before and during treatment, with the greater cost of treatment for the study treatment offset by lower inpatient and ER costs. At 18-month follow-up, however, annual health care costs for patients in the partial hospitalization group were only one-fifth of those in the psychiatric general care control group. |

## Summary of studies on psychotherapy of borderline personality disorder *(continued)*

| Article | Patients | Treatment | Outcome |
|---|---|---|---|
| **Individual and group psychoanalytic psychotherapy** *(continued)* | | | |
| Bateman and Fonagy 2008 | 38 patients with BPD. | Psychoanalytic psychotherapy; individual and group in a partially hospitalized setting for up to 18 months *vs.* the control treatment of standard psychiatric care patients assigned in a randomized controlled design. | At 5-year follow-up after mentalization-based treatment, patients had some impaired social functioning, but far superior clinical outcomes compared with TAU patients with respect to suicidality (23% *vs.* 74%), diagnostic status (13% still diagnosable with BPD compared with 87%), psychiatric outpatient service use (2 years *vs.* 3.5 years), use of medication (0.02 *vs.* 1.90 years using 3 or more medications), global function above 60 (45% *vs.* 10%), and vocational status (employed or in school 3.2 years *vs.* 1.2 years). |

# 4 | Psychotherapy in the Treatment of Posttraumatic Stress Disorder

Susan G. Lazar, M.D.
William Offenkrantz, M.D.

**P**osttraumatic stress disorder (PTSD) is a debilitating and costly illness that occurs in veterans and in crime, trauma, and abuse victims. Its incidence is approximately 1% in the general population and much higher in those exposed to war, abuse, and natural disasters. Patients suffer from significantly increased health complaints and medical costs, work disability, and marital and family problems. Although there are few data specific to the cost-effectiveness of psychotherapy of PTSD, the high costs associated with the illness, taken with the efficacy of psychotherapy demonstrated in research studies, are highly suggestive of the cost-effectiveness of psychotherapy for this disorder.

## Search Methodology

A MEDLINE search between January 1984 and December 2007 was done using the following terms: "PTSD + psychotherapy + cost" and "PTSD + cost-effectiveness + psychotherapy." In addition, relevant articles about the epidemiology and costs of PTSD, relevant review articles, and selected older articles on the efficacy of psychotherapy for PTSD have been included for background information. Articles on eye movement desensitization and reprocessing (EMDR) for PTSD were not included because it was felt that this treatment for PTSD does not fit the definition of psychotherapy used for the purposes of this volume and is more akin to psychobiological techniques such as biofeedback.

# The Illness

According to DSM-IV-TR (American Psychiatric Association 2000), PTSD is an illness subsequent to a trauma, or an event with a perceived or actual threat that has aroused an extreme emotional response of intense fear, helplessness, or horror. There are three groups of symptoms: 1) a reexperiencing of the trauma in intrusive thoughts, nightmares, flashbacks, emotional distress when reminded of the trauma, or physiological arousal when reminded of the trauma; 2) at least three avoidance symptoms such as avoidance of thinking about the traumatic event, avoidance of people or situations associated with the trauma, inability to recall an important aspect of the trauma, a loss of interest in activities, detachment from others, a restriction in the range of affect, or a sense of a foreshortened future; and 3) two arousal symptoms such as sleep disturbance, irritability, difficulty concentrating, hypervigilance, or an exaggerated startle response.

# Epidemiology

According to the National Comorbidity Survey Replication, the lifetime prevalence of PTSD is 6.8% (Kessler et al. 2005a) and the 12-month prevalence is 3.5% (Kessler et al. 2005b). Other surveys of the general population indicate that PTSD affects 15% to 24% of those exposed to trauma. While more men than women are exposed to trauma, nonetheless, the ratio of female-to-male lifetime prevalence of PTSD is 2:1 (Breslau 2001a). In a study of 1,007 young adults in Michigan, the rate of PTSD in those exposed to trauma was 23%. Despite the lower prevalence of exposure to trauma among women, those women who were exposed developed PTSD at a rate of 30.7%, compared with 14% of men exposed to trauma. Besides being female, an increased vulnerability to the development of PTSD after trauma is associated with early separation from parents, preexisting psychiatric disorder and family history of anxiety, depression, psychosis, and antisocial behavior (Breslau et al. 1991)

In addition, patients with PTSD are three times as likely to have serious problems with alcohol, drugs, or both compared with those without PTSD

(Brady 2001; Resnick et al. 1993). Among those with PTSD, the increased risk for drug abuse or dependence is highest for prescribed psychoactive drugs (Breslau 2001b).

# Veterans

In the United States, the National Vietnam Veterans Readjustment Study, based on 3,000 in-depth interviews in every state, revealed that 15% of all male Vietnam combat veterans had PTSD in 1987. It also estimated that 31% would eventually be diagnosed with PTSD (Kulka et al. 1990). Compared with veterans without PTSD, those with PTSD were five times as likely to be unemployed and two to six times more likely to be substance abusers. Seventy percent were divorced compared with 35% in the comparison group; 55% had significant parenting problems; 35% had been homeless or vagrant at some time; 50% had been arrested at least once; and 37% had six or more violent acts in the year of the study. Of veterans with PTSD, 26% had four or more chronic medical conditions (four times that of the comparison group), 40% reported high levels of expressed hostility, and 56% had high scores of psychological distress compared with 10% of the comparison group. In all of the above-mentioned categories, the incidence of abnormal findings was two times or more the incidence of that found in the comparison groups. Another slightly earlier study had also found that compared with the families of Vietnam veterans without PTSD, the families of those veterans suffering from PTSD experience significantly more problems with parenting, as well as in marital and family adjustment (Jordan et al. 1992). Those with PTSD were found to be twice as likely to have never married, and if married, were twice as likely to have been divorced. The families of these with PTSD were six times more likely than families of veterans without PTSD to have the most extreme parental problems and 2½ times more likely to have the most severe problems of family adjustment, including a significantly higher incidence of family violence. In addition, the children of Vietnam veterans suffering from PTSD were also much likelier to be disturbed.

Beckham et al. (1998) found an even higher rate of self-reported health problems for combat veterans with PTSD than did the National Vietnam Veterans Readjustment Study. Greater physical health problems were associated with the presence and severity of PTSD. Those veterans with PTSD had higher ratings on all health status measures than did those without PTSD and had a greater number of total illnesses from a broader range of medical categories. The PTSD patients had both more somatization and more health problems. The severity of PTSD was also associated with poorer health status.

For returning Iraq and Afghanistan war veterans, 14% screen positive for PTSD and 14% for major depression and only about half of these have sought help from a physician or a mental health provider for their mental health problem in the past year (Tanielian and Jaycox 2008).

# Morbidity of Trauma and Rape in Women Patients

The scope of criminal violence against women is such that one in five are the victims of completed rape and one in four have been physically battered (Koss et al. 1991). The victimization of women also leads to increased health-related complaints and medical costs. Koss et al. found that severely victimized women reported more distress and visited physicians twice as frequently as nonvictims with 2½ times the outpatient costs. Women who have been multiply victimized visit their physicians 6.9 times per year or twice as often as nonvictims. The greater the severity of criminal victimization over a woman's lifetime, the worse she perceives her state of health and the higher her medical expenses and the number of physician visits. In fact, the severity of criminal victimization is a more accurate predictor of medical visits and outpatient medical costs than age and known health hazards.

In a study of 131 patients with a history of childhood sexual abuse seen in a general medical practice, Felitti (1991) found that even decades after the abuse, these patients had much higher levels of chronic depression, morbid obesity, marital instability, high utilization of medical care, psychosomatic complaints, chronic gastrointestinal distress, and recurrent headaches. Compared with a national average of 4.3 doctor office visits per year, 22% of this study group had 10 or more doctor visits per year. Most outstanding was the presence of chronic significant depression.

In a review of the literature, Harvey and Herman (1992) reported that depending on the sample, one in three to one in eight women have experienced rape or attempted rape, many prior to age 18, and a significant number prior to age 11. Thirty-one percent of all rape victims develop rape-related PTSD at some point in their lifetimes. Rape puts women at an increased risk for alcohol and substance abuse and for major depression. Few seek care of any kind immediately after rape.

A study by Walker et al. (2003) of health care costs of a large group of women members of a major health maintenance organization (HMO) found that women with PTSD symptoms have significantly higher total and component health care costs, even after controlling for depression and chronic medical illness. PTSD patients in the most symptomatic group had greater mean unadjusted total annual health care costs in all categories measured and significantly higher odds of nonzero costs, including total outpatient, specialty care, primary care, pharmacy, and mental health care costs. These most symptomatic patients were 13 times more likely to use ambulatory services than those with a low level of symptoms. Total annual costs were more than twice as high in women with the greatest symptoms and 38% higher in those with moderate symptoms, compared with women with a low level of PTSD symptoms. The increases were in every cost component measured, and only a small portion of the increased costs was due to mental health costs (Walker et al. 2003).

# Efficacy of Psychotherapy

Although there are a few systematic studies investigating the cost-effectiveness of psychotherapy for PTSD, combining what is known about the prevalence of PTSD and the high costs associated with the illness with what is known about the efficacy of treatments, it becomes clear that effective treatments are quite likely to be cost-effective. Some studies of the efficacy of psychotherapy for PTSD are discussed below and summarized in the review table at the end of this chapter. (A useful summary and discussion of the PTSD psychotherapy literature can also be found in Hamblen et al. 2009.) In addition, there are several more recent studies of psychotherapy for PTSD that address cost-effectiveness more directly that are discussed in what follows.

A study comparing psychodynamic psychotherapy, hypnotherapy, systematic desensitization, and a wait-list control group (Brom et al. 1989) found that the psychodynamic group achieved a greater reduction in avoidance symptoms but a lesser change in intrusion symptoms. Patients treated with either hypnotherapy or desensitization showed the reverse, with a greater reduction in intrusive symptoms and less improvement in avoidance symptoms. Overall, each of the treatment conditions yielded similar rates of improvement. Sixty percent of treated patients and 26% of the untreated control group had clinically significant improvements.

One study of a cognitive approach called stress inoculation training or SIT (using muscle relaxation, thought stopping, breath control, and "guided self-dialogue," practiced under stressful conditions) found SIT to be most effective immediately after treatment in reducing symptoms compared with flooding, supportive counseling, and wait-list controls (Foa et al. 1991). However, when patients were assessed 3.5 months later, flooding was found to have produced the greatest effect. In addition, in Foa et al.'s study, both supportive counseling and wait-list patients showed improvement in arousal symptoms of PTSD but not in intrusion and avoidance symptoms.

In a study of psychotherapy for chronic combat-related PTSD, Frueh et al. (1996) assessed trauma management therapy consisting of 29 treatment sessions that combined elements of intensive exposure therapy, including sessions planned and conducted by the patients themselves, in addition to social and emotional skills training. The subjects were 15 chronic Veterans Affairs patients who were assessed with a comprehensive battery of measures both before and after treatment administered by clinicians as well as by patient self-assessment measures. The treatment was found to be effective in treating many of the symptoms of chronic combat-related PTSD. Although there were no conclusive findings with respect to cost-effectiveness, there was an implication of potential cost-effectiveness by virtue of the fact that none of the patients required psychiatric hospitalization during the course of their treatment. The findings from this study are limited in their generalizability because of the small number of subjects and the absence of follow-up measures.

An article by Foa (1997) found that 3 months after assault, the prevalence of PTSD was 48% in rape victims and 25% in nonsexual crime victims. In this study, both SIT and prolonged exposure (reliving and recounting the traumatic memory) were found to be effective alone or in combination in the treatment of chronic PTSD. Efficacy was maintained for 3 months of follow-up.

In a study of trauma and grief-focused brief psychotherapy, Goenjian et al. (1997) evaluated the effect of the psychotherapy for 64 early adolescents in Armenia after the 1988 earthquake. Posttraumatic stress and depressive reactions were assessed by using the Child PTSD Reaction Index before and after the intervention as well as at 18 months and 3 years after the earthquake for those treated and for 29 untreated controls. Posttraumatic stress reactions were significantly decreased in treated subjects, whereas those in the untreated subjects increased significantly. The improvement in PTSD symptoms in those treated were in all three symptom categories of intrusion, avoidance, and arousal. There was no change in depressive symptoms in subjects treated, whereas depressive symptoms in those untreated worsened significantly over time.

In a study of 15 noninjured women exposed to a terrorist attack in Israel, all of the women participated in psychological debriefing therapy consisting of group debriefing with brief group psychotherapy (Amir et al. 1998). The treatment consisted of six meetings during the first 2 months after the event. At three intervals (2 days after the attack, 2 months after, and 6 months after), the women were administered a PTSD diagnostic scale, the Impact of Event Scale (IES), and the Hopkins Symptom Checklist–90, a self-report measure of psychiatric symptoms for the 2 weeks prior to the assessment period. The IES showed significant decrease, but the other scales showed no difference. At 6 months, 4 women (27%) satisfied all of the diagnostic criteria for PTSD, a rate similar to untreated survivors of trauma. The authors concluded that intervention had little if any effect.

In a study of psychoeducational group therapy for PTSD, Lubin et al. (1998) studied the effectiveness of a 16-week trauma-focused cognitive-behavioral group psychotherapy using assessments of group members, at baseline, at 1-month intervals during treatment, at termination, and at 6-month follow-up. At termination, patients showed significant improvement in all three clusters of PTSD symptoms (reexperiencing, avoidance, and hyperarousal) and in depressive symptoms. These improvements were sustained at 6-month follow-up.

For children and adolescents with PTSD after a single-incident stressor, March et al. (1998) studied an 18-week, group-administered cognitive-behavioral protocol and found that it led to resolution of PTSD in 57% of the 17 subjects immediately posttreatment, with additional improvement on 6-month follow-up such that 86% were free of PTSD.

A Scottish study of the long-term outcome, 2–14 years after the original treatment, for patients in eight controlled clinical trials of cognitive-behavior therapy (CBT) for anxiety disorders assessed the effectiveness and cost-effectiveness of CBT for these conditions (Durham et al. 2005). For all of the anxiety disorder diagnoses, there was a somewhat better initial long-term outcome for patients treated with CBT compared with non-CBT interventions in that they had improved overall in symptom severity, but not in diagnostic status. However, the patients with PTSD did especially poorly. The positive effects that were found eroded over time with no evidence of cost-effectiveness of CBT versus non-CBT.

In a study of 13 patients with severe PTSD after extensive exposure to the World Trade Center attacks, virtual reality enhanced exposure therapy provided significantly superior improvement compared with a wait-list control group (Difede et al. 2007). The virtual reality enhancement was delivered by carefully titrated, increasingly intense computer-generated 3-D sequences of the World Trade Center attacks. The large effect size of the study intervention compared with control was especially impressive because half of the treated patients had previously been unsuccessfully treated for their PTSD.

In a study comparing self-management therapy (a CBT group psychotherapy) with active-control therapy (a strictly educational therapy provided in a group) for male veterans with comorbid chronic PTSD and depressive disorder, 101 patients were randomly assigned to one of these treatments to evaluate the efficacy and cost-effectiveness of the self-management therapy against the active-control therapy (Dunn et al. 2007). Both therapies were highly structured 1.5-hour weekly group sessions meeting for 14 weeks. Medical and psychiatric service utilization and costs were also measured for both conditions. While self-management therapy yielded slightly greater improvement on depressive symptoms, this difference disappeared on follow-up. However, psychiatric outpatient utilization and overall outpatient costs were lower with self-management therapy, and this decrease was maintained through the 1-year follow-up. Thus, while the CBT group psychotherapeutic approach to depressed veterans with PTSD demonstrated no greater efficacy clinically than a nonpsychotherapeutic group approach, the group psychotherapy treatment did lead to decreased overall outpatient costs over time.

# Review Articles

A review of 255 English language reports of PTSD treatments for all types of traumatized populations found 11 studies, including 6 involving psychotherapy that were conducted with randomized clinical trials (Solomon et al. 1992). The studies examining systematic desensitization, or flooding, showed improvement in the level of intrusive symptoms, although caution is advised because complications have also been reported with flooding.

In a review article of exposure therapies for PTSD, Foa et al. (2003) found that exposure therapy is effective for the majority of PTSD patients including Vietnam War veterans with PTSD and sexual and nonsexual assault victims with PTSD. Exposure therapy augments the effectiveness of other treatments such as cognitive restructuring (CR). However, adding CR or SIT to exposure therapy does not augment the effectiveness of exposure therapy alone.

An Australian study (Issakidis et al. 2004) compared the burden and economic efficiency of current and optimal treatment for the anxiety disorders by calculating the direct health care costs of treatment and the outcome as the averted years lived with disability (YLD). The cost per YLD averted was compared for those already in treatment for a mental health problem with a hypothetical optimal care package of evidence-based treatment for the same patient group. For PTSD patients, the increased efficacy of optimal care would be achieved by increasing the rate of psychotherapeutic treatment to current care rates with psychotropic medication. For all the anxiety disorders studied, evidence-based care would result in a one-and-a-half to twofold increase in efficacy, a 40%–60% increase in YLDs averted—a 54% increase—compared with current care, at a similar or lower overall cost (Issakidis et al. 2004).

# Case Vignette

Miss A, a 28-year-old graduate student, was referred for psychotherapy following the sexual exploitation and abuse by her graduate advisor who had used threats and intimidation to force her compliance. She had PTSD with intense anxiety, nightmares about the abuse, and a depressed mood. Once-weekly psychodynamic psychotherapy over 3 years was arduous and difficult, going over the details of the trauma and linking it with prior abuse in her childhood that had made her vulnerable to the current situation of exploitation. Because of the intensity of focus, depth of inquiry, and length of the treatment, the patient recovered from the trauma and acquired new strengths in self-assertiveness she had not previously possessed.

# Conclusion

Victims of trauma and abuse and veterans of war are all at risk for the development of PTSD, a highly costly illness to society both financially and in terms of human suffering and pain. The one-quarter of those exposed to trauma who develop PTSD are at increased risk for substance and prescription drug abuse. Veterans with PTSD are at particular risk of enormously increased rates of unemployment, substance abuse, divorce, homelessness, violence, arrest, and chronic medical conditions. The 20% of women who have been raped and 25% who have been physically battered have greatly increased health problems, depression, obesity, marital instability, medical visits, and medical costs. With some exceptions (Amir et al. 1998), specialized exposure therapies that desensitize to trauma as well as psychodynamic and cognitive-behavioral psychotherapies have all been shown to be effective for PTSD. With one negative report of the cost-effectiveness of psychotherapy for PTSD (Durham et al. 2005) and little direct positive evidence of its cost-effectiveness, there are nonetheless many studies demonstrating psychotherapy's efficacy for this condition. It is clear that any psychotherapy that has been demonstrated to be effective for this disorder will also ultimately be cost-effective.

# References

American Psychiatric Association: Diagnostic and Statistical Manual of Mental Disorders, 4th Edition, Text Revision. Washington, DC, American Psychiatric Association, 2000

Amir M, Weil G, Kaplan Z, et al: Debriefing with brief group psychotherapy in a homogenous group of non-injured victims of a terrorist attack: a prospective study. Acta Psychiatr Scand 98:237–242, 1998

Beckham JC, Moore SD, Feldman ME, et al: Health status, somatization, and severity of posttraumatic stress disorder in Vietnam combat veterans with posttraumatic stress disorder. Am J Psychiatry 155:1565–1569, 1998

Brady K: Comorbid posttraumatic stress disorder and substance use disorders. Psychiatr Ann 31:313–319, 2001

Breslau N: The epidemiology of posttraumatic stress disorder: what is the extent of the problem? J Clin Psychiatry 62 (suppl 17):16–22, 2001a

Breslau N: Outcomes of posttraumatic stress disorder. J Clin Psychiatry 62 (suppl 17):55–59, 2001b

Breslau N, Davis GC, Andreski P, et al: Traumatic events and posttraumatic stress disorder in an urban population of young adults. Arch Gen Psychiatry 48:216–222, 1991

Brom D, Kleber RJ, Defares PB: Brief psychotherapy for posttraumatic stress disorders. J Consult Clin Psychol 57:607–612, 1989

Difede J, Cukor J, Jayasinge N, et al: Virtual reality exposure therapy for the treatment of posttraumatic stress disorder following September 11, 2001. J Clin Psychiatry 68:1639–1647, 2007

Dunn NJ, Rehm LP, Schillaci JS, et al: A randomized trial of self-management and psychoeducational group therapies for comorbid chronic posttraumatic stress disorder and depressive disorder. J Trauma Stress 20:221–237, 2007

Durham RC, Chambers JA, Power KG, et al: Long-term outcome of cognitive behaviour therapy clinical trials in central Scotland. Health Technol Assess 9:1–174, 2005

Felitti VJ: Long-term medical consequences of incest, rape, and molestation. South Med J 84:328–331, 1991

Foa EB: Trauma and women: course, predictors, and treatment. J Clin Psychiatry 58 (suppl 9):25–28, 1997

Foa EB, Rothbaum BO, Riggs DS, et al: Treatment of posttraumatic stress disorder in rape victims: a comparison between cognitive-behavioral procedures and counseling. J Consult Clin Psychol 59:715–723, 1991

Foa EB, Rothbaum BO, Furr JM: Augmenting exposure therapy with other CBT procedures. Psychiatr Ann 33:47–53, 2003

Frueh BC, Turner SM, Beidel DC, et al: Trauma management therapy: a preliminary evaluation of a multicomponent behavioral treatment for chronic combat-related PTSD. Behav Res Ther 34:533–543, 1996

Goenjian AK, Karayan I, Pynoos RS, et al: Outcome of psychotherapy among early adolescents after trauma. Am J Psychiatry 154:536–542, 1997

Hamblen J, Schnurr P, Rosenberg A, et al: A guide to the literature on psychotherapy for PTSD. Psychiatr Ann 39:348–354, 2009

Harvey M, Herman J: The trauma of sexual victimization: feminist contributions to theory, research and practice. PTSD Research Quarterly 3:1–7, 1992

Issakidis C, Sanderson K, Corry J, et al: Modelling the population cost-effectiveness of current and evidence-based optimal treatment for anxiety disorders. Psychol Med 34:19–35, 2004

Jordan BK, Marmar CR, Fairbank JA, et al: Problems in families of male Vietnam veterans with posttraumatic stress disorder. J Consult Clin Psychol 60:916–926, 1992

Kessler RC, Berglund P, Demler O, et al: Lifetime prevalence and age-of-onset distributions of DSM-IV disorders in the national comorbidity survey replication. Arch Gen Psychiatry 62:593–602, 2005a

Kessler RC, Chiu WT, Demler O, et al: Prevalence, severity, and comorbidity of 12-month DSM-IV in the national comorbidity survey replication. Arch Gen Psychiatry 62: 617–627, 2005b

Koss MP, Koss PG, Woodruff WJ: Deleterious effects of criminal victimization on women's health and medical utilization. Arch Intern Med 151:342–347, 1991

Kulka RA, Schlenger WE, Fairbank JA, et al: Trauma and the Vietnam War Generation: Report of Findings from the National Vietnam Veterans Readjustment Study. New York, Brunner/Mazel, 1990

Lubin H, Loris M, Burt J, et al: Efficacy of psychoeducational group therapy in reducing symptoms of posttraumatic stress disorder among multiply traumatized women. Am J Psychiatry 155:1172–1177, 1998

March JS, Amaya-Jackson L, Murray MC, et al: Cognitive-behavioral psychotherapy for children and adolescents with posttraumatic stress disorder after a single-incident stressor. J Am Acad Child Adolesc Psychiatry 37:585–593, 1998

Resnick HS, Kilpatrick DG, Dansky BS, et al: Prevalence of civilian trauma and posttraumatic stress disorder in a representative national sample of women. J Consult Clin Psychol 61:984–991, 1993

Solomon SD, Gerrity ET, Muff AM: Efficacy of treatments for posttraumatic stress disorder. An empirical review. JAMA 268:633–638, 1992

Tanielian T, Jaycox LH (eds): Invisible Wounds of War: Psychological and Cognitive Injuries, Their Consequences, and Services to Assist Recovery. Santa Monica, CA, Rand Center for Military Health Policy Research, 2008

Walker EA, Katon W, Russo J, et al: Health care costs associated with posttraumatic stress disorder symptoms in women. Arch Gen Psychiatry 60:369–374, 2003

## Summary of studies on psychotherapy of posttraumatic stress disorder

| Article | Patients | Treatment | Outcome |
| --- | --- | --- | --- |
| Brom et al. 1989 | 112 patients with serious posttraumatic stress disorder (PTSD) from traumatic events within past 5 years (bereavement, acts of violence, traffic accidents, acute or chronic illness, loss of loved one after suicide or homicide). | Patients randomly assigned to trauma desensitization, hypnotherapy, brief psychodynamic therapy, or untreated control condition, mean length of treatments was 15 sessions. | Treated case patients showed similar rates of improvement, 60%, compared with 26% for untreated group. Brief psychodynamic psychotherapy improved avoidance symptoms; trauma desensitization and hypnotherapy improved intrusion symptoms. |
| Foa et al. 1991 | 45 rape victims with PTSD. | 1. Stress inoculation training (SIT) 2. Prolonged exposure (PE), flooding 3. Supportive counseling (SC) 4. Wait-list control (WL) | All groups improved on all measures. SIT led to significantly more improvement than did SC and WL immediately after treatment. PE produced superior outcome on PTSD symptoms at follow-up. |
| Frueh et al. 1996 | 15 Veterans Affairs patients with chronic combat-related PTSD. | 29 treatment sessions combining intensive exposure therapy and social and emotional skills training. | Patients were assessed before and after treatment, and treatment was found to be effective. Implied cost-effectiveness since none of the patients required hospitalization during treatment. |

## Summary of studies on psychotherapy of posttraumatic stress disorder *(continued)*

| Article | Patients | Treatment | Outcome |
|---|---|---|---|
| Foa 1997 | 96 female patients with chronic PTSD after sexual or aggravated assault. | Patients were randomly assigned to nine sessions conducted over 5 weeks of<br><br>1. Prolonged exposure treatment<br>2. Stress inoculation training<br>3. A combination of the above<br><br>or to<br><br>4. Wait-list control | 1. After prolonged exposure treatment, only 32 % still had full PTSD.<br>2 and 3.<br>Patients treated with these therapies produced similar results as above.<br>4. All control subjects still retained PTSD diagnosis.<br>At 3-month follow up, patients treated retained their gains.<br>Almost half of patients treated with exposure met more stringent criteria of 50% decrease in PTSD symptoms and normal scores on depression and anxiety scales. The other treated patients showed smaller gains, although their results approached those for exposure at follow up at 10.7 months. |
| Goenjian et al. 1997 | 64 Armenian adolescents with PTSD and depressive reactions after an earthquake. | Trauma- and grief-focused brief psychotherapy given to 35 patients; 29 patients served as untreated controls. | Symptoms assessed before and after treatment, at 18 months, and at 3 years for those treated and 29 untreated controls. All categories of PTSD symptoms were decreased in those treated, increased in untreated. Depressive symptoms unchanged in those treated, worse in untreated. |

**Summary of studies on psychotherapy of posttraumatic stress disorder *(continued)***

| Article | Patients | Treatment | Outcome |
|---|---|---|---|
| Amir et al. 1998 | 15 noninjured women exposed to a terrorist attack. | 6 sessions of group debriefing with brief group psychotherapy. | At 6 months 27% of subjects developed PTSD. Intervention was assessed as ineffective. |
| Lubin et al. 1998 | 29 traumatized women with chronic PTSD. | 16-week trauma-focused cognitive-behavioral group therapy. | Significant reductions in depressive and all types of PTSD symptoms at termination. Near significant reductions in general psychiatric and dissociative symptoms. All improvements sustained at 6-month follow-up. |
| March et al. 1998 | 17 children and adolescents with PTSD after single-incident stressor. | 18-week cognitive-behavioral group treatment. | Resolution of PTSD in 57% immediately posttreatment and in 86% on 6-month follow-up. |
| Durham et al. 2005 | Participants in eight randomized controlled clinical trials of cognitive-behavior therapy (CBT) for anxiety disorders (and two randomized controlled clinical trials of CBT for schizophrenia) conducted between 1985 and 2001. | Follow-up interviews 2–14 years after original treatment to assess diagnosis, comorbidity, and severity of remaining symptoms. Examination of case note reviews of health care resources for 2 years prior to treatment and for the 2 years prior to follow-up interviews. | Patients with PTSD did particularly poorly with a 40% increase in health care costs over the two time periods, mainly due to increased use of medications. |

**Summary of studies on psychotherapy of posttraumatic stress disorder *(continued)***

| Article | Patients | Treatment | Outcome |
|---|---|---|---|
| Difede et al. 2007 | Male disaster workers with PTSD consequent to the World Trade Center attacks of September 11, 2001, were assigned to a virtual reality treatment ($n = 13$) or to a wait-list control ($n=8$). | 6-to-14 weekly 75-minute (of which 45 minutes are spent in virtual world) treatment sessions of exposure virtual reality treatment of gradually increasing intensity recreating the sights and sounds of the September 11 trauma. Patients closely followed by a therapist who titrates the progression of intensity according to the patient's responses, asking about the patient's experiences until habituation is achieved. | Patients given the virtual reality treatment had both statistically and clinically significant improvement compared with wait-list control group. Prior to virtual reality treatment, half of patients with severe PTSD had participated in other treatment, including imaginal exposure therapy, without improvement. |
| Dunn et al. 2007 | 101 male veterans with chronic combat-related PTSD and depressive disorder. | Patients were randomly assigned to self-management therapy, a CBT group treatment, or active-control therapy, a strictly educational group therapy. | There was initially a greater improvement from self-management therapy that disappeared on follow-up, but psychiatric outpatient utilization and overall outpatient costs were lower with self-management therapy including in the year after the treatment. |

## Summary of studies on psychotherapy of posttraumatic stress disorder *(continued)*

| Article | Patients | Treatment | Outcome |
|---------|----------|-----------|---------|
| **Review articles** | | | |
| Solomon et al. 1992 | | A review of 255 English language reports of PTSD treatments for all types of PTSD patients; 11 studies including 6 involving psychotherapy with randomized clinical trials. | Systematic desensitization provides improvement in intrusive symptoms. |
| Foa et al. 2003 | | A review of studies using exposure therapy with and without cognitive restructuring, stress inoculation training, supportive counseling, and cognitive processing therapy. | Exposure therapy augments other treatment approaches. Adding other treatments to exposure therapy does not augment its effectiveness. |
| Issakidis et al. 2004 | | A large-scale cost-effectiveness study to calculate the economic efficiency of current and optimal treatment for the major mental disorders, this publication reports on the anxiety disorders including PTSD. | For PTSD patients, total health expenditure under evidence-based optimal care would be similar to that under current care, but with costs shifted from the general health to the mental health sector with increased rates of psychological treatment and the rates of pharmacological treatment remaining the same under current care. |

# 5 | Psychotherapy in the Treatment of Anxiety Disorders

Allan Rosenblatt, M.D.

Anxiety disorder is the most common of mental health problems. It is also one of the most expensive, accounting for 31% of total mental health costs and totaling an estimated $46.6 billion in 1 year. Treatment with cognitive-behavioral therapy (CBT), as well as brief dynamic psychotherapy combined with medication, is more effective in the treatment of panic disorder than medication alone and can be cost-effective, as demonstrated by the reduction of medical utilization, with a resulting cost offset. Obsessive-compulsive disorder (OCD) is also more responsive to combination pharmacotherapy and CBT than to medication alone. The cost of untreated OCD is significantly greater than the cost of effective treatment. Similarly, the cost of effective treatment of generalized anxiety disorder can be shown to be significantly less than that of the untreated disorder. Although it has been demonstrated that phobic disorder can be effectively treated by psychotherapy, there are no cost-effectiveness data at present.

## Epidemiology and Costs

The most prevalent psychiatric illness is the group of anxiety disorders that affect 18.1% of adult Americans every year (Kessler et al. 2005b) and 28.8%

of the population at some time during their lifetime (Kessler et al. 2005a). Over 30 million Americans have suffered at some point from an anxiety disorder, the most common of mental health problems (Eaton et al. 1994; Karno and Golding 1991). Not only the most common but also the most expensive disorder, it accounts for 31% of total mental health costs, compared with 22% for mood disorders and 20% for schizophrenia (Rice and Miller 1993). According to the Epidemiological Catchment Area (ECA) surveys (Regier et al. 1984; Robins and Regier 1991; Robins et al. 1984), the total direct and indirect costs of anxiety disorders are estimated to have been $46.6 billion in 1990 (DuPont et al. 1995).

Another study (Greenberg et al. 1999) estimated the annual cost of anxiety disorders in 1990 at $42.3 billion, or $1,542 per patient, with $23 billion (54% of the total) in nonpsychiatric medical costs, $13.3 billion (31%) in psychiatric care costs, $4.1 billion (10%) in indirect workplace costs, $1.2 billion (3%) in mortality costs, and $0.8 billion (2%) in prescription drug costs. Of the $256 in workplace costs per worker with anxiety, 88% is due to lost productivity at work as opposed to absenteeism. In the 1990s, it is calculated that anxiety disorders cost the health care system approximately $63.1 billion annually in 1998 dollars. Nonpsychiatric direct medical costs were 54% of total costs.

The indirect costs stem from the social morbidity, as well as the indirect health costs associated with anxiety disorders. Indirect health costs include increased mortality rates (Coryell et al. 1982), increased prevalence of attempted suicide (Weissman 1990), excess risk for stroke (Weissman et al. 1990), and increased utilization of both psychiatric and medical care (Markowitz et al. 1989). Social morbidity includes a considerably elevated rate of financial dependence, unemployment (60% of men with panic disorder, for example), substance abuse, and dependence (Leon et al. 1995).

# Search Methodology

As with other chapters in this volume, a search of the literature was conducted for the years 1984 through 2007 using the terms "psychotherapy + cost + panic disorder" and repeated for "obsessive-compulsive disorder," "phobic disorder," and "generalized anxiety disorder." Other studies that related to epidemiology and to efficacy of psychotherapy were also included as they permit extrapolations of cost-effectiveness (for summary of studies, see review table at the end of this chapter).

# Panic Disorder

The National Comorbidity Survey, a psychiatric epidemiologic survey of the entire U.S. population, found that American adults between the ages of 15 and 54 years have a 15% occurrence of a panic attack over their lifetimes and a 3% occurrence of a panic attack in the preceding month, and 1% meet diagnostic criteria for panic disorder in the preceding month. Panic attacks and panic disorder are associated with the female sex and lower educational achievement (Eaton et al. 1994). The updated National Comorbidity Survey Replication found lifetime prevalence rates of 22.7% for isolated panic attacks without agoraphobia and 0.8% for panic attacks with agoraphobia but without panic disorder, 3.7% for panic disorder without agoraphobia, and 1.1% for panic disorder with agoraphobia. All four subgroups are significantly comorbid with other lifetime DSM-IV (American Psychiatric Association 1994) disorders. Twelve-month treatment that meets treatment guideline standards for these patients is low (54.9% for panic disorder with agoraphobia—18.2% for panic attacks only), although lifetime treatment is high (96.1% for panic disorder with agoraphobia—61.1% for panic attacks only) (Kessler et al. 2006).

In the past 15 years, the efficacy of cognitive-behavioral modalities of treatment for panic disorder has been widely documented, and the American Psychiatric Association (2006) has issued guidelines for the treatment of panic disorder that cites cognitive-behavioral therapy (CBT) as a first-line treatment. A number of studies indicate that CBT is at least as effective as pharmacotherapy alone and suggest that relapse rates are lower (see Barlow et al. 2000; Beck et al. 1992; Clarke et al. 1994; Klosko et al. 1990; Marks et al. 1993; Sharp et al. 1997). Moreover, in addition to the highly controlled efficacy research, several studies demonstrated the feasibility and effectiveness of administering CBT in a community mental health center (see Stuart et al. 2000; Wade et al. 1998).

Controlled studies show that CBT eliminates panic attacks in more than 80% of patients who suffer from panic disorder (Laberge et al. 1993), although the rate of remission may be lower when high end-state functioning is assessed rather than mere cessation of panics (Rayburn and Otto 2003).

The advantage of combined CBT and pharmacological treatment is as yet not clear. CBT, combined with paroxetine, was reported to be more effective in reducing the number of panic attacks than CBT alone (Oehrberg et al. 1995). However, other studies indicate that the benefit is limited to the acute treatment phase, with CBT alone tending to be as effective as combined treatment over time (see Spiegel and Bruce 1997; Telch and Lucas 1994).

Two studies directly addressed the issue of cost offset as well as cost-effectiveness in the treatment of panic disorder. The first was conducted in Spain (Salvador-Carulla et al. 1995). The treatment given was pharmacological with supportive therapy. A total of 61 patients were studied and followed for 1 year. A 94% reduction in medical utilization was reported for the 12-month period following treatment, compared with the 12-month period prior to the first psychiatric visit. Despite reduction in costs of hospitalization (reduced to zero), medical visits, and laboratory testing, total direct costs increased by 59%, approximately $280 per patient, because of the expense of psychiatric visits and medication. However, demonstrating cost-effectiveness, indirect costs stemming from lost productivity (e.g., number of sick leave days) decreased by 79%, about $684 per patient. Overall, there was about a 30% reduction in total costs. The above figures, however, only calculate the offset for the 12-month posttreatment period. Untreated, such patients would be expected to continue to lose productivity for years, adding to the social costs to be totaled. If one considers the reported effectiveness of CBT, as stated earlier, the above cost-offset results would likely hold true for CBT as well as the supportive therapy used in the study. The average number of visits per patient in the Salvador-Carulla study was 13, and most CBT courses have a duration of 12–15 sessions.

A simple demonstration of cost-effectiveness and cost offset was displayed by a collaborative care intervention that included systematic patient education and approximately two visits with an on-site consulting psychiatrist (Katon et al. 2002). This produced significantly more anxiety-free days than the usual primary care. The total costs were slightly lower, the increased mental health cost being outweighed by the decreased symptom-driven medical visits.

In a third cost-effectiveness study, Otto et al. (2000) examined the costs and outcome of CBT versus medication alone, when delivered in a specialty outpatient clinic. CBT alone was administered to 20 patients, and medication alone was given to another 20 patients. The CBT group attended 10–12 visits during the first 4 months, after which time visits were infrequent, with a mean total of 12.4 visits for the year. The medication group had 5–6 visits during the first 4 months, continuing for a mean total of 13 visits for the year, whereas medication was continued for the year. The total costs per patient for the CBT cohort receiving individual treatment were $1,186 for the first 4 months, whereas the costs per patient of the medication group, including the cost of medication, were $839. When group CBT was administered, the costs were even lower, $518 per patient for the first 4 months. However, after a year, the CBT therapy cohort cost $523 per patient for group therapy and $1,357 for individual therapy, whereas the medication group cost $2,305 per patient. The continued costs of medication were critical. It should be noted that for most clinics or providers, it would be difficult to make available enough patients in the same time period for group treatment to be feasible.

The average annual cost of anxiety disorders is estimated to be $1,542 per sufferer, and panic disorder has one of the highest rates of service use

(Greenberg et al. 1999; Rees et al. 1998). Compared with the cost per patient in this study of $523 and $1,357 per patient for group and individual CBT, respectively, a cost offset even for the first year alone may be inferred. Thereafter, even if the relapse rate were 50% (considerably above estimates), treatment would be cheaper than the cost of no treatment.

Modifications of CBT, using computer-assisted self-study modules and only five to eight therapist sessions, are reported to produce equivalent results. Costs would be significantly lower and cost-effectiveness greater than with full CBT protocols (see Clark et al. 1999; Kenardy et al. 2003; Vincelli et al. 2003).

Brief dynamic psychotherapy (12 weekly sessions) combined with pharmacological treatment is not only more effective than pharmacological treatment alone (100% remission vs. 75% remission after 12 weeks), but the relapse rate was significantly lower (Wiborg and Dahl 1996). Because the duration of treatment is approximately the same, the cost-offset results would apply to this modality as well.

Based on the effect-size calculations from meta-analyses of randomized controlled trials, an Australian study (Heuzenroeder et al. 2004) assessed the incremental cost with CBT and serotonin-norepinephrine reuptake inhibitor (SNRIs). The health benefit was measured as a reduction in disability-adjusted life years (DALYs). Effectiveness of interventions was measured for both panic disorder (treated with CBT, selective serotonin reuptake inhibitors [SSRIs], and tricyclic antidepressants [TCAs]) and generalized anxiety disorder, or GAD (treated costs and benefits were calculated for a period of 1 year for the eligible population based on the prevalence of GAD and panic disorder in the Australian adult population in the year 2000). The CBT intervention was modeled as 12 one-hour consultations plus one general practitioner consultation to a health care provider working privately or on a publicly funded salary. The analysis suggested that CBT was the most effective and cost-effective intervention for panic disorder (and for GAD) particularly if provided by a psychologist on a public salary. It was estimated that CBT results in greater total health benefit than drug intervention for both anxiety disorders.

Another Australian study (Issakidis et al. 2004) compared the burden and economic efficiency of current and optimal treatment for the anxiety disorders by calculating the direct health care costs of treatment and the outcome as the averted years lived with disability (YLDs). The cost per YLD averted was compared for those already in treatment for a mental health problem with a hypothetical optimal care package of evidence-based treatment for the same patient group. For panic disorder, the increased efficacy of optimal care would be achieved by a shift from psychotropic medication to psychotherapeutic treatment. For all the anxiety disorders studied, evidence-based care would result in a one-and-a-half to twofold increase in efficacy, a 40%–60% increase in YLDs averted—a 54% increase—compared with current care, at a similar or lower overall cost.

A review article by Landon and Barlow (2004) of 14 controlled clinical trials of CBT for panic disorder found that CBT was effective and likely to be cost-effective for panic disorder with or without agoraphobia. On average, 40%–90% of patients treated with CBT were panic free at the end of treatment and 75%–87% were panic free at longer term follow-up of 6 months to 2 years. These authors also cited findings that CBT reduces comorbidity (the number and severity of additional diagnoses for which patients meet criteria posttreatment), yields beneficial effects on physical health status with reductions in nonpsychiatric medical symptoms during treatment and at 6-month follow-up, and is effective in patient populations who have been unresponsive to pharmacotherapy.

Very different results are reported, however, by Durham et al. (2005). In their review of the long-term outcome of CBT for patients with anxiety in eight randomized controlled clinical trials in Scotland, they found that while CBT led to better long-term outcome with respect to overall symptom severity than non-CBT treatment, it did not lead to better diagnostic status. Furthermore, in their review, the positive effects of CBT found in the original trials eroded over longer follow-up periods, there was no association between more intensive therapy and more enduring effects of CBT, and CBT was not found to be cost-effective compared with non-CBT. Forty-eight percent of the patients who were originally treated for panic disorder still had a clinical diagnosis at long-term follow-up, with 26% still diagnosable with panic disorder. Irrespective of original anxiety disorder diagnosis, patients originally diagnosed who retained a clinical diagnosis over 2–14 years were likely to have multiple diagnoses and also fluctuated between different disorders. Depression was a common comorbid disorder, found in 43% of those who still had any clinical diagnosis at long-term follow-up. For all anxiety disorder patients, only 7% had no symptoms of anxiety or depression at long-term follow-up, and the proportion of patients achieving clinically significant change on the main outcome measures varied from 20% to just over 60%. While 80% of patients reported some improvement on long-term follow-up, comparison with normative data on measures of symptomatology and health status showed that even those with no clinical diagnosis had poorer scores than population means, and the whole group had means that fell into the worst 12% of the population for symptomatology and the worst 24% for physical health status. Thus, according to this review, although many patients with anxiety disorder reported faring well after treatment, only a small number maintained good levels of recovery.

Reporting sharply contrasting results and even dramatic cost offsets, a study designed to examine the impact on health care utilization of CBT for patients with panic disorder with agoraphobia (PDA) provided one of three empirically supported CBTs (standard, group, or brief) to 84 adult patients meeting diagnostic criteria for PDA (Roberge et al. 2005). Overall health care, mental health care, and medication utilization were measured at baseline, posttreatment, 3-month, 6-month, 9-month, and 1-year follow-up, and associated costs were computed. Results showed both a significant reduction in symptomatology in the three CBT groups compared with wait-list controls and a significant reduction in total and mental health care costs during the 1-year follow-up period after providing an effective CBT treatment for these patients.

Another randomized control trial involved 232 primary care patients with panic disorder from six primary care clinics who were randomly assigned to either treatment as usual or a combined CBT and pharmacotherapy intervention for panic disorder by a mental health therapist in the primary care setting (Katon et al. 2006). Intervention patients had up to six session of CBT in the first 12 weeks and up to six telephone follow-ups over the next 9 months. Compared with usual care, intervention patients had 60.4 more anxiety-free days. Total incremental outpatient costs were $494 higher in intervention versus usual-care patients, with a cost per additional anxiety-free day of $8.40 and a cost per quality-adjusted life year well within the range of other commonly accepted medical interventions such as the use of statins for hypercholesterolemia or the treatment of hypertension. The authors considered the collaborative treatment for panic disorder to be cost-effective by virtue of its providing robust clinical improvement compared with usual care with a moderate increase in ambulatory costs. Although Katon et al.'s study focused primarily on total outpatient costs leading to an assessment of cost-effectiveness just on this cost basis, the additional finding that a significantly higher percentage of usual-care patients had two or more medical hospitalizations compared with intervention patients gave evidence of a total medical cost savings of $240.

A study focused specifically on measuring the relative cost efficacy of empirically supported treatments examined the results from the Multicenter Comparative Treatment Study of Panic Disorder with random patient assignment and calculated cost-efficacy ratios at the end of acute, maintenance, and follow-up phases for CBT alone, imipramine alone, paroxetine alone, and two combination treatments, CBT plus imipramine and CBT plus paroxetine (McHugh et al. 2007). Consistently greater cost efficacy was found for the individual over the combined treatments, imipramine being most cost efficacious at the end of the acute phase and CBT being most cost efficacious both at the end of maintenance treatment and

6 months after treatment termination. These authors concluded that current monotherapies should be considered the first-line treatment of choice for panic disorder and that CBT appears to be the most durable and cost-effective monotherapy.

In a randomized controlled clinical trial of psychoanalytic psychotherapy for panic disorder, Milrod et al. (2007) found that subjects receiving manualized psychodynamic psychotherapy twice weekly for 12 weeks had significantly greater reduction in panic symptoms than panic patients treated with applied relaxation training.

# Obsessive-Compulsive Disorder

Obsessive-compulsive disorder (OCD) affects 2.1% of the population annually, as shown by the ECA surveys of DSM-IV disorders, or 1.0% annually in the National Comorbidity Survey Replication (Kessler et al. 2005b) and 6.3% over a lifetime (Kessler et al. 2005a), and total costs were estimated to have been $8.4 billion in 1990. The cost per individual sufferer can be estimated at about $2,000 per year; without treatment, the disabling condition is chronic and unremitting.

Jenike (1993) concluded, from his review of treatment efficacy for this disorder, that the combination of pharmacotherapy and CBT enables the majority of OCD sufferers to lead relatively normal lives, to work, and to function well in families and in social situations. The percentage of patients who improved range from 60% to 90% in the studies cited. Additional studies not included in his review confirm this conclusion (Abramowitz et al. 2003; Drummond 1993; Greist 1998; Marks 1988; van Balkom et al. 1998). Most outcome studies are primarily of patients with cleaning and checking compulsions, whereas those with other or multiple compulsions, such as exactness, counting, hoarding, or slowness rituals, were underrepresented. Therefore, reported improvement rates may not be generalizable to these patients (Ball et al. 1996).

Although pharmacotherapy has been reported to be effective, relapse rates of 90% have been reported, while CBT alone showed far better maintenance of treatment gains (Jenike 1993). Moreover, according to Jenicke, psychodynamic psychotherapy can be a valuable adjunct in treating the deeply rooted thought patterns that develop in response to obsessive-compulsive behaviors.

Because one-third to one-half of adults develop this disorder during childhood or adolescence (Rasmussen and Eisen 1990), results of treatment of children with OCD are significant. A study of cognitive-behavioral psychotherapy combined with medication for 15 children and adolescents with OCD showed a significant benefit for treatment immediately posttreatment and at follow-up: six patients became asymptomatic, and nine had at least a 50% reduction in symptoms (March et al. 1994). In addition, 31 of 32 investigations, mostly single case reports, reported some benefit for cognitive-behavioral interventions (March 1995).

A review article of psychological treatments versus treatment as usual for OCD examined seven studies with usable data for meta-analyses (Gava et al. 2007). Patients who received any variant of CBT had significantly fewer symptoms after treatment than those receiving treatment as usual, with different types of CBT showing similar differences in effect compared with treatment as usual.

Untreated over a 20-year period, the cost of OCD at $2,000 per year is $40,000 per affected individual. Even if only 50% successful, any treatment that cost less than $20,000 would show a cost offset. Because the onset is often early in life, the disability is usually over a longer period than 20 years, and the cost savings would be greater. From the above-cited studies, it can be inferred that psychotherapy in combination with medication not only is cost-effective in OCD but also is likely to show a cost offset.

# Phobic Disorder

According to the ECA and National Comorbidity Survey, phobic disorder is the most prevalent of the anxiety disorders (Kessler et al. 1994; Schneier et al. 1992). Results from the National Comorbidity Survey show that social phobia has a 12-month prevalence rate of 7.9% and a lifetime prevalence of 14.4%. Agoraphobia has a lifetime prevalence of 6.7% and a 30-day prevalence of 2.3%. Simple phobia has a lifetime prevalence of 11.3% and a 30-day prevalence of 5.5%. For social phobia, the lifetime and 30-day prevalence rates are 13.3% and 4.5%, respectively. Increasing lifetime prevalence rates are found in more recent cohorts (Magee et al. 1996). In the National Comorbidity Survey Replication, social phobia rates are 6.8% annually and 12.1% lifetime, agoraphobia 0.8% annually and 1.4% lifetime, and specific phobia 8.7% annually and 12.5% lifetime (Kessler et al. 2005a, 2005b). As in all the anxiety disorders, the prevalence is twice as great in women as in men. Although the social costs are somewhat less for this disorder, they are still considerable. Men are about one-and-a-half times more likely to be unemployed than those with no Axis I diagnosis, about four times more likely to receive disability payments, almost twice as likely to be on welfare, and about four times as likely to seek help for emotional, drug, or alcohol problems.

There are few explicit studies regarding cost-effectiveness of treatment of phobic disorders. Moreover, some ambiguity exists in the literature regarding the classification of agoraphobia, sometimes included in the panic disorder classification as secondary to panic disorder and sometimes as a phobic disorder.

However, a number of outcome studies have been reported with social phobic patients. One used social effectiveness therapy with 13 patients (Turner et al. 1995), the other used exposure, rational-emotive therapy, and social skills training with 34 patients (Mersch 1995). Results were reported as showing modest but significant improvement, maintained for both groups. A third study included the treatment of 38 agoraphobic patients with psychoanalytically oriented inpatient psychotherapy (Bassler and Hoffmann 1994). An improvement rate of 61.4% was obtained after 12 weeks of hospitalization and treatment. Taylor (1996) reviewed 42 treatment trials of CBTs in a meta-analysis. Although all varieties were significantly better than wait-list controls, only the combined cognitive restructuring and exposure achieved significantly better results than placebo controls. Yet, effectiveness in a public mental health center setting has been demonstrated (Levini et al. 2002; Lincoln et al. 2003).

Cognitive-behavioral group therapy has also been shown to produce significant improvement, greater than that achieved by educational-supportive group therapy (Cottraux et al. 2000; Heimberg et al. 1990), even after a 5-year follow-up (Heimberg 1993). Heimberg and colleagues have also demonstrated the superiority of such therapy to medication with phenelzine (Heimberg et al. 1998).

To compare cognitive-behavioral group therapy and exposure group therapy for 90 patients with social phobia, Hofmann (2004) randomly assigned patients to cognitive-behavioral group therapy, exposure group therapy without explicit cognitive interventions, or a wait-list control. Although both treatments were superior to the wait-list control and led to similar immediate improvement, only the treatment with cognitive intervention led to maintenance of treatment gains at 6-month follow-up. Hofmann speculated that CBT leads to more enduring improvement specifically because of the greater influence on cognitive errors about dreaded social situations that were not explicitly addressed in the exposure therapy treatment.

An above-mentioned Australian study (Issakidis et al. 2004) compared the burden and economic efficiency of current and optimal treatment for the anxiety disorders by calculating both the costs of treatment and the outcome in averted YLDs. The investigators calculated and compared the cost per YLD averted for those anxious patients already in treatment with a hypothetical optimal care treatment approach for the same patient group. For social phobia, the increased efficacy of optimal care would be achieved by increasing the numbers of patients receiving psychotherapeutic treatment in addition to increasing the use of psychopharmacological treatment. For all the anxiety disorders studied, evidence-based care would result in a one-and-a-half to twofold increase in efficacy, a 40%–60% increase in YLDs averted—a 54% increase—compared with current care, at a similar or lower overall cost (Issakidis et al. 2004).

# Generalized Anxiety Disorder

Because the initial diagnostic category of GAD in DSM-III (American Psychiatric Association 1980) represented a residual diagnosis with low reliability, data regarding its national prevalence and the social costs were not nationally projected in the ECA study. However, the diagnostic criteria were refined in DSM-III-R (American Psychiatric Association 1987), and an epidemiological survey of this category, as part of the National Comorbidity Survey of psychiatric disorders, found a 12-month prevalence rate of 3.1% (Wittchen et al. 1994). In that study a substantial comorbidity was found, of 65.0% for current comorbidity and 89.8% for lifetime comorbidity, using DSM-III-R criteria. The National Comorbidity Survey Replication found annual rates of GAD of 3.1% and lifetime of 5.7% (Kessler et al. 2005a, 2005b). Thus GAD in pure form is a relatively rare disorder. However, because at least a third of those with a current diagnosis of GAD had no other current or recent diagnosis, the validity of GAD as an independent diagnostic entity is supported.

It should be noted that GAD is common in children, adolescents, and the elderly. A 1-year prevalence rate of 2.9% was found for overanxious anxiety, the childhood equivalent of GAD (Anderson et al. 1987), and in adolescents it was found to be 7.3% (Kashani and Orvaschel 1988). In the elderly, GAD accounts for the majority of anxiety disorders, with prevalence rates ranging from 0.7% to 7.1% (Flint 1994).

Bassler and Hoffmann (1994) reported a study of psychoanalytically oriented inpatient psychotherapy for 85 hospitalized patients with severe anxiety disorders (GAD, agoraphobia, and panic disorder). An overall improvement rate of 53% was found after hospitalization of approximately 12 weeks. Of those 23 patients diagnosed with GAD, 40% were reported as improved, whereas about 21% failed to improve. It bears repeating that these patients were severely enough disabled to require hospitalization.

Barlow et al. (1984) reported a 12-week cognitive therapy program that included relaxation training and electromyography feedback. The treatment group, compared with a wait-list control, improved significantly more and continued to improve 3 months following treatment. Butler et al. (1987) treated a larger group with a similar CBT package and reported significantly greater improvement than a wait-list control group. It should be noted that Butler et al.'s study reported benefits greater than did a study of the short-term effects of benzodiazepines on generalized anxiety (Harvey and Rapee 1995).

In the aforementioned Australian study (Heuzenroeder et al. 2004) to assess the incremental cost-effectiveness of interventions for GAD (CBT and SNRIs) and panic disorder (CBT, SSRIs, and TCAs), the health benefit was measured as a reduction in DALYs. The costs and benefits were calculated for a period of 1 year for the eligible population based on the year 2000 prevalence of GAD (and panic disorder) in the Australian adult population. The analysis suggested that CBT was both the most effective and cost-effective intervention for GAD (and panic disorder) particularly if provided by a psychologist on a public salary. CBT was estimated to result in greater total health benefit than drug intervention for both anxiety disorders.

Another previously cited Australian study (Issakidis et al. 2004) compared the burden and economic efficiency of current and optimal treatment for the anxiety disorders by calculating and comparing the cost per YLD averted for those anxious patients already in treatment with a hypothetical optimal evidence-based treatment for the same patient group. For GAD patients, the increased efficacy of optimal care would be achieved by increased rates of psychotherapeutic treatment while maintaining similar rates of psychopharmacological treatment as in current care. For all the anxiety disorders studied, evidence-based care would result in a one-and-a-half to twofold increase in efficacy, a 40%–60% increase in YLDs averted—a 54% increase—compared to current care, at a similar or lower overall cost.

Despite the positive findings of some of the above studies and estimates, it is sobering to consider the previously mentioned Durham et al. (2005) analysis of eight randomized controlled trials of CBT for patients with anxiety disorder in central Scotland. For the GAD patients, 52% had at least one clinical diagnosis at long-term follow-up with 34% still diagnosable with GAD. In this group, there were also fairly high levels of depression (25%), agoraphobia (19%), dysthymia (18%), panic disorder (17%), and social phobia (15%.) While 80% of the treated patients with anxiety disorder reported some improvement at long-term follow-up, as a group they fell into the worst 12% of the population in more objective measures of symptomatology and the worst 24% in measures of physical health status. Thus, although many with anxiety disorders appear to have achieved significant improvement immediately after CBT treatment, only a relatively small number maintain good levels of recovery over the long term according to this review.

A number of the studies cited above for the various categories of anxiety disorder have included randomized controlled clinical trials. A word of caution is therefore in order in extrapolating such efficacy studies to effectiveness in clinical practice (see Morrison et al. 2003). In clinical practice many, if not most, patients present with multiple diagnoses, which increase treatment length (e.g., see Williams and Falbo 1996, regarding the effect of agaraphobic disability on outcome of panic disorder treatment). Even so, cost-effectiveness and offset, though likely somewhat diminished in practice, would still be quite significant.

# Case Vignette

The following is an example of a patient with an anxiety disorder that was successfully treated by psychotherapy along with medication.

> Mr. G is a 38-year-old married professional man referred for psychiatric consultation because of a long history of generalized anxiety, hypochondriacal fears, and a phobia of crowds since late adolescence. He had been seen in emergency rooms on a number of occasions for chest pain and had been observed for possible cardiac pathology. No organic pathology was discovered, and repeated 24-hour Holter monitor observations revealed no cardiac arrhythmias. Anxiolytic medication had provided only limited control of his symptoms. His professional life was significantly impaired by his anxiety and phobic symptoms. Noteworthy were the patient's inhibited affects and compliant behavior.
>
> The diagnosis of GAD with phobic and hypochondriacal features was made, and twice-weekly psychotherapy with antianxiety medication was conducted for a period of 21 months. The patient's fear of crowds, especially where he could not easily and inconspicuously leave, was occasioned by the fear that he would vomit or otherwise humiliate himself before he could escape from public scrutiny.
>
> As therapy progressed, it became apparent to the patient and therapist that his episodes of anxiety were occasioned by any interpersonal exchange that might provoke anger, which he could not allow himself to feel. It also became clear that the phobic anxiety appeared primarily when he was in a theater or other gathering where someone had the spotlight. Such circumstances would evoke an angry, yet extremely shameful fantasied demand of, "Look at me, I'm just as important!," which he would put out of his mind. He recalled as an adolescent, shortly before the onset of his symptoms, going on one of his first dates. During intermission, he attempted to be "cool" in front of his date by smoking a cigarette and inhaling for the first time. He choked and fell down the steps, to his intense embarrassment. When he recounted this misadventure to his mother, to whom he confessed everything, her comment was, "It served you right for showing off."
>
> His fear of and shame about any strong emotion, especially anger and needs for attention, were linked to family experiences. His hypochondriacal mother, who blatantly favored his younger sister, would react to any display of rebellion or temper by the patient as a mortal wound, possibly provoking (she would claim) a heart attack.
>
> At the conclusion of therapy, the patient had discontinued all anxiolytic medication and was mostly symptom free, experiencing only occasional ep-

isodes of mild anxiety, which he was able to control. He no longer visited emergency rooms and physician's offices fearing he was having a heart attack. He returned 4 years later because of a recurrence of phobic symptoms after the birth of a baby son. Seven sessions were sufficient to help him understand the relationship between his recurrence and shameful angry feelings about his wife's greater maternal attention to the baby son, and the symptoms abated.

# Conclusion

Although there are increasing data that specifically measure the cost-effectiveness of psychotherapy for the anxiety disorders, a strong case can be made for the cost-effectiveness of psychotherapy (alone or in combination with pharmacotherapy) simply by considering the available data documenting the high costs of these illnesses and data indicating the cost of effective treatment. Yet, of the more than six million visits to a primary care physician with a recorded anxiety disorder diagnosis, only 60% resulted in treatment for anxiety being offered. Almost 2.5 million patients went untreated. Moreover, the use of psychotherapy decreased over this time period in visits both to primary care physicians and to psychiatrists. It seems apparent that underrecognition and undertreatment constitute a significant problem, and medication is being substituted for psychotherapy (Harman et al. 2002).

Considering the prevalence rates of each of the categories of anxiety disorder, even if the total social costs of the disorders other than OCD are only one-half of those of OCD (and they are likely greater), the cost savings over a 20-year period for each category would be considerable. Provision for adequate treatment of these disorders would not only significantly increase overall productivity in the United States but also provide tangible dollar savings to federal programs as well as in insurance costs.

# References

Abramowitz JS, Foa EB, Franklin ME: Exposure and ritual prevention for obsessive-compulsive disorder: effects of intensive versus twice-weekly sessions. J Consult Clin Psychol 71:394–398, 2003

Anderson JC, Williams S, McGee R, et al: DSM-III disorders in preadolescent children. Prevalence in a large sample from the general population. Arch Gen Psychiatry 44:69–76, 1987

American Psychiatric Association: Diagnostic and Statistical Manual of Mental Disorders, 3rd Edition. Washington, DC, American Psychiatric Association, 1980

American Psychiatric Association: Diagnostic and Statistical Manual of Mental Disorders, 3rd Edition, Revised. Washington, DC, American Psychiatric Association, 1987

American Psychiatric Association: Diagnostic and Statistical Manual of Mental Disorders, 4th Edition. Washington, DC, American Psychiatric Association, 1994

American Psychiatric Association: Quick Reference to the American Psychiatric Association Practice Guidelines for the Treatment of Psychiatric Disorders: Compendium 2006. Washington, DC, American Psychiatric Press, 2006

Ball SG, Baer L, Otto MW: Symptom subtypes of obsessive-compulsive disorder in behavioral treatment studies: a quantitative review. Behav Res Ther 34:47–51, 1996

Barlow DH, Cohen AS, Waddell MT, et al: Panic and generalized anxiety disorders: nature and treatment. Behavior Therapy 15:431–449, 1984

Barlow DH, Gorman JM, Shear MK, et al: Cognitive-behavioral therapy, imipramine, or their combination for panic disorder: a randomized controlled trial. JAMA 283:2529–2536, 2000

Bassler M, Hoffmann SO: [Inpatient psychotherapy of anxiety disorders—a comparison of therapeutic effectiveness in patients with generalized anxiety disorder, agoraphobia and panic disorder]. Psychother Psychosom Med Psychol 44:217–225, 1994

Beck AT, Sokol L, Clark DA, et al: A crossover study of focused cognitive therapy for panic disorder. Am J Psychiatry 149:778–783, 1992

Butler G, Cullington A, Hibbert G, et al: Anxiety management for persistent generalised anxiety. Br J Psychiatry 151:535–542, 1987

Clark DM, Salkovskis PM, Hackmann A, et al: A comparison of cognitive therapy, applied relaxation and imipramine in the treatment of panic disorder. Br J Psychiatry 164:759–769, 1994

Clark DM, Salkovskis PM, Hackmann A, et al: Brief cognitive therapy for panic disorder: a randomized controlled trial. J Consult Clin Psychol 67:583–589, 1999

Coryell W, Noyes R, Clancy J: Excess mortality in panic disorder. A comparison with primary unipolar depression. Arch Gen Psychiatry 39:701–703, 1982

Cottraux J, Note I, Albuisson E, et al: Cognitive behavior therapy versus supportive therapy in social phobia: a randomized controlled trial. Psychother Psychosom 69:137–146, 2000

Drummond LM: The treatment of severe, chronic, resistant obsessive-compulsive disorder. An evaluation of an in-patient programme using behavioural psychotherapy in combination with other treatments. Br J Psychiatry 163:223–229, 1993

DuPont RL, Rice DP, Shiraki S, et al: Economic costs of obsessive-compulsive disorder. Med Interface 8:102–109, 1995

Durham RC, Chambers JA, Power KG, et al: Long-term outcome of cognitive behaviour therapy clinical trials in central Scotland. Health Technol Assess 9:1–174, 2005

Eaton WW, Kessler RC, Wittchen HU, et al: Panic and panic disorder in the United States. Am J Psychiatry 151:413–420, 1994

Flint AJ: Epidemiology and comorbidity of anxiety disorders in the elderly. Am J Psychiatry 151:640–649, 1994

Gava A, Barbui C, Aguglia E, et al: Psychological treatments versus treatment as usual for obsessive compulsive disorder (OCD). Cochrane Database Syst Review April 18:CD005333, 2007

Greenberg PE, Sisitsky T, Kessler RC, et al: The economic burden of anxiety disorders in the 1990s. J Clin Psychiatry 60:427–435, 1999

Greist JH: The comparative effectiveness of treatments for obsessive-compulsive disorder. Bull Menninger Clin 62:A65–81, 1998

Harman JS, Rollman BL, Hanusa BH, et al: Physician office visits of adults for anxiety disorders in the United States, 1985–1998. J Gen Intern Med 17:165–172, 2002

Harvey AG, Rapee RM: Cognitive-behavior therapy for generalized anxiety disorder. Psychiatr Clin North Am 18:859–870, 1995

Heimberg R, Hope D, Dodge C, et al: DSM-III-R subtypes of social phobia: comparison of generalized social phobics and public speaking phobics. J Nerv Ment Dis 178:172–179, 1990

Heimberg RG, Salzman D, Holt CS, et al: Cognitive behavioral group treatment of social phobia: effectiveness at 5-year follow-up. Cogn Ther Res 17:325–339, 1993

Heimberg R, Liebowitz M, Hope D, et al: Cognitive behavioral group therapy vs phenelzine therapy for social phobia: 12 week outcome. Arch Gen Psychiatry 55:1133–1141, 1998

Heuzenroeder L, Donnelly M, Haby MM, et al: Cost-effectiveness of psychological and pharmacological interventions for generalized anxiety disorder and panic disorder. Aust N Z J Psychiatry 38:602–612, 2004

Hofmann S: Cognitive mediation of treatment change in social phobia. J Consult Clin Psychol 72:393–399, 2004

Issakidis C, Sanderson K, Corry J, et al: Modelling the population cost-effectiveness of current and evidence-based optimal treatment for anxiety disorders. Psychol Med 34:19–35, 2004

Jenike MA: Obsessive-compulsive disorder: efficacy of specific treatments as assessed by controlled trials. Psychopharmacol Bull 29:487–499, 1993

Karno M, Golding JM: Obsessive-compulsive disorder, in Psychiatric Disorders in America: The Epidemiological Catchment Area Study. Edited by Robins LN, Regier DA. New York, Free Press, 1991, pp 204–219

Kashani JH, Orvaschel H: Anxiety disorders in mid-adolescence: a community sample. Am J Psychiatry 145:960–964, 1988

Katon WJ, Roy-Byrne P, Russo J, et al: Cost-effectiveness and cost offset of a collaborative care intervention for primary care patients with panic disorder. Arch Gen Psychiatry 59:1098–1104, 2002

Katon WJ, Russo J, Sherbourne C, et al: Incremental cost-effectiveness of a collaborative care intervention for panic disorder. Psychol Med 36:353–363, 2006

Kenardy JA, Dow MG, Johnston DW, et al: A comparison of delivery methods of cognitive-behavioral therapy for panic disorder: an international multicenter trial. J Consult Clin Psychol 71:1068–1075, 2003

Kessler RC, McGonagle KA, Zhao S, et al: Lifetime and 12-month prevalence of DSM-III-R psychiatric disorders in the United States. Results from the National Comorbidity Survey. Arch Gen Psychiatry 51:8–19, 1994

Kessler RC, Berglund P, Demler O, et al: Lifetime prevalence and age-of-onset distributions of DSM-IV disorders in the national comorbidity survey replication. Arch Gen Psychiatry 62:593–602, 2005a

Kessler RC, Chiu WT, Demler O, et al: Prevalence, severity, and comorbidity of 12-month DSM-IV in the national comorbidity survey replication. Arch Gen Psychiatry 62: 617–627, 2005b

Kessler RC, Chiu WT, Jin R, et al: The epidemiology of panic attacks, panic disorder, and agoraphobia in the national comorbidity survey replication. Arch Gen Psychiatry 63:415–424, 2006

Klosko JS, Barlow DH, Tassinari R, et al: A comparison of alprazolam and behavior therapy in treatment of panic disorder. J Consult Clin Psychol 58:77–84, 1990

Laberge B, Gauthier JG, Cote G, et al: Cognitive-behavioral therapy of panic disorder with secondary major depression: a preliminary investigation. J Consult Clin Psychol 61:1028–1037, 1993

Landon T, Barlow D: Cognitive-behavioral treatment for panic disorder: current status. J Psychiatr Pract 10:211–226, 2004

Leon AC, Portera L, Weissman MM: The social costs of anxiety disorders. Br J Psychiatry Suppl:19–22, 1995

Levini D, Piacentini D, Campana A: Effectiveness of cognitive-behavioral therapy of panic disorder with secondary major depression: a preliminary investigation. Epidemiol Psichiatri Soc 11:127–133, 2002

Lincoln TM, Rief W, Hahlweg K, et al: Effectiveness of an empirically supported treatment for social phobia in the field. Behav Res Ther 41:1251–1269, 2003

Magee WJ, Eaton WW, Wittchen HU, et al: Agoraphobia, simple phobia, and social phobia in the National Comorbidity Survey. Arch Gen Psychiatry 53:159–168, 1996

March JS: Cognitive-behavioral psychotherapy for children and adolescents with OCD: a review and recommendations for treatment. J Am Acad Child Adolesc Psychiatry 34:7–18, 1995

March JS, Mulle K, Herbel B: Behavioral psychotherapy for children and adolescents with obsessive-compulsive disorder: an open trial of a new protocol-driven treatment package. J Am Acad Child Adolesc Psychiatry 33:333–341, 1994

Markowitz JS, Weissman MM, Ouellette R, et al: Quality of life in panic disorder. Arch Gen Psychiatry 46:984–992, 1989

Marks IMl: Drug vs behavioral treatment of obsessive-compulsive disorder. Biol Psychiatry 28:1072–1073, 1988

Marks IM, Swinson RP, Basoglu M, et al: Alprazolam and exposure alone and combined in panic disorder with agoraphobia. A controlled study in London and Toronto. Br J Psychiatry 162:776–787, 1993

McHugh RK, Otto MW, Barlow DH, et al: Cost-efficacy of individual and combined treatments for panic disorder. J Clin Psychiatry 68:1038–1044, 2007

Mersch PP: The treatment of social phobia: the differential effectiveness of exposure in vivo and an integration of exposure in vivo, rational emotive therapy and social skills training. Behav Res Ther 33:259–269, 1995

Milrod B, Leon A, Busch F, et al: A randomized controlled clinical trial of psychoanalytic psychotherapy for panic disorder. Am J Psychiatry 164:265–272, 2007

Morrison KH, Bradley R, Westen D: The external validity of controlled clinical trials of psychotherapy for depression and anxiety: a naturalistic study. Psychol Psychother 76:109–132, 2003

Oehrberg S, Christiansen PE, Behnke K, et al: Paroxetine in the treatment of panic disorder: a randomised, double-blind, placebo-controlled study. Br J Psychiatry 167:374–379, 1995

Otto MW, Pollack MH, Maki KM: Empirically supported treatments for panic disorder: costs, benefits, and stepped care. J Consult Clin Psychol 68:556–563, 2000

Rasmussen SA, Eisen JL: Epidemiology of obsessive compulsive disorder. J Clin Psychiatry 51 Suppl:10–13; discussion 14, 1990

Rayburn NR, Otto MW: Cognitive-behavioral therapy for panic disorder: a review of treatment elements, strategies, and outcomes. CNS Spectr 8:356–362, 2003

Rees CS, Richards JC, Smith LM: Medical utilisation and costs in panic disorder: a comparison with social phobia. J Anxiety Disord 12:421–435, 1998

Rice DP, Miller LS: The economic burden of affective disorders. Adv Health Econ Health Serv Res 14:37–53, 1993

Roberge P, Marchand A, Reinharz D, et al: Healthcare utilization following cognitive-behavioral treatment for panic disorder with agoraphobia. Cognitive Behaviour Therapy 34:79–88, 2005

Robins LN, Regier DA: Psychiatric Disorders in America. New York, The Free Press, 1991

Robins LN, Helzer JE, Weissman MM, et al: Lifetime prevalence of specific psychiatric disorders in three sites. Arch Gen Psychiatry 41:949–958, 1984

Regier D, Myers JK, Kramer M, et al: The NIMH Epidemiologic Catchment Area program: historical context, major objectives, and study population characteristics. Arch Gen Psychiatry 41:934–941, 1984

Salvador-Carulla L, Segui J, Fernandez-Cano P, et al: Costs and offset effect in panic disorders. Br J Psychiatry Suppl:23–28, 1995

Schneier FR, Johnson J, Hornig CD, et al: Social phobia. Comorbidity and morbidity in an epidemiologic sample. Arch Gen Psychiatry 49:282–288, 1992

Sharp DM, Power KG, Simpson RJ, et al: Global measures of outcome in a controlled comparison of pharmacological and psychological treatment of panic disorder and agoraphobia in primary care. Br J Gen Pract 47:150–155, 1997

Spiegel DA, Bruce TJ: Benzodiazepines and exposure-based cognitive behavior therapies for panic disorder: conclusions from combined treatment trials. Am J Psychiatry 154:773–781, 1997

Stuart GL, Treat TA, Wade WA: Effectiveness of an empirically based treatment for panic disorder delivered in a service clinic setting: 1-year follow-up. J Consult Clin Psychol 68:506–512, 2000

Taylor S: Meta-analysis of cognitive-behavioral treatments for social phobia. J Behav Ther Exp Psychiatry 27:1–9, 1996

Telch MJ, Lucas RA: Combined pharmacological and psychological treatment of panic disorder: current status and future directions, in Treatment of Panic Disorder. Edited by Wolfe BE, Maser JD. Washington, DC, American Psychiatric Press, 1994, pp 177–197

Turner SM, Beidel DC, Cooley-Quille MR: Two-year follow-up of social phobias treated with social effectiveness therapy. Behav Res Ther 33:553–555, 1995

van Balkom AJ, de Haan E, van Oppen P, et al: Cognitive and behavioral therapies alone versus in combination with fluvoxamine in the treatment of obsessive compulsive disorder. J Nerv Ment Dis 186:492–499, 1998

Vincelli F, Anolli L, Bouchard S, et al: Experiential cognitive therapy in the treatment of panic disorders with agoraphobia: a controlled study. Cyberpsychol Behav 6:321–328, 2003

Wade WA, Treat TA, Stuart GL: Transporting an empirically supported treatment for panic disorder to a service clinic setting: a benchmarking strategy. J Consult Clin Psychol 66:231–239, 1998

Weissman MM: The hidden patient: unrecognized panic disorder. J Clin Psychiatry 51(suppl):5–8, 1990

Weissman MM, Markowitz JS, Ouellette R, et al: Panic disorder and cardiovascular/cerebrovascular problems: results from a community survey. Am J Psychiatry 147:1504–1508, 1990

Wiborg IM, Dahl AA: Does brief dynamic psychotherapy reduce the relapse rate of panic disorder? Arch Gen Psychiatry 53:689–694, 1996

Williams SL, Falbo J: Cognitive and performance-based treatments for panic attacks in people with varying degrees of agoraphobic disability. Behav Res Ther 34:253–264, 1996

Wittchen HU, Zhao S, Kessler RC, et al: DSM-III-R generalized anxiety disorder in the National Comorbidity Survey. Arch Gen Psychiatry 51:355–364, 1994

**Summary of studies addressing cost-effectiveness in the treatment of anxiety disorders**

| Article | Patients | Treatment | Outcome |
|---|---|---|---|
| **Panic disorders** | | | |
| Laberge et al. 1993 | 8 patients with panic disorder and major depression. 7 patients with panic disorder without major depression. | All patients treated with information-based therapy followed by cognitive-behavioral therapy (CBT). | CBT was significantly superior to information-based therapy in reducing panic attacks. There were no significant differences between depressed and nondepressed patients. |
| Oehrberg et al. 1995 | 120 patients with panic disorder. | Patients randomly assigned to treatment with paroxetine (20, 40, or 60 mg) or to placebo and cognitive therapy given to all patients. | Paroxetine treatment resulted in statistically significant superior results in 50% reduction in total number of panic attacks and in number of panic attacks reduced to one or zero over the study period. There was a positive trend in favor of paroxetine in the mean change in total number of attacks from baseline. Paroxetine plus cognitive therapy was significantly more effective than placebo plus cognitive therapy for panic disorder. |

## Summary of studies addressing cost-effectiveness in the treatment of anxiety disorders *(continued)*

| Article | Patients | Treatment | Outcome |
|---|---|---|---|
| **Panic disorders** *(continued)* | | | |
| Salvador-Carulla et al. 1995 | 61 patients with panic disorder. | An average of 13 sessions of supportive therapy plus medication. | Patients were studied and followed for 1 year. When functioning and costs in the 12-month period following treatment were compared with those in the 12 months prior to treatment, hospitalization costs were reduced to zero, medical visits and lab costs were reduced, but total direct costs increased 59% ($280 per patient) due to psychiatric visits and medication. However, indirect costs from lost productivity and sick days decreased by 79% ($684 per patient), resulting in a 30% reduction in overall costs, demonstrating cost-effectiveness for the 12-month posttreatment period. |
| Wiborg and Dahl 1996 | Patients with panic disorder. | Brief dynamic psychotherapy (12 weekly sessions) combined with medication. | Combined treatment is more effective than medication alone (100% remission vs. 75% remission after 12 weeks) and has a significantly lower relapse rate. |
| Spiegel and Bruce 1997 | Patients with panic disorder. | A review of studies combining benzodiazepines and exposure-based CBT. | The strongest support for combined treatment is for the addition of CBT to pharmacotherapy for patients with agoraphobia, and for those whose benzodiazepine treatment is being discontinued. |

## Summary of studies addressing cost-effectiveness in the treatment of anxiety disorders *(continued)*

| Article | Patients | Treatment | Outcome |
| --- | --- | --- | --- |
| **Panic disorders *(continued)*** | | | |
| Clark et al. 1999 | 43 patients with panic disorder. | Patients were randomly assigned to full cognitive therapy (FCT) with up to 12 one-hour sessions, brief cognitive therapy (BCT) of 5 sessions (both of these treatments had up to 2 booster sessions), or a 3-month wait list. | FCT and BCT were superior to wait list, with treatment gains maintained at 12-month follow up and no significant differences between FCT and BCT. |
| Barlow et al. 2000 | 312 patients with panic disorder. | Patients randomly assigned to receive imipramine only, CBT only, placebo only, CBT plus imipramine, or CBT plus placebo for 3 months; responders then seen monthly for 6 months, then followed up for 6 months. | Both imipramine and CBT were significantly superior to placebo for the acute treatment phase. At follow-up, patients treated with CBT alone maintained their improvement significantly better than those treated with imipramine alone. After 6 months of maintenance, combined treatment with imipramine and CBT were significantly more effective than placebo but not significantly more effective than CBT plus placebo. |

## Summary of studies addressing cost-effectiveness in the treatment of anxiety disorders *(continued)*

| Article | Patients | Treatment | Outcome |
|---|---|---|---|
| **Panic disorders** *(continued)* | | | |
| Otto et al. 2000 | 80 patients with panic disorder. | 20 patients had already been on some medication and initiated pharmacotherapy as a part of the study, 20 had been medication free and initiated medication as a part of the study, 20 had been medication free and received CBT alone, 20 were already on medication and initiated CBT as a part of the study. Half of the CBT was given in an individual format and half in a group format. | Regardless of previous medication status, treatment with CBT provided patients with short-term benefits at least equal and possibly superior to that from pharmacotherapy. Group CBT was the lowest cost treatment, followed by pharmacologic treatment and then individual CBT. |
| Katon et al. 2002 | 115 primary care patients with panic disorder. | Patients randomly assigned either to a collaborative care intervention that included systematic patient education and approximately two visits with an on-site consulting psychiatrist or to usual primary care. | The intervention led to significantly more anxiety-free days than usual primary care, with total costs slightly lower and increased mental health costs outweighed by decreased symptom-driven medical visits, demonstrating both cost offset and cost-effectiveness. |

## Summary of studies addressing cost-effectiveness in the treatment of anxiety disorders *(continued)*

| Article | Patients | Treatment | Outcome |
|---|---|---|---|
| **Panic disorders** *(continued)* | | | |
| Kenardy et al. 2003 | 186 patients with panic disorder from two sites in Scotland and Australia. | Patients randomly assigned to 12 sessions of therapist-delivered CBT (CBT12), 6 sessions of therapist-delivered CBT (CBT6), computer-augmented CBT (CBT6-CA), or wait-list control. | CBT12 was significantly more effective than CBT6, and CBT6-CA fell between CBT12 and CBT6 but was not statistically distinguishable from either. None of the three active treatments differed statistically at 6-month follow-up. |
| Vincelli et al. 2003 | 12 patients with panic disorder with agoraphobia. | Patients randomly assigned to 8 sessions of experiential-cognitive therapy (ECT) integrating virtual reality with CBT, 12 sessions of traditional CBT, or wait-list control. | Both CBT and ECT significantly reduced number of panic attacks, level of depression, and state and trait anxiety. ECT obtained these results using 33% fewer sessions than CBT. |
| Landon and Barlow 2004 | Patients with panic disorder from14 different controlled clinical trials of CBT. | 14 different trials of CBT compared with a variety of control conditions including supportive therapy, placebo, alprazolam, wait list, fluvoxamine, imipramine, applied relaxation, and emotion-focused therapy. | A review of 14 studies found CBT effective and likely cost-effective for panic disorder with or without agoraphobia; 40%–90% of patients treated with CBT were panic free at end of treatment and 75–87% were panic free at follow-up of 6 months to 2 years. CBT reduces comorbidity, yields benefits in physical health status and reductions in nonpsychiatric medical symptoms during treatment and at 6-month follow-up, and is effective in patient populations unresponsive to pharmacotherapy. |

## Summary of studies addressing cost-effectiveness in the treatment of anxiety disorders *(continued)*

| Article | Patients | Treatment | Outcome |
|---|---|---|---|
| **Panic disorders** *(continued)* | | | |
| Roberge et al. 2005 | 84 adult patients meeting diagnostic criteria for panic disorder with agoraphobia. | Patients assigned to one of three empirically supported CBT treatments (standard: 14 one-hour sessions with a therapist, group: 14 one-hour sessions, or brief: 7 one-hour sessions with a therapist over a 15-week period). | Overall health care, mental health care, and medication utilization were measured at baseline, posttreatment, 3-month, 6-month, 9-month, and 1-year follow-up and associated costs computed. Results showed both a significant reduction in symptomatology in the three CBT groups compared with wait-list controls and a significant reduction (23%) in total and mental health care costs during the 1-year follow-up period after providing an effective CBT treatment for these patients. |
| Katon et al. 2006 | 232 primary care patients with panic disorder from six primary care clinics. | Patients randomly assigned to either treatment as usual or a combined CBT and pharmacotherapy intervention for panic disorder by mental health therapist in primary care setting with up to six sessions of CBT in the first 12 weeks and up to six telephone follow-ups over the next 9 months. | Compared with usual care (UC) patients, intervention patients had 60.4 more anxiety-free days (AFDs). Total incremental outpatient costs were $494 higher in intervention vs. UC patients, with a cost per additional AFD of $8.40 and a cost per quality adjusted life-year well within the range of that of other commonly accepted medical interventions. Collaborative treatment for panic disorder is cost-effective, providing robust clinical improvement compared with UC, with moderate increase in ambulatory costs. Study focused primarily on total outpatient costs, finding cost-effectiveness just on this basis; significantly higher percentage of UC patients had two or more medical hospitalizations compared with intervention patients, demonstrating cost offset of $240 total medical cost savings. |

**Summary of studies addressing cost-effectiveness in the treatment of anxiety disorders** *(continued)*

| Article | Patients | Treatment | Outcome |
|---|---|---|---|
| **Panic disorders** *(continued)* | | | |
| McHugh et al. 2007 | 312 patients with panic disorder. | Empirically supported treatments from the Multicenter Comparative Treatment Study of Panic Disorder with random patient assignment, including CBT alone, imipramine alone, paroxetine alone, and two combination treatments, CBT plus imipramine and CBT plus paroxetine. | Relative cost-efficacy ratios for the different interventions were measured by examining the results at the end of acute, maintenance, and follow-up phases. Consistently greater cost efficacy was found for the individual over the combined treatments, imipramine being most cost efficacious at end of the acute phase and CBT being most cost efficacious both at end of maintenance treatment and 6 months after treatment termination. Current monotherapies should be considered the first-line treatment of choice for panic disorder; CBT appears to be the most durable and cost-effective monotherapy. |
| Milrod et al. 2007 | 49 adult patients with panic disorder. | Patients randomly assigned to panic-focused psychodynamic psychotherapy or applied relaxation training in twice-weekly sessions for 12 weeks. | Patients receiving psychodynamic psychotherapy had superior reduction in severity of both panic symptoms and functional impairment. |

## Summary of studies addressing cost-effectiveness in the treatment of anxiety disorders *(continued)*

| Article | Patients | Treatment | Outcome |
|---|---|---|---|
| **Obsessive-compulsive disorder (OCD)** | | | |
| Jenike 1993 | Patients with OCD. | A review of treatment efficacy studies. | The combination of pharmacotherapy and CBT enables most OCD patients to work and function well; the percentage of patients improved ranges from 60% to 90%. Pharmacotherapy alone is effective but relapse rates can be as high as 90%. Psychodynamic psychotherapy can be a valuable adjunct. |
| March et al. 1994 | 15 child and adolescent patients with OCD. | CBT plus medication. | Significant improvement immediately posttreatment and at follow-up. 6 patients became asymptomatic, and 9 had at least a 50% reduction in symptoms. |
| March 1995 | Patients with OCD from 32 studies. | CBT. | 31 of 32 investigations, mostly single case reports, reported some benefit from CBT. |
| Gava et al. 2007 | Patients with OCD from seven studies of psychological treatments vs. treatment as usual. | A review article of psychological treatments vs. treatment as usual for OCD from seven studies with usable data for meta-analyses. | Patients who received any variant of CBT had significantly fewer symptoms after treatment than those receiving treatment as usual, with different types of CBT showing similar differences in effect compared with treatment as usual. |

---

**Summary of studies addressing cost-effectiveness in the treatment of anxiety disorders *(continued)***

| Article | Patients | Treatment | Outcome |
| --- | --- | --- | --- |
| **Phobic disorders** | | | |
| Mersch 1995 | 34 patients with social phobia. | Patients were treated with either exposure in vivo or an integrated treatment consisting of rational-emotive therapy, social skills training, and exposure in vivo; there was also a wait-list control group. | Integrated treatment was not superior to exposure in vivo alone. Long-term effectiveness of both treatments was equally good. |
| Turner et al. 1995 | 13 patients with social phobia. | Patients were treated with social effectiveness therapy, a behavioral treatment. | 8 patients who completed the treatment study were available for follow-up. Treatment gains were maintained over the 2-year follow-up period with some indication of further improvement since that at posttreatment. |
| Taylor 1996 | Patients with social phobia. | A meta-analysis of 25 studies with 42 treatment outcome trials. Six treatment conditions were compared: waitlist control, placebo, exposure (EXP) (within session and as homework), cognitive therapy (CT) (cognitive restructuring without exposure exercises), CT + EXP, and social skills training. | All interventions, including placebo, had larger effect sizes than waitlist control. Only CT + EXP led to a larger effect size than placebo. Effects of treatment tended to increase during follow-up period. |

## Summary of studies addressing cost-effectiveness in the treatment of anxiety disorders *(continued)*

| Article | Patients | Treatment | Outcome |
|---|---|---|---|
| **Phobic disorders** *(continued)* | | | |
| Heimberg et al. 1998 | 133 patients with social phobia. | 12 weeks of cognitive behavioral group therapy (CBGT), phenelzine therapy, pill placebo, or educational-supportive group therapy. | Phenelzine therapy and CBGT led to marked positive response, phenelzine being superior to CBGT on some measures, both more efficacious than the other two treatment groups. |
| Cottraux et al. 2000 | 67 patients with social phobia. | Patients randomly assigned to either: Group 1: CBT of 8 one-hour sessions of individual cognitive therapy for 6 weeks followed by 6 weekly two-hour sessions of group social skills training; Group 2: 6 half-hour sessions of supportive therapy (ST) for 12 weeks and then switched to CBT. Patients were not medicated during the trial. | At both week 6 and week 12, group 1 had superior improvement, even after group 2 was switched to CBT. At follow-up both groups had sustained improvement. CBT was more effective than ST and demonstrated long-lasting effects. |
| Hofmann 2004 | 90 patients with social phobia. | Patients randomly assigned to CBGT of 12 weekly sessions, exposure group therapy without explicit cognitive interventions of 12 weekly sessions, or wait-list control. | Both treatments were equally superior to wait-list control in reducing social anxiety at posttest, but only CBT showed continued improvement at 6-month follow-up, suggesting that cognitive intervention leads to better maintenance of treatment gains. |

## Summary of studies addressing cost-effectiveness in the treatment of anxiety disorders *(continued)*

| Article | Patients | Treatment | Outcome |
|---|---|---|---|
| **Generalized anxiety disorder (GAD)** | | | |
| Butler et al. 1987 | 45 patients with GAD. | Anxiety management (teaches relaxation, with cognitive and exposure elements) given immediately or after a 12-week waiting period (average 8.7 sessions). | Highly significant improvement in anxiety, depression, and problem ratings that were replicated when the wait-list patients also were treated. Gains maintained by both groups for 6 months. |
| **Mixed diagnoses** | | | |
| Bassler and Hoffmann 1994 | 23 patients with GAD, 38 patients with agoraphobia, 24 patients with panic disorder. | Psychoanalytically oriented inpatient psychotherapy, both individual and group four times weekly for 12 weeks. | 40% of GAD patients improved; 21.2% did not. 61.4% of agoraphobia patients improved; 6.3% did not. 52.5% of panic disorder patients improved; 6.5% did not. |
| Heuzenroeder et al. 2004 | Based on the prevalence of GAD and panic disorder in the Australian population in 2000, effect size calculations were made of the outcome of different interventions for these disorders. | Meta-analyses of randomized controlled trials of both CBT and treatment with serotonin-norepinephrine reuptake inhibitor for GAD and of CBT, selective serotonin reuptake inhibitor, and tricyclic antidepressants for panic disorder. CBT intervention modeled as 12 one-hour consultations + one general practitioner consultation for referral to mental health care providers working privately or on a publicly funded salary. | Based on estimation of the reduction in disability adjusted life years, CBT would be the most effective and cost-effective for both GAD and panic disorder especially if provided by a psychologist on a public salary. CBT would result in greater total health benefit than psychotropic medication intervention for both GAD and panic disorder. |

## Summary of studies addressing cost-effectiveness in the treatment of anxiety disorders *(continued)*

| Article | Patients | Treatment | Outcome |
|---|---|---|---|
| **Mixed diagnoses** *(continued)* | | | |
| Issakidis et al. 2004 | Patients with the major categories of anxiety disorders including panic disorder with or without agoraphobia, social phobia, and GAD. | A large-scale cost-effectiveness study to calculate and compare the economic efficiency of current and optimal treatment for the major mental disorders, this publication reports on the anxiety disorders. | Outcomes were calculated as averted years lived with disability (YLDs) and direct health care costs in Australian dollars. Cost per YLD averted was compared for patients currently in mental health care and for a hypothetical optimal care based on evidence-based treatment, which it was estimated would produce substantial health gain (40%–60% increase in YLDs averted and one-and-a-half to twofold increase in efficacy) at a similar cost as current care and thus much greater cost-effectiveness for the anxiety disorders studied. For panic disorder, increased efficacy is achieved by a shift from pharmacologic to psychological treatment (with cost savings of 80%); for GAD, increased rates of psychological treatment would be required with current levels of pharmacological treatment (at similar costs to those of current care). Social phobia would require increased outpatient care that would ultimately yield substantial savings due to decreased inpatient costs. All of the anxiety disorders would require an increase in psychological treatments for optimal care. |

**Summary of studies addressing cost-effectiveness in the treatment of anxiety disorders *(continued)***

| Article | Patients | Treatment | Outcome |
|---|---|---|---|
| *Mixed diagnoses (continued)* | | | |
| Durham et al. 2005 | Participants in eight randomized controlled clinical trials of CBT for anxiety disorders conducted between 1985 and 2001. | Follow-up interviews 2 to 14 years after original treatment to assess diagnosis, comorbidity, and severity of remaining symptoms. Examination of case note reviews of health care resources for 2 years prior to treatment and for the 2 years prior to follow-up interviews. | 52% of GAD patients had at least one clinical diagnosis at long-term follow-up with 34% still diagnosable with GAD, fairly high levels of depression (25%), agoraphobia (19%), dysthymia (18%), panic disorder (17%), and social phobia (15%).<br><br>80% of treated anxiety-disordered patients had some improvement at long-term follow-up but were in worst 12% of the population in objective measures of symptomatology and worst 24% in physical health status. Anxiety-disorder patients had significant improvement immediately after CBT, but only a few maintained recovery over long term. While CBT led to better outcome in symptom severity, positive effects eroded over time and CBT not cost-effective compared with non-CBT. |

# 6 | Psychotherapy in the Treatment of Depression

## Susan G. Lazar, M.D.

Depression is the leading diagnosis among American primary care patients, is experienced by one-fifth of all Americans at some point during their lifetimes, and costs the country $83.1 billion per year in medical costs and losses stemming from disability, lost productivity, and suicide. Depression is more disabling than many of the most common chronic medical illnesses and is a leading cause of disability in the world. Both antidepressant medication and psychotherapy are effective in treating depression. Psychotherapy augments the effectiveness of medication, is invaluable for patients who cannot take medication, and is helpful as a primary treatment for certain subgroups of depressed patients, such as those with perfectionistic character structures. Psychotherapy has been demonstrated to be cost-effective for patients in primary care with major depression, for depressed medical patients, and for patients with manic-depressive illness, schizoaffective disorder, and major depression. Savings result from decreased disability, reduced hospitalization, and other medical costs.

As the studies cited in this chapter indicate, depression is a monumental public health problem worldwide. A common illness afflicting millions of individuals during their lifetimes, it also contributes to enormous social costs through disability and lowered productivity, pain and suffering, exacerbation of the symptoms and costs of medical illnesses, and greatly increased medical expenses. The significant loss of life through depression-related suicide and the emotional toll of its impact on the families of survivors are impossible to quantify adequately. Not only is depression more disabling than many purely physical illnesses, it also complicates and increases the disability of medical illnesses. Depression is extremely common, but also commonly unrecognized and consequently untreated. The lack of accurate diagnosis is all the more tragic because depression is often highly treatable. For depressed patients taking antidepressant medication, studies demonstrate that psychotherapy can have an augmenting therapeutic effect and is also both effective and often cost-effective when used as the sole approach.

# Search Methodology

A MEDLINE search was conducted from 1984 to 2007 using the terms "depression + psychotherapy + cost" and "depression + psychotherapy + cost-effectiveness" and studies were selected from which cost-effective data could be extracted. In addition, relevant literature on the direct and indirect costs of depression, on the epidemiology of depression, and on the efficacy of psychotherapy for depression were included.

# Epidemiology and Costs

According to one study, in the United States 9.5% of the adult population is afflicted with affective disorders each year. Two-thirds of those patients have major depression, one-sixth suffer from dysthymia, and one-quarter have bipolar disorder (Kessler et al. 2005b). In 2002, the lifetime prevalence of major depressive disorder for U.S. adults was 16.2% and for 12 months was 6.6%. Of the 12-month cases, 10.4% of cases were mild, 38.6% were moderate, 38.0% were severe, and 12.9% were very severe. The mean episode duration was 16 weeks with nearly 60% of the 12-month cases experiencing severe to very severe role impairment. Of the 12-month cases of major depressive disorder, only 51.6% were treated, and only 41.9% of those treated received adequate treatment, resulting in only 21.7% of all patients with major depressive disorder in the 12 months receiving adequate care (Kessler et al. 2003). For all mood disorders, the National Comorbidity Survey Replication found prevalences of 9.5% annually (Kessler et al. 2005b) and 20.8% over a lifetime (Kessler et al. 2005a). Although depression is the most common diagnosis found in primary care, Katon and Sullivan (1990) found that primary care physicians miss the diagnosis 50% of the time.

Greenberg and his colleagues at the Massachusetts Institute of Technology estimated the overall cost of depression in the United States by both measuring direct costs of medical treatments to all patients with depression and estimating indirect morbidity costs related to absenteeism, reduced productivity, and the mortality costs of lost human resources from suicide (Greenberg et al. 1993). They found that in 1990, depression, dysthymia, and bipolar illness cost the country $43 billion. The estimated cost of direct treatment was only $12.4 billion. In a 10-year update of this study, Greenberg et al. (2003) found that while the treatment rate of depression increased by over 50%, its economic burden rose only 7%, from $77.4 billion in 1990 (inflation-adjusted dollars) to $83.1 billion in 2001. Of the total cost, $26.1 billion (31%) were direct medical costs, $5.4 billion (7%) were suicide-related mortality costs, and $51.5 billion (62%) were losses in the workplace.

While depression is extremely costly to society, the subgroup of at least 20% of depressed patients who are treatment resistant are particularly so (Crown et al. 2002). Not only difficult to treat effectively, they have significantly greater health care costs than other depressed patients, being at least twice as likely to be hospitalized both for depression and general medical admissions and having at least 12% more outpatient visits and 1.4 to 3 times more psychotropic medications. Patients in the hospitalized treatment-resistant group had over six times the mean total medical costs of non-treatment-resistant depressed patients, with total depression-related costs 19 times greater than non-treatment-resistant patients.

In a study of 2,980 participants in the National Institute of Mental Health Epidemiologic Catchment Area Study in North Carolina, Broadhead et al. (1990) found that those with major depression had a 4.78 times greater risk of disability than nondepressed controls. Those with minor depression had a 1.55 times greater risk. Because of its prevalence in the community, those with minor depression had 51% more disability days than those with major depression.

Suicide accounts for 1,000 deaths a day worldwide or 0.9% of all deaths. Two-thirds of suicides are committed by people with depressive disorders. Of patients with depressive disorders, 18% to 21% attempt suicide (Sartorius 2001). In 1996, a 5-year international study under the auspices of the World Health Organization concluded that mental illness is currently a leading cause of "disease burden." Their measure of disease burden—the disability-adjusted life year or DALY—is a quantitative measure of years lost from a healthy life by disability or premature death. According to this study, in 1990, unipolar depression caused more disability than most chronic medical illnesses with the possible exception of myocardial infarction (Murray and Lopez 1996). In the World Health Organization 2004 survey, unipolar depressive disorders were the greatest cause of disability worldwide for both men and women in low-, middle-, and high-income countries (World Health Organization 2008).

# Studies Comparing Depression With Common Chronic Medical Conditions

In a study from the RAND Corporation, a comparison of depression with eight of the most common chronic medical illnesses, including chronic obstructive pulmonary disease, hypertension, diabetes mellitus, chronic inflammatory bowel disease, acute myocardial infarction, and rheumatoid arthritis, found that those who suffered depression were more disabled not only with regard to their social functioning (fulfilling their roles as parent, spouse, employee, etc.) but also with regard to their physical functioning. In addition, there was more pain associated with depression than with seven of the eight illnesses (Wells et al. 1989). In another RAND publication, Hays et al. (1995) compared a 2-year observational study of 1,790 adult outpatients with depression, diabetes, hypertension, recent myocardial infarction, and/or congestive heart failure. The change in functional states and well-being was compared for depressed patients versus those with the chronic medical illnesses. Over the 2 years of follow-up, while the limitations in functioning and well-being improved somewhat for the depressed patients, their level of limitation was still substantial and similar to or worse than that associated with the chronic medical illnesses.

Judd et al. (1996) found significantly more depressed subjects versus those who were nondepressed who reported high levels of household strain, financial strain, irritability, limitations in physical and job functioning, restricted activity days, number of days in bed, and poor health status. Except for self-reports of health status, there were no significant differences between subjects with subsyndromal depression and those with major depression. The authors concluded that subsyndromal depressive symptoms and major depression are associated with significant disability that has an important negative impact on society and the economy.

Wells and Sherbourne (1999) found that primary care patients with depressive conditions have poorer mental health and poorer emotional role and social functioning than patients with the common chronic medical conditions of asthma, diabetes, hypertension, arthritis, chronic lung disease, neurological disease, heart disease, gastrointestinal tract disease, back problems, eye problems, and migraine. In addition, patients with depression had worse physical functioning than patients with four of the common chronic medical conditions but better physical functioning than patients with four other conditions. And an assessment of disability in major life roles as part of the National Comorbidity Survey Replication found that musculoskeletal disorders and major depression had the greatest effects on disability days (Merikangas et al. 2007).

# The Disability and Health Care Costs of Depression

A study of 18,000 employees of First Chicago Corporation between 1989 and 1992 found that the average length of a disability period for the depressive disorders was longer for depression (40 days) than for low back pain (37 days), heart disease (37 days), other mental health disorders (32 days), hypertension (27 days), and diabetes (26 days). Furthermore, employees with depressive disorders were significantly more likely to have a recurrence of their disability within a 12-month period than employees with the other conditions. Thus depressive disorders not only produced longer periods of disability than the other common conditions but also resulted in a significantly increased rate of relapse. In addition, depressive disorders resulted in the largest medical plan costs of all behavioral health diagnoses (Conti and Burton 1994).

In a study of the health and disability costs of depression in a major American corporation, Druss et al. (2000) examined the records of 15,153 employees to compare the mental health costs, medical costs, sick days, and total health and disability costs associated with depression and four other conditions, including ischemic heart disease, diabetes, hypertension, and back problems. The combined health and disability costs for depressed employees were $5,415, significantly more than the cost for hypertension and comparable with the cost for the other three medical conditions. The annual health care costs alone for depressed employees was $4,373, which was comparable with that of employees with the other conditions but significantly higher than the annual costs of $949 for employees without any of the other medical conditions. The health care costs for depressed employees included $1,341 for mental health care costs. Their other medical costs were $3,032, which was significantly higher than the non-mental health care costs for patients without any of the four comparison medical conditions. Depressed employees who also suffered from any of the other conditions had costs 1.7 times more than those with the medical conditions alone. Depressed employees had a mean of 9.86 annual sick days, which was significantly more than for any of the other conditions. In addition to their sick days, one must also consider that depressed employees may be more vulnerable to errors at work, decreased productivity, and accidents. Thus, the authors noted that the true economic impact of depressed employees on work-related costs may be higher than those measured in their report. In addition, they pointed out that within the corporation studied, reductions in mental health expenditures over a period of 3 years were followed by an increase both in medical costs and in lost work days in employees with mental disorders. They speculated that the decrease in mental health benefits may have been an important factor driving up disability and health costs reported in this study.

Surveys estimate that 1.8% to 3.6% of workers in the U.S. labor force suffer from major depression and that 37% to 48% of depressed workers experience short-term disability (Goldberg and Steury 2001). In 2002, patients with major depressive disorder reported a mean of 35.2 days in the past year when they were totally unable to work or carry out their normal activities (Kessler et al. 2003). Stewart et al. (2003) studied lost productive time (LPT) costs from depression among employed individuals screened in a depressive disorders study in 2002. Workers with depression had significantly more total health-related LPT than those without depression (5.6 hours per week compared with 1.5 hours per week). Eighty-one percent of the LPT costs were due to reduced performance. According to this study, extrapolation of these results and self-reported annual incomes to the entire population of U.S. workers suggests that U.S. workers with depression cost employers an estimated $44 billion a year in LPT, $31 billion more than the LPT of workers without depression. Nonetheless, the workers' compensation system and the courts have been slow to recognize depression as a work-related disability contributing to the fact that employers have few incentives to treat and prevent workplace depression (Goldberg and Steury 2001).

The medical consequences and intrinsic pain of depression lead patients to seek medical care at much higher rates than patients without depression. Simon and his colleagues in Seattle, Washington, compared 6-month medical treatment costs for health maintenance organization (HMO) patients who screened positively for anxiety or depressive disorders with patients without these diagnoses. Those primary care patients with DSM-III-R (American Psychiatric Association 1987) anxiety or depressive disorders were found to have a mean semiannual health care cost of $2,390 compared with $1,397 for those without anxiety or depression (Simon et al. 1995a). Significant cost differences persisted even after adjustment for medical morbidity. In addition, less than 10% of the total costs for the anxious and depressed patients was related to mental health care, demonstrating that the cost differences reflected a higher utilization of general medical services for this group. In a second study of primary care patients, Simon et al. (1995b) found that patients with recognized depression had much higher annual medical costs ($4,246) compared with nondepressed controls ($2,371). Specialty mental health care costs accounted for 10% of total costs for the depressed patients and accounted for only one-fifth of the difference in total health care costs between depressed and nondepressed patients. In every other category of medical care, the depressed group had approximately 1.5 times the annual medical costs of the nondepressed group. And while the depressed patients in this study had more treated chronic medical disease than the comparison group, adjusting for this difference did not fully account for their greater utilization of health care services. The authors speculated that depression may increase the depressed patients' experience of pain and other physical symptoms leading to more medical visits, more diagnostic evaluations, and more prescribed treatments in response to the depressed patients' reported distress.

# Studies of Efficacy

Numerous studies have demonstrated the efficacy of various psychotherapeutic approaches for depression. A number of these are summarized below.

The National Institute of Mental Health Treatment of Depression Collaborative Research Program compared patients in 16 weeks of randomly assigned treatment with cognitive-behavior therapy (CBT), interpersonal psychotherapy, imipramine hydrochloride plus clinical management, or placebo plus clinical management. The percentage of patients who recovered and remained well during follow-up did not differ significantly among the four treatments, and relapse rates over 18 months were high, ranging between 33% and 50%. The investigators concluded that 16 weeks of these treatments is insufficient for most patients to achieve full recovery and lasting remission (Shea et al. 1992). Another follow-up study of depressed patients who had responded to combined short-term and continuation treatment with imipramine hydrochloride and interpersonal psychotherapy was designed to determine whether a maintenance form of interpersonal psychotherapy alone or in combination with medication would prevent recurrence (Frank et al. 1990). Three-year outcomes for maintenance treatment compared once-monthly interpersonal psychotherapy, high-dose imipramine hydrochloride (200 mg daily) both with and without interpersonal psychotherapy, and placebo plus clinical management. The best outcome was achieved with the combination of imipramine and interpersonal psychotherapy, followed by imipramine alone. Significantly, interpersonal psychotherapy at the frequency of only once per month helped depressed patients maintain remission nearly twice as long as placebo and clinical management (82 weeks compared with 45 weeks).

Addressing the fact that depression and anxiety are the most common psychiatric disorders in ambulatory medical patients, a review of randomized controlled trials conducted in primary care settings generally supports the efficacy of psychosocial treatments for these patients (Brown and Schulberg 1995). All studies using manualized treatments found that psychotherapy produced significantly greater reductions in symptoms than usual care provided by a general practitioner, no treatment, or pharmacotherapy.

Studies by Fava et al. (1994, 1996, 1998) demonstrate the efficacy of CBT for depression. In the first study (Fava et al. 1994), 40 patients with major depression were successfully treated with antidepressant medication and then randomly assigned to CBT or to standard clinical management. Both groups had their medication tapered and then discontinued. The group given the psychotherapy had significantly less residual symptomatology as well as a nonstatistically significant lower rate of relapse (15%) at a 2-year follow-up than the clinical management group (35%). A second investigation (Fava et al. 1996) extended the follow-up period to 4 years and demonstrated a more statistically significant lower relapse rate in the CBT group (35%) compared with the clinical management group (70%). In a subsequent study (Fava et al. 1998), after successful treatment with antidepressants, 40 depressed patients were randomly assigned either to CBT of residual depressive symptoms or to clinical management while their medication was tapered and discontinued. The CBT group had significantly fewer residual symptoms after the discontinuation of antidepressant medication compared with the clinical management group. In addition, at 2-year follow-up, the CBT group had a significantly lower rate of relapse (25%) compared with 80% in the clinical management group. These authors concluded that CBT is a viable alternative to maintenance pharmacotherapy for some depressed patients.

In another study designed to assess the efficacy of sertraline and group CBT, alone or in combination, for primary dysthymia, 97 dysthymic patients were given sertraline or placebo in a double-blind design for 12 weeks (Ravindran et al. 1999). Weekly group CBT was also given to a subgroup of 49 of these patients. Patients given sertraline alone or sertraline plus group therapy experienced similar levels of improvement, greater than that seen in the group therapy alone or in the placebo group. Nonetheless, the group CBT was found to augment the beneficial effects of the antidepressant medication.

In another study of patients with major depression seen in primary care settings, a psychotherapeutic approach—problem-solving treatment—was compared with antidepressant medication and combined treatment (Mynors-Wallis et al. 2000). Problem-solving treatment was found to be effective for depressive disorders in primary care. Combining this psychotherapy with medication was no more effective than either treatment alone.

For those depressed patients unwilling or unable to take antidepressant medication, psychotherapy is an important treatment modality. Among these are often pregnant women and nursing mothers who constitute an important subgroup of depressed patients since the incidence of major depression is two to three times as great in women as in men, with a peak incidence in the childbearing years (Weissman 1993). In fact, a study of interpersonal psychotherapy for postpartum depression compared 60 postpartum women with major depression given 12 weeks of interpersonal psychotherapy with 60 similar patients who served as a waiting-list control group (O'Hara et al. 2000). A significantly greater proportion of women who received interpersonal psychotherapy recovered from their depressive episode compared with women in the control group. The authors concluded that interpersonal psychotherapy is an effective treatment for postpartum depression and provides an alternative to pharmacotherapy, especially for breastfeeding mothers.

A study of 228 depressed patients seen in four large primary care clinics of a major HMO randomly assigned patients to usual care or to specialty care that often (but not always) included psychotherapy as part of its intervention (Walker et al. 2000). Most patients in the usual-care group and all patients in the intervention group were treated with antidepressant medication. Those in the intervention group also received at least two visits with a psychiatrist, more visits as needed clinically, monitoring of adherence to medication, and referral to psychotherapy for those with severe psychosocial stressors. Although both intervention and usual-care patients improved, intervention patients in the lower severity group were significantly more likely to improve compared with usual-care patients. Intervention patients who were more severely ill had a more significant change in the first 3 months, but the difference between them and the usual-care group had disappeared at 6 months. The investigators concluded that the more severely depressed patients may require more intensive clinician follow-up and/or psychotherapy to achieve sustained improvement from depressive symptoms.

A group psychotherapy intervention, mindfulness-based cognitive therapy, was compared with treatment as usual for 145 recently recovered recurrently depressed patients who were randomly assigned to one of the two treatments (Teasdale et al. 2000). For patients with three or more previous episodes of depression, the mindfulness-based cognitive therapy significantly reduced their risk of relapse by almost half compared with treatment as usual. For patients with only two previous episodes, the recurrence rate was not reduced. Although no cost data were reported, the investigators concluded that the group treatment might offer a cost-efficient psychological approach to preventing depressive relapse in recovered recurrently depressed patients.

Patients with major depression who have achieved remission with a brief course of cognitive psychotherapy have been shown to be at substantial risk of recurrence. A study on the efficacy of continuation-phase cognitive therapy (10 sessions given over 8 months to depressed patients who had responded to acute-phase cognitive psychotherapy) showed significantly reduced relapse rates in those treated compared with control patients who had not received the additional treatment (10% vs. 31%) (Jarrett et al. 2001).

For patients with bipolar disorder who were treated with mood-stabilizing medications, those given a more intensive course of psychotherapy (up to 50 weekly sessions of integrated family and individual therapy, IFIT) did better than similar patients who receive medications, crisis management, and two family educational sessions. The patients in the IFIT group had a longer time without relapsing than those in the other group. Those given IFIT also had greater reductions in their depressive symptoms over the 1 year of their treatment compared with their baseline levels (Miklowitz et al. 2003).

In a review of a number of studies of chronic depression lasting 2 years or longer, Arnow and Constantino (2003) concluded that for chronic major depression, combined treatment of medication and psychotherapy is superior to either treatment alone. There was a less robust but similar finding for patients with chronic dysthymia.

Bolton et al. (2003), in a randomized controlled clinical trial of 223 depressed patients in rural Uganda, found that 16 weeks of group interpersonal psychotherapy was significantly more effective for those receiving the group treatment compared with depressed control patients who did not receive it.

Investigating a very different kind of question, Blatt and his colleagues studied the impact of character structure on treatment outcome for depressed patients. In a reexamination of data from the National Institute of Mental Health Treatment of Depression Collaborative Research Program, Blatt et al. (1995) found that perfectionistic patients did especially poorly in all brief treatments and that there was no direct correspondence between perfectionism and any particular type of brief treatment. On the other hand, earlier work (Blatt 1992) did indicate that perfectionistic patients fare better in more intensive, long-term psychoanalytic therapy than in less intensive long-term psychotherapy.

# Cost-Effectiveness of Psychotherapy for Depression

By combining what is known about the enormous social and financial costs of depression with what is known about the efficacy of psychotherapy, one can form an impression of its likely cost-effectiveness. The reports of studies that are briefly summarized below (and in the review table at the end of this chapter) examine the potential cost-effectiveness of a variety of psychotherapeutic approaches more directly by assessing their impact on cost-sensitive outcome measures. Most of the studies document the efficacy of the psychotherapy interventions, and many also illustrate some measure of cost-effectiveness as well by virtue of decreased disability (Kamlet et al. 1992; Mynors-

Wallis 1996; Schoenbaum et al. 2005; Smit et al. 2006), significantly greater efficacy and compliance with treatment at similar or small additional cost over other treatment approaches (Bower et al. 2000; Chisholm 2005; Friedli et al. 2000; King et al. 2000; Lave et al. 1998; Leff et al. 2000; Schoenbaum et al. 2005; Tutty et al. 2000; Von Korff et al. 1998), or a decrease in days spent in the hospital (Huxley et al. 2000; Retzer et al. 1991; Rosset and Andreoli 1995; Verbosky et al. 1993). Other studies demonstrate the cost-effectiveness of psychotherapy according to the older and more stringent standard of cost offset, in terms of reduction in medications (Hengeveld et al. 1988) or decreased total health care costs (Browne et al. 2002; Dunn et al. 2007; Edgell et al. 2000). Several studies did not find psychotherapy to be cost-effective (Bosmans et al. 2007; Petrou et al. 2006).

In an investigation of the impact of psychiatric consultations for depressed medical inpatients (Hengeveld et al. 1988), a randomized controlled study was done with a random sample of 33 depressed medical inpatients who were given the consultation and compared with a matched control group of 35 depressed medical inpatients who did not receive it. As measured by the Beck Depression Inventory, the group receiving the psychiatric consultation had a significant improvement in their depression whereas the control group did not. Furthermore, the number of patients receiving no analgesic and/or psychotropic medication in the consult group was significantly greater than that in the control group. The consult group patients who did receive psychotropic and/or analgesic medication were given far fewer prescriptions than patients in the control group. Other significant reductions in medical care expenses and length of hospital stay were not demonstrated between the two groups, probably because the patient sample was too heterogeneous with too low a prevalence of mental disorders.

In a theoretical study to examine the impact of the treatment of depression on costs, Kamlet et al. (1992) calculated that interpersonal psychotherapy leads both to an improved quality of life for depressed patients and to reduced treatment costs because of fewer depressive episodes. If one looks only at direct costs, interpersonal psychotherapy is expensive. However, if one includes indirect costs such as lost income from work absenteeism, the authors of this study estimate that interpersonal psychotherapy alone as a maintenance treatment yields a lifetime savings of $9,000. In addition, the lifetime probability of suicide declines from 8.8% to 4%. By combining interpersonal psychotherapy with antidepressant medication, the lifetime savings are estimated at $11,540.

In a study of the impact of family therapy, Retzer et al. (1991) studied 30 patients with manic-depressive and schizoaffective psychoses who were used as their own controls. Hospital admissions per year were measured before and after the provision of family therapy. With an average course for family treatment of 6.6 sessions, the hospital admissions per patient per year declined from 1.5 to 0.3.

In another study by Scott and Freeman (1992), 121 patients with major depression were assigned to one of four treatment groups: 1) amitriptyline prescribed by a psychiatrist, 2) CBT administered by a psychologist, 3) counseling administered by a social worker, and 4) routine care by a general practitioner that might include counseling, medication, or referral to another agency. Although all of the groups improved markedly over a period of 16 weeks, the individual counseling by a social worker was statistically significant in superiority to the care by a general practitioner. In addition, the psychological treatments, especially the counseling by the social worker, were most highly valued by patients. Because the care by the general practitioner was half as costly, the investigators felt that this treatment approach outweighed the advantages of specialty care. Nonetheless, they speculated that if specialist treatment were shown to prevent recurrences over a longer period of time, their cost-benefit conclusion might be different.

Several studies demonstrate that psychotherapy in conjunction with medication is a cost-effective treatment for depression. In a study by Verbosky et al. (1993), a brief psychotherapy intervention in conjunction with psychotropic medication was given to 15 of 18 depressed medical inpatients. The length of hospital stay for the treated group was 31.8 days shorter than that of the depressed medical patients who did not receive treatment, a highly cost-saving intervention. Another study by Rosset and Andreoli (1995) of 122 subjects with major depression compared 1) specialized inpatient care for 3 weeks followed by 8 weeks of medication; 2) standard hospital treatment with limited staffing, careful observation, and medication; and 3) specialized crisis intervention consisting of 1 week of daily supportive psychotherapy and medication followed by approximately 8 weeks of clomipramine, two to three psychotherapy sessions per week, and family support. Although treatment duration and costs were high for all groups, the specialized crisis intervention considerably reduced the duration of hospitalization and its associated costs.

In a report of three studies of a brief psychotherapy, problem-solving treatment (PST), provided to patients in a primary care setting, Mynors-Wallis (1996) found PST to be as effective for patients with major depression as antidepressant medication and superior to placebo. For patients with more broadly defined emotional disorders, many of whom had depressive features, PST proved to be cost-effective by virtue of the economic benefit of decreased absenteeism in the PST group compared with patients given usual care by a general practitioner.

In a report of two randomized controlled trials by Von Korff et al. (1998), usual care delivered to depressed patients in primary care settings was compared with collaborative care by psychologists in conjunction with primary care management of medication. In the first trial, 217 depressed patients were randomly assigned to a regimen of medication and brief psychoeducational interventions or to usual care. In the second trial, 153 depressed patients received medication, patient education and brief CBT, or usual care. This study is notable for its careful attention to cost-effectiveness in distinction to cost offset, both of which were measured. Treatment cost was defined as the average direct and overhead costs to the HMO of providing treatment services for depressive illness. Cost offset was defined as the mean costs of health care services among intervention patients minus the mean costs of those services among patients who received usual care. Cost-effectiveness was defined as the average depression treatment costs divided by the measure of treatment effectiveness and was estimated by dividing the average annual costs of treating depression by the proportion of patients successfully treated. The resulting figure provides an estimate of the average annual costs of depression treatment per patient successfully treated. Using these definitions and computations, the authors showed that while the cost of collaborative care was greater than usual care, the cost-effectiveness of collaborative care was greater for patients with major depression, although not for minor depression.

In another randomized controlled study of primary care patients with major depression by Lave et al. (1998), cost-effectiveness for three different treatment approaches was compared. Pharmacotherapy with nortriptyline for 91 patients, interpersonal psychotherapy for 93 patients, and a primary care physician's usual care for 92 patients were compared using two outcome measures of depression-free days and "quality-adjusted" days (calculated by a scoring of treatment effectiveness by measuring days free of depression and days in which there is a lifting of depression). The costs of care were calculated, and cost-effectiveness of each approach was computed by comparing the incremental outcomes with the incremental costs for the different treatments. While patients treated with medication did slightly better than those receiving psychotherapy, both the treatment with nortriptyline and the interpersonal psychotherapy provided better outcomes than usual care by a primary physician. There were no cost-offset effects; in fact, both the treatment with antidepressant medication and the treatment with interpersonal psychotherapy were more expensive than usual care. This study illustrates the more appropriate standard of cost-effectiveness of treatment for psychiatric illness. In this case, interpersonal psychotherapy was found to be almost as efficacious and similarly cost-effective as antidepressant pharmacotherapy for major depression. Both were clearly superior to usual care given by primary physicians.

In a study by Friedli et al. (2000), nondirective counseling was compared with routine general practice care for 136 patients with emotional problems, mainly depression. Seventy patients were given 1 to 12 weeks of weekly counseling, and 66 patients were cared for by their general practitioners. Direct medical costs of outpatient appointments, length of inpatient stays, and medications were assessed, as well as indirect costs such as sick days off of work, travel costs, and child-care costs. In terms of direct plus indirect costs, counseling was no more clinically effective or expensive than general practice care over a 9-month period. While the counselor group was at first more costly to treat and had greater direct and indirect expenses for the first 3 months, over the next 6 months the counselor group had lower costs than the general practice group. The reversal of direct costs, becoming greater for the general practice group during the last 6 months, was largely because the general practice group had a greater number of outpatient appointments and inpatient stays during the entire 9-month study period. The authors speculated that a 9-month follow-up may be too brief to get beyond the initial, expensive counselor costs and that a longer follow-up period may lead to a conclusion for greater cost-effectiveness for the counselor care.

A pilot study for depressed adults in primary care compared 28 patients begun on antidepressant medication who were given telephone counseling with 94 depressed patients given usual care (Tutty et al. 2000). The telephone group received written educational materials and six weekly counseling and support sessions by phone by a therapist with cognitive-behavioral strategies for self-monitoring and self-management. Those receiving the psychotherapy had significantly lower depressive symptoms than did the controls at both 3 months and 6 months and were twice as likely to adhere to antidepressant medication with adequate dose thresholds (25% vs. 13%). They were also half as likely to meet criteria for major depression than controls, although these differences were not statistically significant. The overall cost per patient ($150) and total outpatient visits for depression treatment between groups did not differ. The telephone counseling was a more cost-effective treatment, yielding a significantly greater improvement of depression outcome for the same costs.

Two publications describe a study of depressed patients and patients with mixed anxiety and depression and report the outcome of a randomized controlled comparison of nondirective counseling, CBT, and usual general practitioner care (Bower et al. 2000; King et al. 2000). A total of 464 patients either were treated with brief psychological therapy (a maximum of 12 sessions) of nondirective counseling or CBT or were given routine general practitioner care. At 4 months, both groups given psychological treatment had improved to a significantly greater degree than those receiving usual care and had scores that were four to five points lower on the Beck Depression Inventory, demonstrating superior cost-effectiveness of the CBT at this time interval. At 12 months, the patients in all three groups had improved to the same extent. Direct costs of providing care and indirect costs of productivity and societal costs did not differ between the three groups. At 12 months, the patients who had received nondirective counseling were more satisfied that those in the other two groups.

In a randomized controlled study of antidepressant drugs versus couple therapy for 77 depressed patients living with a critical partner, depression improved significantly for both treatment groups (Leff et al. 2000). Of the patients given the drug treatment, 56.8% dropped out, whereas of those receiving couple therapy, 15% dropped out. According to scores on the Beck Depression Inventory at the end of treatment and at the 2-year follow-up, couple therapy showed a significant advantage. While the cost of the two treatments did not differ, the couple therapy was much more acceptable to patients than the drugs and at least as effective, if not more so, without being any more expensive.

A review article of 32 peer-reviewed reports involving 1,052 patients with bipolar disorder included 14 studies of group therapy, 13 studies on couple or family therapy, and 5 studies on individual psychotherapy (Huxley et al. 2000). All patients were also treated with standard pharmacotherapy. Despite methodological limitations, objective measures demonstrated that the various psychotherapuetic treatments led to improved clinical stability, functional and psychosocial benefits, and reduced rehospitalization (a highly cost-sensitive measure).

Insurance claims data were used to compare patients given no therapy, psychotherapy, drug therapy, or a combination in a study to examine the economic outcome associated with initial treatment choice after a diagnosis of depression (Edgell et al. 2000). Total and mental health care costs were estimated. A significantly greater total cost was found for those given combination treatment compared with those given psychotherapy alone. Total health care costs may be higher in those who initiated therapy with drug therapy and combination therapy as opposed to no therapy or psychotherapy alone. Also, those initially receiving psychotherapy alone tended to have higher mental health care costs but lower total health care costs than other patients, perhaps because the psychotherapy has an impact on comorbid illness with a subsequent reduction on total health care costs.

In a study of adults with dysthymic disorder, with or without past and/or current major depression, Browne et al. (2002) randomly assigned 707 patients to treatment with sertraline alone (50–200 mg), 10 sessions of interpersonal therapy (IPT) alone, or the combination over a course of 6 months. There was an additional 18-month follow-up phase during which patients were assessed for effectiveness of treatment, and costs of treatment, social services, and other medical expenses were measured. At 2 years, there was no significant difference between sertraline alone and sertraline plus IPT in symptom reduction. Both of these treatments were more effective than IPT alone. There was a statistically significant difference between groups in costs of health and social services. Of the two more effective treatments, patients who received sertraline plus IPT had lower health and social service costs by $480 per person over the 2 years. These findings emphasize the impact and cost-effectiveness of combining psychotherapy and pharmacotherapy

In a review of 12 studies of depressed patients seen in primary care settings, Schulberg et al. (2002) found that a depression-specific psychotherapy is more effective for major depression than usual primary care and similar to effectiveness as psychotropic medication. For patients with dysthymia, the effectiveness of psychotherapy compared with usual care is more equivocal. Although providing psychotherapy is more expensive than usual care, psychotherapy's greater effectiveness for major depression makes it cost-effective.

In a study designed to compare the cost-effectiveness of psychotherapy with antidepressant medication for depressed patients, Miller et al. (2003) found that psychotherapy treatment is a dominant cost-effective strategy for a small proportion of patients with mild to moderate depression. For a larger proportion of patients, the antidepressant intervention is the dominant cost-effective strategy.

Pirraglia et al. (2004) examined selected articles regarding cost-utility analysis of depression management from the Harvard Center for Risk Analysis Cost-Effectiveness Registry. Of the 539 cost-utility analyses in the registry, 9 were of depression management. Psychotherapy, care management alone, and psychotherapy plus care management all had lower costs per QALY than usual care. Cost-utility analyses examine the effects of interventions on both quantity and quality of life, allowing a comparison of many interventions for the same condition. They are a subset of cost-effective analysis, a technique in which the cost and effects of an intervention and an alternative are presented in a ratio of incremental cost to incremental effect. A cost-utility analysis combines both the quality of life and the mortality benefits of an intervention in one common metric, QALY. In this review, psychotherapy alone or as part of a case management effort was superior to usual care per QALY, while maintenance imipramine had a favorable cost per QALY compared with maintenance psychotherapy plus placebo. Psychotherapy had a lower cost per QALY than usual care. Pharmacologic treatment either alone or in combination with psychotherapy had a lower cost per QALY than psychotherapy alone.

A study from the World Health Organization (Chisholm 2005) addressed the question of how much the enormous international disease burden of psychiatric disorders could be averted by the increased implementation of effective interventions. The study estimated the avertable burden of a particular disease arising from the use of an evidence-based set of interventions and the relative cost of their implementation for a target patient population. This research report provided an overview of the mental health component of the World Health Organization's CHOICE Project, the goal of which is generating cost-effectiveness evidence for a large number of interventions for various illnesses in a range of geographical and epidemiological settings around the world. Expected costs and effects of effective pharmacological and psychosocial interventions were modeled for four disorders: schizophrenia, bipolar disorder, depression, and panic disorder. It was predicted that the addition of psychosocial treatment to pharmacotherapy is projected to have a far greater benefit than switching from older to newer psychotropic agents for both schizophrenia and bipolar disorder. The relatively modest additional cost of psychosocial treatment for schizophrenia and bipolar disorder yields significant health gains and is more cost-effective than pharmacotherapy alone. Newer antidepressants in combination with brief psychotherapy in Latin America, the Caribbean, Europe, and Central Asia are three to four times more cost-effective than episodic treatment with antidepressant drugs alone.

A study investigating the cost-effectiveness of interventions for major depressive disorder in low-income minority women randomly assigned 267 women to one of three treatment groups: 1) pharmacotherapy with either paroxetine or bupropion, 2) CBT, or 3) community referral (Revicki et al. 2005). The main outcome measures were intervention and health care costs, depression-free days, and QALYs. Cost-effectiveness ratios compared patient outcomes and costs for pharmacotherapy relative to community referral and for CBT relative to community referral. Compared with community referral patients, the pharmacotherapy patients had significantly improved depression from the 3rd month through the 10th month of the study, as did the CBT group from the 5th month through the 10th month. There were significantly more depression-free days in both the pharmacotherapy and the CBT groups compared with the community referral group. The cost per additional depression-free day was $24.65 for pharmacotherapy and $27.04 for CBT compared with community referral. The pharmacotherapy and CBT interventions were cost-effective relative to community referral for the health care system. While all health care costs were measured in this study, indirect costs and benefits were not measured, including foster care placement for children, increased work productivity, reduced work lost days, and potential improved health outcome and school performance benefits for children of depressed women.

Schoenbaum et al. (2005) compared two approaches to increased effectiveness of depression treatment in primary care settings, including the different impact on male and female patients. Matched primary clinics in the United States were randomly assigned to either usual care or one of two quality improvement (QI) interventions: 1) QI-Meds to facilitate medication management or 2) QI-Therapy to facilitate psychotherapy. For QI-Therapy, local psychotherapists were trained to provide 8- to 12-session courses of individual and group CBT. Patients and clinicians could choose the type of treatment or none. The study examined 46 clinics, 6 nonacademic managed care organizations, and 181 primary care providers and 375 male and 981 female patients with depression. Compared with usual care, QI-Therapy significantly reduced depression burden and increased employment for both genders but QI-Meds significantly reduced depression only among women. Average health care costs increased $429 in QI-Meds and $983 in QI-Therapy among men; corresponding costs increases were $424 and $275 for women. For women, QI-Meds and QI-Therapy had comparable effects on depression burden and quality of life. The relative cost-effectiveness for both interventions was well within the range for other accepted medical interventions, especially for QI-Therapy because of its relatively small effect on costs. QI-Meds was not effective and therefore not cost-effective for men. The positive effects of QI-Therapy were particularly large for men in that compared with usual care, it yielded more than 7 work weeks over 2 years. For women, QI-Therapy yielded 3 work weeks.

Vos et al. (2005) examined and summarized the potential cost-effectiveness results of a range of interventions for depression, schizophrenia, attention-deficit/hyperactivity disorder, and anxiety disorders and estimated the impact on total expenditures if recommended mental health interventions for depression and schizophrenia were to be implemented in Australia. The authors concluded that underutilized cost-effective treatment options for mental disorders include CBT for depression and anxiety and family therapy interventions for schizophrenia. Providing all those seeking care for their depression in the year 2000 with drug maintenance would cost $312 million (Australian) over 5 years and $160 million (Australian) for maintenance CBT. Both treatments are estimated to reduce the disease burden of depression by approximately 50%.

Petrou et al. (2006) reported the cost-effectiveness of a preventive intervention of counseling and support for the mother-infant relationship targeting women at high risk for postnatal depression. Women identified as high risk for developing postnatal depression were randomly assigned to either preventive intervention (*n*=74) or routine primary care (*n*=77). The women treated were visited antenatally, then on days 3, 7, and 17 postnatally, and then weekly for up to 8 weeks and provided counseling and other support. The outcome measures were the duration of postpartum depression during the first 18 months and the impact of the intervention on health and social care costs. A nonsignificant increase in the mean number of months free of postnatal depression and a nonsignificant increase in health and social care costs were demonstrated. The 18-month time horizon for the economic evaluation was felt to have underestimated the long-term cost-effectiveness of the preventive intervention in terms of health status and health service utilization over the mother's and infant's lifetime. Adopting a broader societal perspective would have captured other direct non-medical costs, including lost productivity and intangible costs of fear, pain, and suffering of postnatal depression.

Smit et al. (2006) examined 363 primary care adult patients from 19 general practices in the Netherlands with subthreshold depression who were assigned either to minimal contact psychotherapy or to usual care. The psychotherapy was cognitive-behavioral using a self-help manual with the addition of six short telephone calls with a prevention worker. In the measuring of outcomes, a societal perspective was taken including the costs of all types of health services and costs stemming from work absenteeism and reduced efficiency. The risk of developing a full-blown depressive disorder decreased from 18% to 12% in the intervention group. In addition to the greater efficacy of the treatment of the minimal contact psychotherapy in preventing major depression, the intervention patients had less work loss. Depending on the acceptability of the increased costs of the intervention over 1 year (on average 423 euros), minimal contact psychotherapy has a 70% probability of being more cost-effective than usual care alone.

In a randomized controlled trial involving 12 general practices in and around Amsterdam, depressed patients age 55 years and older were given 10 sessions of IPT over 5 months and compared with care as usual (CAU) (Bosmans et al. 2007). A full economic evaluation was done to assess cost-effectiveness in which outcomes were measured at 2, 6, and 12 months after baseline. Cost data were collected from a societal perspective over 12 months. Of the 69 patients assigned to the IPT group and the 74 to the CAU group, 60% of the IPT patients and 42% of the CAU patients had recovered at 6 months, a difference of recovery rate just short of statistical significance. At 12-month follow-up, the recovery rate in both groups was the same at 45%. While the mean total costs were higher in the IPT group, the differences were not statistically significant. At 6 months, the IPT group experienced 19% more recoveries than the CAU group; however, after 12 months, the IPT group had 6% fewer remissions than the CAU group. Because the IPT patients had greater costs, there was a negative incremental cost-effectiveness ratio at 12 months for the IPT group. Based on these results, provision of IPT in primary care to elderly depressed patients was not cost-effective in comparison with CAU. While Lave et al. (1998) found that IPT was significantly more effective and expensive than usual care, in their study patients were offered a maximum of 20 IPT sessions by experienced therapists, whereas in Bosman et al.'s study patients were offered a maximum of 10 IPT sessions by less experienced therapists. In addition, Lave et al. studied more severely depressed patients. It is likely that otherwise effective treatments are less effective in mild than in severe depressions because the room for improvement is limited. Also, in the Bosmans et al. study, the effects of IPT in comparison with CAU were somewhat greater at 6 months than at 12 months. It is possible that IPT is more effective than CAU in the short term but that this effect dissipates at 1-year follow-up, possibly because depression in elderly people often has a chronic and recurrent course. Future trials should investigate maintenance treatments to sustain gains made in the acute treatment phase. With respect to costs, because more mildly depressed patients have lower overall health care costs than severely depressed patients, the high costs of IPT itself will have a more negative effect on total costs for less depressed patients.

A study by Dunn et al. (2007) compared self-management therapy (a CBT group psychotherapy) with active-control therapy (a strictly educational therapy provided in a group) for male veterans with comorbid chronic posttraumatic stress disorder and depressive disorder. Both therapies were highly structured 1.5-hour weekly group sessions for 14 weeks. One hundred and one patients were randomly assigned to one of these treatments to evaluate the efficacy and cost-effectiveness of the self-management therapy against the active-control therapy as the active control. Medical and psychiatric service utilization and cost were also measured for both conditions. While self-management therapy yielded slightly greater improvement in depressive symptoms, this difference disappeared on follow-up. However, psychiatric outpatient utilization and overall outpatient costs were lower with self-management therapy, and this decrease was maintained through the 1-year follow-up.

Wells et al. (2007) studied a total of 746 primary care patients with 12-month depressive disorder and 502 patients with subthreshold depression in a randomized controlled trial. Matched clinics were randomly assigned to enhanced usual care or one of two QI interventions that provided education to manage depression over time and resources to facilitate access to medication management or psychotherapy for 6 to 12 months. The medication QI provided support for medication adherence through monthly visits or telephone contacts for 6 to 12 months. In the therapy QI, therapists provided individual and group CBT for 6 months. In all conditions, patients could receive medication, therapy, both, or neither. The effects on depression-burden days, measure of days worked in each 6-month follow-up, intervention costs, and health care costs were all assessed. The costs of the intervention were much smaller for patients with subthreshold depression. The interventions were found to be as cost-effective for patients with subthreshold depression as are many widely used medical therapies as well as for patients with depressive disorders.

# Case Vignette

A 32-year-old mother of a 2-year-old and a 10-week-old newborn presented with major depression. She was nursing her new baby, tending to the 2-year-old, and working full time. She felt hopeless, trapped, fatigued, and angry in a family situation in which she was the major breadwinner. Due to the severity of her depression, a clinical decision was made to recommend that she discontinue breastfeeding so that antidepressant medication could be given. Shortly after the institution of the antidepressant, the patient was distressed to learn that she had again become pregnant. The medication was discontinued and weekly psychotherapy was begun with occasional couple's sessions attended by the patient with her husband. Difficult aspects of the patient's characteristic coping style and of the marital relationship were explored, particularly the greater dependency of the family on the patient's income and her longstanding suppression of anger toward her husband. The patient became much more aware of and able to express her longing for more support and her despair about obtaining it, all of which had become especially intense in the context of her pregnancy, delivery, full-time work, and management of two young children. Despite the difficult circumstances of the family, the couple, and the new pregnancy, the patient's major depression lifted and was resolved with psychotherapy alone over the course of her pregnancy and immediate postpartum period.

# Conclusion

Depression presents an international public health challenge of monumental proportions and leads to great and essentially incalculable costs in financial terms as well as in human suffering. Depression is a seriously disabling condition in itself, from depression-related suicide and for medical illness complicated by depression. Its social costs include lost productivity from sick days as well as lowered efficiency from employees who are depressed on the job. Depressed patients also have significantly increased medical costs.

There are many studies that illustrate the efficacy of psychotherapy for depression, and given the enormous direct and indirect costs of depression, the cost-effectiveness of all effective therapeutic approaches can be confidently assumed. In addition, there are a number of studies that investigate and demonstrate directly the cost-effectiveness of psychotherapy for depression. This literature includes studies of psychiatric consultation and psychotherapy for medical inpatients and family therapy for manic-depressive and schizoaffective patients that yield cost savings by virtue of decreased hospitalization. A variety of psychotherapeutic interventions are cost saving by reducing depression-related disability. Other studies of psychotherapy for depression do not indicate cost savings directly but demonstrate, nonetheless, that it is cost-effective by virtue of its superior efficacy compared with treatment as usual and other approaches (and thus saves more of the depression-related medical, disability, and other costs). A few studies do not find psychotherapeutic interventions to be cost-effective (Bosmans et al. 2007; Friedli et al. 2000; Scott and Freeman 1992); the investigators in these studies have suggested that a longer course of treatment and a more complete accounting of the depression-related societal costs might yield a different conclusion.

With the exception of one study (Mynors-Wallis et al. 2000), psychotherapy for depression generally augments the efficacy of antidepressant medication alone; one factor seems to be an increased compliance with the medication regimen. One review article explored this hypothesis by examining 16 trials in which the combined subjects totaled 932 depressed patients randomly assigned to pharmacotherapy alone and 910 to combined treatment with both medication and psychotherapy and found that combined treatment is in fact generally more effective and that patients in treatment for longer than 12 weeks also showed a significant reduction of dropouts (Pampallona et al. 2004).

Except for one report finding a comparably significant cost-effective impact for subthreshold depression (Wells et al. 2007), most of the studies find a more robustly cost-effective impact of psychotherapy in the treatment of major depression compared with dysthymia and less severe depressive states. In addition, psychotherapy is especially important for perfectionistic depressed patients and for pregnant and nursing women who would prefer to avoid psychotropic medication.

For the many studies of effectiveness and cost-effectiveness summarized and discussed in the chapter, it is important to acknowledge the enormous range of study conditions and the inherent difficulties comparing these "apples" and "oranges" to glean conclusions confidently from the large and disparate literature. In looking for the evidence of cost-effectiveness of any kind of psychotherapeutic intervention, one notes that not only are different kinds and lengths of psychotherapeutic regimens studied in various depressed populations against various alternative treatments and control conditions, but also that the examination of costs measured is widely disparate, generally becoming more sophisticated in more recent research designs. While many of the earlier studies yield a strong indirect suggestion of cost-effectiveness from improved work functioning, lowered hospitalization and medical costs, and so on, the more recent studies measure the cost-effectiveness of treatments directly, for example, with a cost-utility analysis that combines the quality of life and mortality benefits of an intervention in the metric of QALY. More recent cost-effectiveness literature also uses the much more appropriate standard of acceptable thresholds for effective treatments, in other words, the cost considered acceptable for any medical treatment in terms of QALY value gained. Thus "cost-effective" does not necessarily mean "cheap" or "money saving"; it should signify both the cost and the value of one treatment approach compared with others in lieu of the double standard of "cost-offset," in which psychotherapy is valued only if it leads to savings in other (presumably more inherently valuable and unchallengeable) medical treatments.

# References

American Psychiatric Association: Diagnostic and Statistical Manual of Mental Disorders, 3rd Edition, Revised. Washington, DC, American Psychiatric Association, 1987

Arnow BA, Constantino MJ: Effectiveness of psychotherapy and combination treatment for chronic depression. J Clin Psychol 59:893–905, 2003

Blatt SJ: The differential effect of psychotherapy and psychoanalysis with anaclitic and introjective patients: the Menninger Psychotherapy Research Project revisited. J Am Psychoanal Assoc 40:691–724, 1992

Blatt SJ, Quinlan DM, Pilkonis PA, et al: Impact of perfectionism and need for approval on the brief treatment of depression: the National Institute of Mental Health Treatment of Depression Collaborative Research Program revisited. J Consult Clin Psychol 63:125–132, 1995

Bolton P, Bass J, Neugebauer R, et al: Group interpersonal psychotherapy for depression in rural Uganda: a randomized controlled trial. JAMA 289:3117–3124, 2003

Bosmans JE, van Schaik DJ, Heymans MW, et al: Cost-effectiveness of interpersonal psychotherapy for elderly primary care patients with major depression. Int J Technol Assess Health Care 23:480–487, 2007

Bower P, Byford S, Sibbald B, et al: Randomised controlled trial of non-directive counselling, cognitive-behaviour therapy, and usual general practitioner care for patients with depression. II: cost effectiveness. BMJ 321:1389–1392, 2000

Broadhead WE, Blazer DG, George LK, et al: Depression, disability days, and days lost from work in a prospective epidemiologic survey. JAMA 264:2524–2528, 1990

Brown C, Schulberg HC: The efficacy of psychosocial treatments in primary care. A review of randomized clinical trials. Gen Hosp Psychiatry 17:414–424, 1995

Browne G, Steiner M, Roberts J, et al: Sertraline and/or interpersonal psychotherapy for patients with dysthymic disorder in primary care: 6-month comparison with longitudinal 2-year follow-up of effectiveness and costs. J Affect Disord 68:317–330, 2002

Chisholm D: Choosing cost-effective interventions in psychiatry: results from the CHOICE programme of the World Health Organization. World Psychiatry 4:37–44, 2005

Conti DJ, Burton WN: The economic impact of depression in a workplace. J Occup Med 36:983–988, 1994

Crown WH, Finkelstein S, Berndt E, et al: The impact of treatment-resistant depression on health care utilization and costs. J Clin Psychiatry 63:963–971, 2002

Druss BG, Rosenheck RA, Sledge WH: Health and disability costs of depressive illness in a major U.S. corporation. Am J Psychiatry 157:1274–1278, 2000

Dunn NJ, Rehm LP, Schillaci JS, et al: A randomized trial of self-management and psychoeducational group therapies for comorbid chronic posttraumatic stress disorder and depressive disorder. J Trauma Stress 20:221–237, 2007

Edgell ET, Hylan TR, Draugalis JR, et al: Initial treatment choice in depression: impact on medical expenditures. Pharmacoeconomics 17:371–382, 2000

Fava GA, Grandi S, Zielezny M, et al: Cognitive behavioral treatment of residual symptoms in primary major depressive disorder. Am J Psychiatry 151:1295–1299, 1994

Fava GA, Grandi S, Zielezny M, et al: Four-year outcome for cognitive behavioral treatment of residual symptoms in major depression. Am J Psychiatry 153:945–947, 1996

Fava GA, Rafanelli C, Grandi S, et al: Prevention of recurrent depression with cognitive behavioral therapy: preliminary findings. Arch Gen Psychiatry 55:816–820, 1998

Frank E, Kupfer DJ, Perel JM, et al: Three-year outcomes for maintenance therapies in recurrent depression. Arch Gen Psychiatry 47:1093–1099, 1990

Friedli K, King MB, Lloyd M: The economics of employing a counsellor in general practice: analysis of data from a randomised controlled trial. Br J Gen Pract 50:276–283, 2000

Goldberg R, Steury S: Depression in the workplace: costs and barriers to treatment. Psychiatr Serv 52:1639–1643, 2001

Greenberg PE, Stiglin LE, Finkelstein SN, et al: The economic burden of depression in 1990. J Clin Psychiatry 54:405–418, 1993

Greenberg PE, Kessler RC, Birnbaum HG, et al: The economic burden of depression in the United States: how did it change between 1990 and 2000? J Clin Psychiatry 64:1465–1475, 2003

Hays RD, Wells KB, Sherbourne CD, et al: Functioning and well-being outcomes of patients with depression compared with chronic general medical illnesses. Arch Gen Psychiatry 52:11–19, 1995

Hengeveld MW, Ancion FA, Rooijmans HG: Psychiatric consultations with depressed medical inpatients: a randomized controlled cost-effectiveness study. Int J Psychiatry Med 18:33–43, 1988

Huxley NA, Parikh SV, Baldessarini RJ: Effectiveness of psychosocial treatments in bipolar disorder: state of the evidence. Harv Rev Psychiatry 8:126–140, 2000

Jarrett RB, Kraft D, Doyle J, et al: Preventing recurrent depression using cognitive therapy with and without a continuation phase: a randomized clinical trial. Arch Gen Psychiatry 58:381–388, 2001

Judd LL, Paulus MP, Wells KB, et al: Socioeconomic burden of subsyndromal depressive symptoms and major depression in a sample of the general population. Am J Psychiatry 153:1411–1417, 1996

Kamlet MS, Wade M, Kupfer DJ, et al: Cost-utility analysis of maintenance treatment for recurrent depression: a theoretical framework and numerical illustration, in Economics of Mental Health. Edited by Frank RG, Manning WG Jr. Baltimore, MD, Johns Hopkins University Press, 1992, pp 267–291

Katon W, Sullivan MD: Depression and chronic medical illness. J Clin Psychiatry 51 (suppl):3–11; discussion 12–14, 1990

Kessler RC, Berglund P, Demler O, et al: The epidemiology of major depressive disorder: results from the National Comorbidity Survey Replication (NCS-R). JAMA 289:3095–3105, 2003

Kessler RC, Berglund P, Demler O, et al: Lifetime prevalence and age-of-onset distributions of DSM-IV disorders in the national comorbidity survey replication. Arch Gen Psychiatry 62:593–602, 2005a

Kessler RC, Chiu WT, Demler O, et al: Prevalence, severity, and comorbidity of 12-month DSM-IV in the national comorbidity survey replication. Arch Gen Psychiatry 62: 617–627, 2005b

King M, Sibbald B, Ward E, et al: Randomised controlled trial of non-directive counselling, cognitive-behaviour therapy and usual general practitioner care in the management of depression as well as mixed anxiety and depression in primary care. Health Technol Assess 4:1–83, 2000

Lave JR, Frank RG, Schulberg HC, et al: Cost-effectiveness of treatments for major depression in primary care practice. Arch Gen Psychiatry 55:645–651, 1998

Leff J, Vearnals S, Brewin CR, et al: The London Depression Intervention Trial. Randomised controlled trial of antidepressants v. couple therapy in the treatment and maintenance of people with depression living with a partner: clinical outcome and costs. Br J Psychiatry 177:95–100, 2000

Merikangas KR, Ames M, Cui L, et al The impact of comorbidity of mental and physical conditions on role disability in the US adult household population. Arch Gen Psychiatry 64:1180–1188, 2007

Miklowitz DJ, Richards JA, George EL, et al: Integrated family and individual therapy for bipolar disorder: results of a treatment development study. J Clin Psychiatry 64:182–191, 2003

Miller P, Chilvers C, Dewey M, et al: Counseling versus antidepressant therapy for the treatment of mild to moderate depression in primary care: economic analysis. Int J Technol Assess Health Care 19:80–90, 2003

Murray C, Lopez A: The Global Burden of Disease: A Comprehensive Assessment of Mortality and Disability from Diseases, Injuries, and Risk Factors in 1990 and projected to 2020. Cambridge, MA, Harvard School of Public Health on behalf of the World Health Organization and the World Bank, 1996

Mynors-Wallis L: Problem-solving treatment: evidence for effectiveness and feasibility in primary care. Int J Psychiatry Med 26:249–262, 1996

Mynors-Wallis LM, Gath DH, Day A, et al: Randomised controlled trial of problem solving treatment, antidepressant medication, and combined treatment for major depression in primary care. BMJ 320:26–30, 2000

O'Hara MW, Stuart S, Gorman LL, et al: Efficacy of interpersonal psychotherapy for postpartum depression. Arch Gen Psychiatry 57:1039–1045, 2000

Pampallona S, Bollini P, Tibaldi G, et al: Combined pharmacotherapy and psychological treatment for depression. A systematic review. Arch Gen Psychiatry 61:714–719, 2004

Petrou S, Cooper P, Murray L, et al: Cost-effectiveness of a preventive counseling and support package for postnatal depression. Int J Tech Assess Health Care 22:443–453, 2006

Pirraglia PA, Rosen AB, Hermann RC, et al: Cost-utility analysis studies of depression management: a systematic review. Am J Psychiatry 161:2155–2162, 2004

Ravindran AV, Anisman H, Merali Z, et al: Treatment of primary dysthymia with group cognitive therapy and pharmacotherapy: clinical symptoms and functional impairments. Am J Psychiatry 156:1608–1617, 1999

Retzer A, Simon FB, Weber G, et al: A follow-up study of manic-depressive and schizoaffective psychoses after systemic family therapy. Fam Process 30:139–153, 1991

Revicki DA, Siddique J, Frank L, et al: Cost-effectiveness of evidence-based pharmacotherapy or cognitive behavior therapy compared with community referral for major depression in predominantly low-income minority women. Arch Gen Psychiatry 62:868–875, 2005

Rosset N, Andreoli A: Crisis intervention and affective disorders: a comparative cost-effectiveness study. Soc Psychiatry Psychiatr Epidemiol 30:231–235, 1995

Sartorius N: The economic and social burden of depression. J Clin Psychiatry 62 (suppl 15):8–11, 2001

Schoenbaum M, Sherbourne C, Wells K: Gender patterns in cost effectiveness of quality improvement for depression: results of a randomized, controlled trial. J Affect Disord 87:319–325, 2005

Schulberg HC, Raue PJ, Rollman BL: The effectiveness of psychotherapy in treating depressive disorders in primary care practice: clinical and cost perspectives. Gen Hosp Psychiatry 24:203–212, 2002

Scott AI, Freeman CP: Edinburgh primary care depression study: treatment outcome, patient satisfaction, and cost after 16 weeks. BMJ 304:883–887, 1992

Shea MT, Elkin I, Imber SD, et al: Course of depressive symptoms over follow-up. Findings from the National Institute of Mental Health Treatment of Depression Collaborative Research Program. Arch Gen Psychiatry 49:782–787, 1992

Simon G, Ormel J, VonKorff M, et al: Health care costs associated with depressive and anxiety disorders in primary care. Am J Psychiatry 152:352–357, 1995a

Simon GE, VonKorff M, Barlow W: Health care costs of primary care patients with recognized depression. Arch Gen Psychiatry 52:850–856, 1995b

Smit F, Willemse G, Koopmanschap M, et al: Cost-effectiveness of preventing depression in primary care patients: randomised trial. Br J Psychiatry 188:330–336, 2006

Stewart WF, Ricci JA, Chee E, et al: Cost of lost productive work time among US workers with depression. JAMA 289:3135–3144, 2003

Teasdale JD, Segal ZV, Williams JM, et al: Prevention of relapse/recurrence in major depression by mindfulness-based cognitive therapy. J Consult Clin Psychol 68:615–623, 2000

Tutty S, Simon G, Ludman E: Telephone counseling as an adjunct to antidepressant treatment in the primary care system. A pilot study. Eff Clin Pract 3:170–178, 2000

Verbosky LA, Franco KN, Zrull JP: The relationship between depression and length of stay in the general hospital patient. J Clin Psychiatry 54:177–181, 1993

Von Korff M, Katon W, Bush T, et al: Treatment costs, cost offset, and cost-effectiveness of collaborative management of depression. Psychosom Med 60:143–149, 1998

Vos T, Haby MM, Magnus A, et al: Assessing cost-effectiveness in mental health: helping policy-makers prioritize and plan health services. Aust N Z J Psychiatry 39:701–712, 2005

Walker EA, Katon WJ, Russo J, et al: Predictors of outcome in a primary care depression trial. J Gen Intern Med 15:859–867, 2000

Weissman M: The rationale for psychotherapy as a maintenance treatment for major depression. Presented to the Mental Health Work Group of the White House Task Force for National Health Care Reform, Washington, DC, April 23, 1993

Wells KB, Sherbourne CD: Functioning and utility for current health of patients with depression or chronic medical conditions in managed, primary care practices. Arch Gen Psychiatry 56:897–904, 1999

Wells KB, Stewart A, Hays RD, et al: The functioning and well-being of depressed patients. Results from the Medical Outcomes Study. JAMA 262:914–919, 1989

Wells KB, Schoenbaum M, Duan N, et al: Cost-effectiveness of quality improvement programs for patients with subthreshold depression or depressive disorder. Psychiatr Serv 58:1269–1278, 2007

World Health Organization: Global Burden of Disease: 2004 Update. Geneva, World Health Organization, 2008

## Summary of studies addressing cost-effectiveness in the treatment of depression

| Article | Patients | Treatment | Outcome |
|---|---|---|---|
| Hengeveld et al. 1988 | 68 depressed medical inpatients. | Nonspecific, supportive psychiatric consultation for 33 patients; 35 matched control patients received no consultation. | Significant difference in the number in consult group receiving no analgesic and/or psychotropic meds (39%) compared with controls (17%). Significant decrease in Beck Depression Index for consult group (from 20 to 13), nonsignificant decrease in controls (from 19 to 16). No significant reduction in medical care costs or length of hospital stay. |
| Kamlet et al. 1992 | 230 depressed patients. | Three maintenance treatments for depression: 1. Interpersonal therapy (IPT-M) 2. Imipramine drug therapy (Drug) 3. Combination of above | Both IPT-M and IPT-M plus Drug improve lifetime health. By estimating improvements in absenteeism and the lowering of suicide rate, lifetime savings are between $9,000 and $11,540. |
| Retzer et al. 1991 | 30 patients with manic-depressive and schizoaffective psychoses. | 6.6 sessions of family therapy given to patients who served as own controls. Hospital admissions per year measured before and after family therapy. | Number of hospital admissions declined from 1.5 to 0.3 per patient per year. |
| Scott and Freeman 1992 | 121 patients with major depression. | 1. Amitriptyline given by psychiatrist. 2. Cognitive-behavioral therapy (CBT) by psychologist. 3. Counseling social worker. 4. Routine care by general practitioner. | All groups improved in 16 weeks. Best and most valued outcome was social worker counseling. General practitioner care cost half as much. |

**Summary of studies addressing cost-effectiveness in the treatment of depression *(continued)***

| Article | Patients | Treatment | Outcome |
| --- | --- | --- | --- |
| Verbosky et al. 1993 | 18 depressed medical inpatients. | Psychiatric consultation with psychotherapy and antidepressant medication given to 15 patients. Psychiatric consultation without psychotherapy or antidepressants given to three patients. | Patients in first group spent 31.8 fewer days in hospital than controls. |
| Rosset and Andreoli 1995 | 122 patients with major depression. | 1. Specialized inpatient care for 3 weeks, then 8 weeks of medication. 2. Standard hospital treatment, observation, medication. 3. Specialized crisis intervention, daily psychotherapy and medication for 1 week, medication and 2–3 psychotherapy sessions per week, family support for 8 weeks. | Specialized crisis intervention greatly reduced hospital duration and hospital costs. |
| Mynors-Wallis 1996 | Three studies of patients in primary care with emotional disorders. | A brief psychotherapy: problem-solving treatment (PST). | For patients with major depression, PST is as effective as antidepressant medication and superior to placebo. For patients with emotional disorders, often including depressive features, PST is cost-effective compared with usual care because of decreased absenteeism. |

## Summary of studies addressing cost-effectiveness in the treatment of depression *(continued)*

| Article | Patients | Treatment | Outcome |
|---|---|---|---|
| Von Korff et al. 1998 | Two separate randomized controlled trials: 217 depressed patients 153 depressed patients | 1. Medication and brief psychoeducational interventions compared with usual care. 2. Medication, patient education, and brief CBT compared with usual care. | For patients with major depression, the cost per patient successfully treated is less for collaborative care than for usual care and therefore collaborative care is cost-effective. For patients with minor depression, collaborative care is not more cost-effective than usual care. |
| Lave et al. 1998 | 276 patients with major depression. | 1. Medication with nortriptyline. 2. Interpersonal psychotherapy. 3. Usual care by primary physician. | Both medication and psychotherapy treatments were more expensive than usual care but were both more cost-effective than usual care by primary physician because of far better outcomes. |
| Friedli et al. 2000 | 136 patients in primary care settings with emotional problems, mainly depression. | 1. 1 to 12 sessions of Rogerian psychotherapy over 12 weeks. 2. Routine general practice care. | Over 9 months, psychotherapy is not more effective or expensive than routine care. Patients receiving counseling had higher costs for therapy during the first 3 months. However, at 9 months, costs for the two groups had reversed with the routine care group having a greater number of outpatient appointments and inpatient stays. It is possible that longer follow-up would show an advantage for the psychotherapy group. |

## Summary of studies addressing cost-effectiveness in the treatment of depression *(continued)*

| Article | Patients | Treatment | Outcome |
|---|---|---|---|
| Tutty et al. 2000 | 122 depressed patients in a primary care setting. | 28 patients received written educational materials and six psychotherapy telephone sessions.<br>94 patients received usual primary care. | Patients receiving psychotherapy telephone sessions were significantly less depressed than controls both at 3- and 6-month follow-up, twice as likely to adhere to antidepressant medication, and half as likely to have major depression than controls. Total outpatient visits for depression treatment were no different between groups. Program costs for psychotherapy telephone sessions were $150 per patient. |
| 1. Bower et al. 2000<br><br>2. King M, et al. 2000 | 464 depressed patients and patients with anxiety and depression. | 1. Brief, nondirective counseling.<br>2. Brief CBT.<br>3. Usual general practitioner care. | At 4 months, both psychotherapy groups significantly improved compared to usual-care group and had scores that were 4 to 5 points lower on Beck Depression Inventory. At 12 months, all three groups improved the same. No difference in costs between the three groups. At 12 months, patients in 1st group were most satisfied. |

## Summary of studies addressing cost-effectiveness in the treatment of depression *(continued)*

| Article | Patients | Treatment | Outcome |
|---|---|---|---|
| Leff et al. 2000 | 77 depressed patients living with a critical partner. | Couple therapy. Antidepressant medication. | Dropouts were 15% from couple therapy compared with 56.8% for medication therapy. Depression improved for both groups but was significantly greater for those patients given couple therapy at end of treatment and 2 years later. No difference in costs of services. |
| Huxley et al. 2000 | Review of 32 studies involving 1,052 patients with bipolar disorder. | 14 studies on group therapy, 13 studies on couples or family therapy, and 5 studies on individual therapy. All patients also received medication. | Increased clinical stability, improved functioning, and decreased rehospitalization associated with psychotherapeutic treatments. |
| Edgell et al. 2000 | 9,110 depressed patients. | Insurance claims data examined retrospectively to compare four groups according to initial treatment choice for depression: 1. No therapy 2. Psychotherapy 3. Medication 4. Psychotherapy + medication | Patients initiating care for depression with medication or combination treatment have higher total health care costs. Patients initially receiving psychotherapy alone have higher mental health care costs but lower total health care costs. |

## Summary of studies addressing cost-effectiveness in the treatment of depression *(continued)*

| Article | Patients | Treatment | Outcome |
|---|---|---|---|
| Browne et al. 2002 | 707 adults with dysthymia and/or major depression. | Random assignment to 6 months of: 1. Sertraline alone at dosage of 50–200 mg 2. 10 sessions of interpersonal therapy (IPT) alone 3. Sertraline and IPT 18-month follow-up phase for all patients. | Sertraline alone or sertraline+IPT was more effective than IPT alone after 6 months. After 2 years, all three treatments are effective although sertraline+IPT are more effective than IPT alone. The patients given sertraline+IPT had lower medical and social service costs by $480 per patient compared with sertraline alone patients over the 2 years. |
| Schulberg et al. 2002 | Review of 12 studies of depressed patients in primary care diagnosed using a structured instrument for major depression, minor depression, or dysthymia. | Patients treated with a depression, specific psychotherapy compared with patients given usual primary care, medication, placebo, or a control group. | For major depression, psychotherapy and pharmacotherapy are similarly effective and superior to usual primary care. For minor depression or dysthymia, psychotherapy's superiority to usual care is equivocal. Despite its higher cost, psychotherapy appears to be cost-effective for patients with major depression because of its greater effectiveness compared with usual care. |

**Summary of studies addressing cost-effectiveness in the treatment of depression (continued)**

| Article | Patients | Treatment | Outcome |
|---|---|---|---|
| Miller et al. 2003 | 323 patients with major depression. | Antidepressant medications versus counseling. | Economic analysis and analysis of clinical outcomes show:<br>1. For a larger proportion of patients, antidepressant medication is a dominant cost-effective strategy.<br>2. For a smaller proportion of patients with mild to moderate depression, counseling is a dominant cost-effective strategy. |
| Pirraglia et al. 2004 | A review of nine articles on the cost-utility analysis of depression management in the Harvard Center for Risk Analysis Cost-Effectiveness Registry. | Psychotherapy, psychotherapy as part of case management, maintenance imipramine, maintenance psychotherapy plus placebo, and usual care. | Psychotherapy had a lower cost per quality-adjusted life year (QALY) than usual care. Pharmacologic treatment either alone or combined with psychotherapy had a lower cost per QALY than psychotherapy alone. |
| Chisholm 2005 | From the mental health component of the World Health Organization CHOICE Project; costs and effects of pharmacological and psychological interventions were modeled for four disorders including bipolar disorder and depression. | Generating cost-effectiveness evidence for a large number of interventions for various illnesses in a range of geographical and epidemiological settings around the world. | The modest additional cost of psychosocial treatment for bipolar disorder yields significant health gains and is more cost-effective than pharmacotherapy alone. Newer antidepressants in combinations with brief psychotherapy in Latin America, the Caribbean, Europe, and Central Asia are three to four times more cost-effective than episodic treatment with antidepressant drugs alone. |

**Summary of studies addressing cost-effectiveness in the treatment of depression *(continued)***

| Article | Patients | Treatment | Outcome |
|---|---|---|---|
| Revicki et al. 2005 | 267 low-income, minority women with major depression. | Random assignment to:<br>1. Pharmacotherapy with either paroxetine or bupropion<br>2. CBT<br>3. Community referral | Compared with community referral patients (3), the pharmacotherapy patients (1) had significantly improved depression from the 3rd month through the 10th month as did the CBT group (2) from the 5th month through the 10th month. Groups 1 and 2 also had more depression-free days compared with group 3. The cost per additional depression-free day was $24.65 for pharmacotherapy and $27.04 for CBT compared with community referral (3). Interventions 1 and 2 were cost-effective for the health care system relative to group 3. All health care costs were measured, indirect costs and benefits were not (increase in work productivity, reduced work lost days, improved health outcomes, impact on costs and functioning for children of depressed women). |

**Summary of studies addressing cost-effectiveness in the treatment of depression *(continued)***

| Article | Patients | Treatment | Outcome |
|---|---|---|---|
| Schoenbaum et al. 2005 | 375 male and 981 female depressed patients from 46 clinics managed by 181 primary care providers. | Two quality improvement (QI) interventions:<br>1. QI-Meds to facilitate medication management<br>2. QI-Therapy by psychotherapists trained to provide 8–12 session courses of individual and group CBT | For women, QI-Meds and QI-Therapy had comparable positive effects on depression burden and quality of life. Over 2 years, cost increases were $424 for QI-Meds and $275 for QI-Therapy, with relative cost-effectiveness for both interventions within the range for other accepted medical treatments, especially QI-Therapy with its smaller impact on costs. QI-Therapy increased work weeks by 3 over 2 years.<br>For men, QI-Therapy significantly reduced depression burden and increased employment by 7 work weeks over 2 years at an increased cost of $983. QI-MEDS increased costs by $429 over 2 years but did not improve depression or work productivity and was therefore not effective or cost-effective. |

**Summary of studies addressing cost-effectiveness in the treatment of depression *(continued)***

| Article | Patients | Treatment | Outcome |
|---|---|---|---|
| Vos et al. 2005 | Estimates made on impact of total expenditures if the recommended mental health treatments for depression were to be implemented for patients in Australia. | 1. Optimum antidepressant drug treatment for depressed patients.<br>2. Maintenance CBT for depressed patients. | 1. Optimum antidepressant drug treatment would cost $312 million (Australian) over 5 years.<br>2. Maintenance cognitive behavioral therapy would cost $160 million (Australian) over 5 years.<br>Both treatments are estimated to reduce the disease burden of depression by approximately 50%. |
| Petrou et al. 2006 | 151 pregnant women at high risk of developing postnatal depression. | 74 women were provided counseling and support for the mother–infant relationship.<br>77 women received routine primary care. | Over 18 months, patients receiving the intervention had a nonsignificant increase in the mean number of months free of postnatal depression and a nonsignificant increase in health and social care costs. The authors felt that a longer follow-up period and a monitoring of other nonmedical costs including lost productivity might have illustrated more cost-effectiveness. |

**Summary of studies addressing cost-effectiveness in the treatment of depression** *(continued)*

| Article | Patients | Treatment | Outcome |
|---|---|---|---|
| Smit et al. 2006 | 363 primary care adult patients with subthreshold depression from 19 general practices in the Netherlands. | 1. Minimal contact psychotherapy consisting of CBT using a self-help manual with six brief telephone calls with a prevention worker.<br>2. Usual care. | Risk of developing a full-blown depressive disorder decreased from 18% to 12% in the intervention group and had lower work-related losses. It was estimated that minimal contact psychotherapy had a 70% probability of being more cost-effective than usual care. |
| Bosmans et al. 2007 | 143 depressed patients ages 55 and older from 12 general practices in and around Amsterdam. | 1. 69 patients were given 10 sessions of IPT over 5 months.<br>2. 74 patients were assigned to care as usual (CAU). | At 6 months, 60% of the IPT patients and 42% of the CAU patients had recovered, a difference just short of statistical significance. At 12 months, the recovery rate in both groups was 45%. Total costs were higher in the IPT group but not statistically significantly. Since the IPT patients had greater costs, there was a negative incremental cost-effectiveness ratio at 12 months for the IPT group and the intervention was not felt to be cost-effective compared with CAU. The authors felt that more depressed patients evidenced more cost-effectiveness in other studies and that their results would have been different with a longer course of treatment by more experienced therapists and with maintenance treatments to sustain gains made in the acute treatment phase. |

## Summary of studies addressing cost-effectiveness in the treatment of depression *(continued)*

| Article | Patients | Treatment | Outcome |
| --- | --- | --- | --- |
| Dunn et al. 2007 | 101 male veterans with comorbid chronic posttraumatic stress disorder and depressive disorder. | 1. Self-management therapy (a cognitive-behavioral group psychotherapy). 2. Active-control therapy (a strictly educational therapy provided in a group). Patients were randomly assigned to one of the two treatment groups, each of which met for 1.5-hour weekly group sessions for 14 weeks. | Self-management therapy patients had slightly greater improvement in depressive symptoms, but this difference disappeared on follow-up. However, these patients also had fewer psychiatric outpatient visits and lower psychiatric and medical/surgical costs during treatment and the year afterward. |
| Wells et al. 2007 | 746 primary care patients with 12-month depressive disorder and 502 with subthreshold depression. | Matched clinics were randomly assigned to provide either 1) enhanced usual care or 2) one of two quality improvement interventions that provided: a) education to manage depression and increased access to medication management; or b) psychotherapy for 6 to 12 months. | Cost-effectiveness of both quality improvement interventions was similar to enhanced usual care both for patients with depressive disorder and subthreshold depression. There were higher total health care costs for depressive disorder patients given medication quality improvement intervention but not for therapy quality improvement intervention. These cost increases were much smaller and statistically insignificant for subthreshold depression patients. |

# 7 | Psychotherapy and Psychosocial Interventions in the Treatment of Substance Abuse

William H. Sledge, M.D.
James Hutchinson, M.D.

While there are many well-conducted scientific studies on the psychotherapy of substance abuse, the biological, psychological, developmental, and social complexity of the topic mean that treatment remains art guided by science even though substantial gains are being made toward the goal of a comprehensive evidence-based approach. Many studies document the extreme medical and social dollar cost of substance abuse. Only a few studies are directed at examining the cost-effectiveness of treatment per se. Outcome and cost-effectiveness studies are most extensive for alcohol and tobacco abuse, less so for cocaine, heroin, and marijuana abuse (Gerstein et al. 1994; Miller et al. 1998). There are great gaps in our understanding of the treatment of stimulant, hallucinogen, designer drug, and inhalant abuse.

There are general trends across several types of addiction. Even addicted with highly addictive substances, many substance abusers try to quit on their own. A small percentage of addicts free themselves of addiction each year without formal treatment. Over time, a substantial number are able to give up drug use on their own, but a steady stream of new addicts replaces them as users (Regier et al. 1993).

Brief interventions by general medical professionals with their substance-abusing patients increase both the numbers who try and those who succeed in quitting. These interventions are cost-effective but not without significant limitations. Many people who are not psychologically or physically addicted to the substances they use still suffer significant medical consequences. This population is particularly benefited by education and brief interventions from primary medical personnel. Brief, focused, repetitively administered psychosocial treatments by mental health professionals are generally highly cost-effective (Moher et al. 2005; Mundt 2006; Saitz 2007; Westmaas et al. 2000).

Dual diagnosis is common (Regier et al. 1990). Affective, anxiety, attentional, and personality disorders (particularly antisocial personality disorder) are common psychiatric comorbid conditions of alcohol, cocaine, and heroin abuse. Good psychiatric treatment for comorbid conditions substantially improves the outcome of substance abuse treatment and is cost-effective. Patients in advanced stages of addiction obtain significantly better clinical outcomes if treatment is multimodal, addressing biological and intrapsychic as well as familial, social, and occupational issues while focusing on the preservation of abstinence (Chen et al. 2006; Kosten et al. 1989; Luborsky et al. 1993).

Given the extraordinary medical and social costs of severe substance abuse even without measuring treatment cost, we can be assured that intensive treatments, if effective, are also likely to be cost-effective. Appropriate outcomes to evaluate the societal costs and benefits of treatment on drug use include criminal activity, capacity to work, capacity to care for dependent children, and physical health. Although many studies have some methodological or design flaw, quite a few find profound reductions in drug use and criminal activity, as well as improvements in physical health after treatment. Those who stay in treatment longer obtain substantially larger benefit. Many studies reveal the multiple social, legal, psychiatric, and medical problems of the population who seek substance abuse treatment in the United States, the generally very small allocation of resources toward treatment, and the rather substantial financial rewards to society from appropriate investment in substance abuse treatment (Crits-Christoph and Siqueland 1996).

# Search Methodology

A MEDLINE search from January 1984 to December 2007 was done using the following terms: "cost + psychotherapy + narcotics," "cost + psychotherapy + alcohol," and "cost + psychotherapy + nicotine." MEDLINE searches of the literature were conducted using the key words "addiction," "treatment," and "cost-effectiveness." Similar searches were conducted using key words "treatment," "cost-effectiveness," and the words "smoking," "tobacco," "nicotine," "alcohol," "cocaine," "marijuana," "hallucinogen," "stimulant," "heroin," and "opiate." Ad hoc references after December 2007 were included as they became known to us. The review table at the end of this chapter includes the citations that address elements of cost or cost-effectiveness as well as selected reviews and reports of effectiveness.

# Costs of Addiction

While tobacco, alcohol, and street drugs are almost universally understood to be a serious health hazard, there is still a sense of shock and disbelief when one looks at the addictive potential and the total dollar cost of substance abuse in the United States. Breslau et al. (2001) gave an excellent account of the epidemiology of nicotine dependence in the United States. They noted, based on the tobacco supplement to the National Comorbidity Study of over 4,000 people, that the lifetime prevalence of nicotine dependence was 24%, with the highest risk for nicotine dependence occurring in the first 16 years after daily smoking began. Reported tobacco use is linked to 400,000 deaths per year, or roughly 10 times the number who die in auto accidents (Centers for Disease Control and Prevention 1993). Smoking is associated with 85% of lung cancer deaths and 30% of all cancer deaths, and there are substantial increases in the risk of cardiovascular disease, osteoporosis, and fetal death or low birth weight infants. These statistics do not include the effects of passive smoke inhalation, which is reported to be as high as 53,000 deaths each year. The statistics do not count those who are burned or die from fires caused by smoking (Centers for Disease Control and Prevention 1993). Over 48 million citizens above the age of 18 smoke over 24 billion packs of cigarettes a year. While the incidence of smoking has decreased in the United States since 1965, women and minorities have been underrepresented in the drop, and there have been ominous increases in teen smoking and dramatic increases in the incidence of cigarette use among Native Americans. The U.S. Public Health Service reported that each pack of cigarettes has been calculated to cost Americans $2.06 in direct health care costs of which the government pays out $89. The direct medical costs were estimated at $50 billion in 1993 (Centers for Disease Control and Prevention 1994). The indirect costs in the same year were estimated at $47.3 billion.

In their review, Anthony et al. (1996) stated that the prevalence of alcohol abuse or dependence in the U.S. population between ages 15 and 54 within the last year was between 8.6% and 11.9% depending on the study. Rice et al. (1990) found the costs of alcohol to society in 1990 were estimated (conservatively) at $99 billion. Roughly 15% of these $99 billion were health care costs; 65% were costs of lost work, disability, or early death; and 20% were non-health-related costs. Alcohol use has been estimated to account for 13% of breast cancers, 40% of traumatic injuries, 41% of seizures, and 72% of pancreatitis. Treno and Holder (1997) stated that alcohol is involved in 70% of traffic accidents that kill those 20 to 25 years old and 50% of fatal accidents overall. There are strong associations between alcohol and burns, falls, drowning, crime, and interpersonal violence. The medical costs of interpersonal violence exceed those of auto accidents. Trauma that is associated with alcohol tends to be serious trauma. Alcohol was found in the blood at admission of 47% of trauma center patients. Anthony et al. (1992) found that 6.8% of the American workforce suffered from alcohol abuse or dependence at the time of the study or within the last year. Harrison and Hoffmann (1989) cited studies that show this population to have higher rates of absenteeism, lateness, work-related injury, disability, and mistakes on the job. Ross et al. (1988) studied psychiatric conditions that are comorbid with alcohol abuse. Up to 80% of alcoholics are reported to suffer from other drug use disorders over their lifetime. Sixty percent of alcoholic men are reported to suffer from anxiety or affective disorders. Approximately 35% of alcoholic women have affective disorders and approximately 67% have anxiety disorders. The reported comorbidity of antisocial personality disorder ranges from 23% to 53%.

The estimates for the medical costs of alcohol may be low. The Institute of Medicine's report on alcohol (Committee on Treatment of Alcohol Problems, Institute of Medicine 1990) states that many drinkers who are not physically or psychologically dependent on alcohol suffer significant medical damage or other negative consequences from their alcohol use. In the 1990s the National Comorbidity Study (Anthony et al. 1994, 1996) found the United States to have the highest incidence of substance abuse among the Western democracies. Over 90% of Americans between the ages of 15 and 54 years had tried alcohol and about 15% of that population, or about 14% of the population as a whole, went on to have an alcohol problem. Three-quarters of Americans had tried tobacco, and about 24% became addicted to cigarettes. Roughly half of this group (46%) tried marijuana, and about 9% of those trying it abused or became dependent on the drug. Tobacco was the drug most likely to lead to dependence, with roughly one-third (32%) of Americans in this age group who tried it becoming dependent. The percentages for heroin, cocaine, and alcohol dependence were 23.1%, 16.7%, and 15.4%, respectively. More recent studies document the lifetime prevalence of any substance use disorder as 14.6% (Kessler et al. 2005a) and the 12-month prevalence as 3.8% (Kessler et al. 2005b). Using different survey instruments, rates published 2 years later showed that a prevalence of 12-month and lifetime drug abuse (1.4% and 7.7%, respectively) exceeded the rates of drug dependence (0.6% and 2.6%, respectively), with 12-month prevalence for all drug use disorders at 2% and lifetime prevalence at 10.3%. Lifetime treatment or help-seeking behavior was not common (8.1% for substance abuse and 37.9% for substance dependence). Most individuals with drug use disorders have never been treated (Compton et al. 2007).

Substance abuse (with the exception of extra medical use of anxiolytics and analgesics) is mainly a disease of the young. In 1992 roughly 7.5% of those ages 12–17 years and 13% of those ages 18–25 years had used illegal drugs in the prior month. Regier et al. (1993) found that 6.72% of pregnant women had used alcohol and 3.49% an illicit drug in the hours or days preceding delivery. This use results in high-risk pregnancies with substantial increases in cost of perinatal medical care of both mothers and infants. Birth defects secondary to substance abuse such as alcohol or crack impose high long-term costs on society. The medical and indirect costs of street drugs were calculated at approximately $67 billion a year. These figures were based on studies conducted before the upsurge of medical and legal costs associated with the HIV and crack epidemics of the late 1980s. Rice et al. (1990) estimated a third of all legal costs are linked to alcohol, substance abuse, or mental illness.

Culture is a powerful force in determining the risk of addiction. One need only compare the low incidence of cigarettes and alcohol addiction among Mormons with the pandemic incidence of alcohol and tobacco use on certain Indian reservations in the United States to be convinced of the point. Different cultures (or even subcultures within a main culture) may encourage or prohibit substance use; they may celebrate, ignore, or severely stigmatize the substance user. Devout Mormons abhor alcohol, tobacco, and caffeine. Devout Muslims abhor alcohol but see tobacco and caffeine as a welcome part of life. To a Mescalaro Indian, mescaline is a sacrament and wine is a dangerous drug; an American of Western European descent might reverse the categories. Psychological consequences, patterns of use, and social consequences of drug use change radically depending on whether one is acting within or outside of the mores of one's culture; medical consequences do not. In England there are addicts who legally use opiates for years without showing evidence of the psychopathology found so often among U.S. heroin addicts.

Margaret Mead's work in the South Pacific conducted after World War II found that those cultures in which old value systems were shattered and support networks had broken down left their members at high risk for substance abuse (Mead 1956). The pandemic and catastrophic use of inhalants in the street children of nondeveloped countries seems to confirm her findings. The powerful influence of culture on treatment and outcome variables suggests researchers should use great caution in generalizing across cultures from their studies.

And yet, while culture has figured predominantly in the consideration of addiction, more and more researchers turn to the biology of inheritance and consider genetic factors and gene×environmental interactions as they struggle with the mysteries and treatments for alcoholism and other forms of addiction (Cloninger 1999; Gelernter 1995; Kendler 2001).

## Case Vignette

Arthur was the youngest of three children of professional parents. He was cared for by a succession of nannies during his early years. When Arthur was 12, the twin traumas of his parents' bitter divorce and an attempted homosexual seduction by a camp counselor ended this period of relative stability. On his return to school, he became moody and rebellious and gravitated toward the aggressive, alienated boys of his class. He began smoking, started to drink beer, and within 18 months of the camp experience was heavily involved in multiple drugs.

His mother did not notice his loss of his healthier friends, his declining grades and truancy, his moodiness, his shift to countercultural dress and music, his sudden insistence on "nontoxic" organic foods, but she did notice ever larger amounts of money missing from her purse. While searching for missing money, she found evidence of Arthur's extensive drug and alcohol use. His violent response to her confrontation led to his involuntary hospitalization. While successfully resisting treatment in the hospital, he befriended two adolescent drug dealers who recruited him as a courier.

After discharge, he lived with his father who tried an authoritarian approach. Arthur took pleasure in defeating his father's restrictions. He lasted 2 weeks at a military school, used any and all available drugs, and as a member of a gang engaged in vandalism, arson, shoplifting, intimidation, and assault. In the absence of intoxication or the excitement of criminal activities, Arthur experienced crushing boredom or despair. Seven juvenile arrests, two auto accidents, and seven court-mandated outpatient treatments had no apparent effect.

However, when a friend was shot in a drug-related incident, Arthur became frightened and actively sought treatment for the first time. He participated in a twelve-step program and cognitive-behavioral therapy arranged for by his father. After 2 years of intensive effort and three painful relapses, he seemed to be in a solid remission from the abuse of street drugs and alcohol. While free of drugs and criminal connections, he remained depressed, anxious, and unable to direct his life. He then sought outpatient psychodynamic psychotherapy. Over several years he resumed his academic career, renewed his interest in drawing, and developed an interest in camping and rock climbing. He made new friends and cautiously began to date. He terminated treatment at the end of 4 years to attend college in another city. He met and married a lively, rather maternal woman. While generally happy together, his continued cigarette smoking was a source of conflict in their marriage. As he became a father for the first time an upsurge of anger and depression led him to return to psychotherapy for a 6-month period. He gradually came to a full recognition of his envy and jealousy of the care his new son received and was able to enjoy a second better childhood vicariously and take pride in his own good parenting. Motivated by his new wish to be a good example for his son, he finally gave up smoking.

# Treatment of Tobacco Addiction

Treatments of smoking addiction were reviewed in April 1996 in a U.S. Department of Health and Human Services (1996) clinical practice guideline. In this study a medical literature search was conducted for 1976 through 1994 evaluating smoking cessation strategies that had objective measures of outcome and a randomized controlled format. Some 3,000 references were obtained and reviewed by a panel selected from those who had derived, studied, and published methods of treating smoking. The literature search for this book described earlier did not add any data that changed the conclusions of this exhaustive review. A number of significant findings were summarized in the reference. Fifty percent of those with a chronic smoking habit eventually give it up. Thirty percent of smokers try to quit each year, but only 10% of this group (3% of all smokers) succeeds in quitting each year. A single episode of friendly advice from a concerned health care professional increases overall quit rates: 30% to 39% of all smokers given such advice are able to quit within the year that the advice is given. Psychotherapy increases quit rates 250%, and 10.5% of all smokers who are given psychotherapy are able to quit within the year of such counseling. Increasing the session length, number of sessions, and duration of the treatment improves outcome. Increasing session length to beyond 10-minute contacts, frequency to 4–7 sessions, and duration of the treatment to over 8 weeks adds substantially to the quit rate. The enormous direct and indirect costs and the inexpensive nature of these interventions led the authors to conclude without measuring treatment costs that such treatments were cost-effective.

Lichtenstein et al. (1996) provided an excellent overview of tobacco cessation models and outcomes. They strongly urged the role of primary care providers and gave an account of the differential efficacy based on different settings. Their approach is deeply ingrained and embedded within the health care system and is consistent with the Agency for Health Care Policy Research interventions.

Law and Tang (1995) provided an encyclopedic overview but did not include cost-effective data in their analysis of the effectiveness of interventions for tobacco cessation. They reviewed the literature of 188 randomized controlled trials spanning personal advice and encouragement from physicians to behavior modification techniques, hypnosis, nicotine replacement therapy (NRT), and other pharmacological approaches. They estimated that when physicians encourage their patients to stop smoking, the effect is a modest 2% effectiveness. However, the cost is quite low at $1,500 per saved life. They also found in their review of the literature that advice and encouragement of smokers at special risk tend to be more effective. Westmaas et al. (2000) also give us an excellent overview, emphasizing the deleterious effect of smoking on cancer. They described the 4 A's protocol of the National Cancer Institute: ask patients about their smoking status; advise them to quit; assist them by recommending pharmacotherapy, counseling, and psychosocial self-help materials; and arrange for follow-up. They noted that the cost-effectiveness of minimal interventions such as brief advice to quit by a physician comes in at a bargain of between $705 and $988 per life gained for men and between $1,200 and $2,060 for women.

West et al. (2000) took the perspective of the oncologist and surgeon in their excellent overview of smoking cessation guidelines for health professionals. They confirmed the good value and cost-effectiveness of the primary care practitioner or general practitioner (GP) opportunistically advising smokers to stop during routine visits and consultations. In another publication, they developed guidelines (West et al. 2000, 2004). Rigotti and Pasternak (1996), in their overview addressing the value of smoking cessation for the expression of mortality and morbidity in coronary artery disease, present data similar to others in that they noted that the health risks of cigarette smoking are extremely high in relationship to coronary artery disease. They gave an excellent account of the barriers to smoking cessation, which include nicotine dependency, behavioral factors, mood disorder, and weight gain. Their review of the treatment approaches is excellent and well organized. Brandon (2001) gave an excellent overview as well on cost-effectiveness data in terms of dealing with the morbidity and mortality of cancer. He noted that the most potent interventions are likely to continue to be multicomponent, intensive behavioral interventions that include pharmacotherapy.

Alterman et al. (2001) reported on a study of three levels of intensity of behavioral treatments and short- and long-term smoking cessation outcomes. This group found that biochemically confirmed abstinent rates at 1 year were 35% for the high-intensity group, 27% for the low-intensity group, and 12% for the moderate-intensity group. The cost of low-intensity treatment was $308 and high-intensity treatment was $582. The low-intensity group entailed one advice and education session with a nurse practitioner and 8 weeks of NRT. The moderate-intensity group had NRT and four advice and education sessions with a nurse practitioner. The high-intensity group received treatment combining NRT, four advice and education sessions, and 12 weeks of individualized cognitive-behavioral therapy (CBT). The authors were puzzled by the relatively disappointing results of the moderate-intensity group and could not account for the differences.

Hall et al. (1998) used nortriptyline and CBT in the treatment of cigarette smoking, based on the fact that a history of major depressive disorder predicted failure to stop smoking. They used a 2 (nortriptyline vs. placebo) $\times 2$ (CBT vs. control)$\times 2$ (history of major depression vs. no history) randomized trial. The results revealed that nortriptyline produced higher abstinence rates than placebo independent of depression history. CBT was more effective for participants with a history of depression, and nortriptyline alleviated a negative affect occurring after smoking cessation. The authors noted that the beneficial effect of nortriptyline is a promising adjunct for smoking cessation, particularly among patients with a history of depression. Klesges et al. (1999) found treatments are clearly useful but not effective for all. The best treatment results are obtained by university-based, multicomponent behavioral programs with treatment manuals and quality control on treatment administered. Such programs have achieved abstinence rates of about 40% during 2- to 6-year follow-up. This means 60% of those receiving current best treatment relapse. Having a life-threatening illness connected with tobacco use improves outcome in efforts to cease tobacco use. Still 50% of those who have life-threatening tobacco-related illness (status post lung removal or status post acute myocardial infarction) are unable to give up smoking. Treatments are clearly still not satisfactory. All effective treatments are clearly cost-effective without measuring treatment costs. Olivier et al. (2007) summarized and discussed evidence of the clinical impact of tobacco smoking in an inpatient psychiatric setting and reviewed some of the literature on the psychiatric and psychological research on smoking cessation within inpatient settings.

West et al. (2000) addressed the issue of smokeless tobacco cessation and concluded that there is insufficient evidence to recommend the use of NRT or bupropion for smokeless tobacco cessation. They called for more research, within the United Kingdom at least, to quantify the personal and population risks and benefits from interventions aimed at smokeless tobacco cessation.

Wolfenden et al. (2005) studied 210 smoking patients in a pre-op clinic for a major teaching hospital in Australia with the aim to assess the efficacy and acceptability as well as the cost of the multifaceted intervention to facilitate smoking cessation in patients scheduled for surgery. They concluded that this approach was accepted by patients as well as staff and seemed to be generally helpful; however, it was not designed to be an effectiveness study.

Halpin et al. (2006) examined three levels of intensity of behavioral treatment through a random-control design of the effectiveness of different benefit designs and discovered that after 8 months, there were no significant increases in quit attempts or quitter rates in the groups with medication and counseling compared with the group with drugs alone. They concluded that the benefit design with the more intensive elements provided no substantial cost-benefit increase over a relatively low-intensity treatment approach.

Moher et al. (2005) and Stead and Lancaster (2005) presented the findings of two different Cochrane Reviews, respectively addressing workplace interventions in smoking cessation and group therapy programs in smoking cessation. There were a total of 31 different studies addressing different aspects of smoking cessation programs. These included group therapy, individual counseling, and self-help materials, as well as NRT. Self-help materials were less effective. Workplace interventions aimed at the workplace as a whole included 14 studies of tobacco bans, 2 studies of social support, 4 studies of environmental support, 5 studies of incentives, and 8 comprehensive multicomponent programs. The authors failed to detect an increase in quit rates from adding social and environmental support to these programs. There was a lack of evidence that comprehensive programs reduce the prevalence of smoking. There was also less evidence that competitions and incentives actually stopped smoking, but they certainly increased attempts at quitting. The review addressing group programs included a total subject population of almost 4,400 patients and found that group programs are more effective than no-intervention controls. There was no evidence that group therapy was more effective than similar intensity of individual counseling, and there was no evidence that adding group therapy to other forms of treatment such as advice from a professional or an NRT provided extra benefit. However, it was clear that one important element seemed to be how the subjects accepted the treatment.

Finally, a comprehensive review of the literature is worth noting. Gordon et al. (2007), in a review of cost-effectiveness of face-to-face behavioral interventions for major risk factors for chronic disease, such as smoking, physical inactivity, poor diet, and alcohol abuse, concluded that there was considerable variation among the studies by target population, intervention components, primary outcome, and economic methods. However, the reported incremental cost effectiveness ratios were consistently low, less than 14,000 euros (in 2006 euros) per quality-adjusted life year (QALY).

# Alcohol Addiction and Psychotherapy

The treatment of alcoholism presents a plethora of choices and strategies. Issues to be considered are the nature of the patients, including the severity of their alcoholism and drinking habits; the presence of complications medically and psychiatrically, such as dually diagnosed patients; modalities of therapy, which include considerations of group therapy or couples therapy; forms of psychotherapy; the concurrent use of psychopharmacology; and the context of the provision of therapy, such as medical versus lay treatments and counseling such as Alcoholics Anonymous (AA) and the twelve-step program.

Also, the treatment of alcoholism offers additional outcome considerations not present in the same way as the treatment of other addictions. Of course, the clinical outcomes include drinking behaviors and the presence or absence of medical and psychological, as well as social complications of drinking. The economic issues include not only QALY but also costs of direct care, cost offset because of changes in the medical morbidity associated with effective treatment of alcoholism, criminal activity, work productivity, and other issues socially and psychologically associated with alcoholism, such as changes in accidents, injuries, arrests, and so on.

Modalities include those noted by Holder et al. (1991) in their review and include treatment approaches such as acupuncture, AA (the twelve-step program), antidipsotropic medication, aversion therapy, behavioral contracting, brief motivational counseling, cognitive therapy, community reinforcement approach, confrontational interventions, counseling, education, group psychotherapy, hypnosis, marital therapy, individual psychotherapy, and other psychotropic medications designed to take away mental states that are believed to be proximate and causal to drinking. Other treatment approaches have included residential milieu therapy, self-control training, social skills training, stress management training, and videotaped self-confrontation. We will only review some of these modalities. However, the presence of so many modalities, some of which have an impressive effectiveness literature behind them, and some of which also have cost-effectiveness studies associated with them, brings up the question of matching of patients with the apparent opportunities presented by so many treatments.

Mattson (2002) reported on the experience of Project MATCH supported by the National Institute on Alcohol Abuse and Alcoholism testing the hypothesis that certain patient characteristics were better treated by specific treatments. A study comparing CBT, twelve-step facilitation, and motivational enhancement found overall that all three were effective; however, twelve-step facilitation was more effective overall on abstinence at a 1-year follow-up. Furthermore, several matching targets were sustained: the low psychiatric severity treated with twelve-step had more abstinence days; motivational enhancement did better with angry patients; patients having a social network supportive of drinking did better in twelve-step than they did in motivational enhancement therapy; and patients who had high alcohol dependence did better in twelve-step, whereas those lower in alcohol dependence did better in CBT. The interactions were more modest than expected but do make sense clinically.

Cisler et al. (1998) attempted to compare the treatment cost of the modalities used in Project MATCH. They found the per-patient contact cost of motivational enhancement therapy (MET) was more than double (mean = $498) that of CBT (mean = $198) and almost double twelve-step facilitation treatment (TSF) (mean = $253). The cost per patient, however, was lower, with MET having a mean cost of $1,700, CBT a mean cost of $1,901, and TSF a mean cost of $1,969. The authors believe that the fact that this was a research project inflated the cost somewhat, although their analysis attempted to take this into consideration. A 2005 study from the United Kingdom found that Project MATCH in the United States is unlikely to support substantial improvements in effective treatment of alcohol problems in terms of the general matching ideas but that the interventions had, in general, established effectiveness.

Miller et al. (1995) presented an extensive examination of the efficacy and cost-effectiveness of various treatments for alcohol abuse. Since 1986, they have confined their reviews to studies with controls and objective measures of outcome. The data cited stem from a computerized database search through 1993 and followed up with a manual literature search of two dozen major journals for studies that included the following: 1) at least one procedure designed to have an impact on problematic drinking; 2) use of a control; 3) use of inferential statistics and control of bias through randomization; and 4) at least one outcome measure. Two hundred and eleven articles were identified that met the criteria for the meta-study. The authors derived a cumulative evidence score (CES) for each modality of treatment. Each study was given an evidence score, which was obtained by multiplying the rating of methodological quality of the study by a measure of the efficacy of the outcome of the treatment in comparison with the control. The CES was the sum of all evidence scores for all treatments in the modality. It should be emphasized that CES will exaggerate the effect of treatments that are brief with short periods of follow-up and simple outcome measures where it is more likely that a positive outcome will be found, where it is easier to get a high mark for methodological aspects of the study, and where multiple studies will have been conducted. Costs of treatment were also estimated. The following four modalities were the highest ranked but not the only studies examined: brief intervention (CES = 239), social skills training (CES = 128), motivational enhancement (CES = 87), and a community reinforcement approach (CES = 80).

This meta-analysis study notes two other findings. Treatments that relied on aggressive confrontation or attempts to shame patients, such as aggressive verbal confrontations of problem drinkers or use of videotapes of patients made while patients were intoxicated, had negative therapeutic effects and consistently had outcomes worse than control. The second interesting finding was the dearth of studies of twelve-step programs. Only two studies of AA met the criteria of the meta-analysis study. Both found AA to be of some benefit. These studies were atypical in that the patient population had been court mandated to attend AA. A meta-analysis of single group evaluation studies conducted by McCrady and Langenbucher (1996) concluded that attendance at AA meetings, when added to professional treatment, increases the probability of decreased drinking and improved psychological functioning.

Holder et al. (1991) found that no benefit was offered by residential treatment over day treatment for alcoholics. They reviewed 10 studies looking at "psychotherapy" as a treatment for alcoholism. Their analysis found it to be the most expensive approach and to affect outcome adversely. Unlike other modalities examined in Holder et al.'s study, no description of what constituted psychotherapy was offered. Two of the studies cited in the meta-study examined the use of LSD to "augment" psychotherapy. One study was a trial of psychotherapy that took place in Harlem, where marked social instability of the patients might be predicted to compromise outcome of a treatment, which depends on continuity. There was no consideration of the impact that dual diagnosis would have on this finding. Holder et al. suggested that society allocate resources for treatment to only those treatments shown effective by their criteria for scientific validity. They also suggested repetitive brief interventions and are dismissive of residential treatment and psychotherapy and are at best lukewarm to twelve-step programs.

Other studies reported on moderately effective programs as well. Powell et al. (1985) found that in three very different treatment approaches (a control or no-treatment group, in which patients were monitored for possible medical complications; a medication-only group, which included disulfiram; and a general supportive therapy group) all groups improved, and there was no statistically significant difference among them. In a study of motivational enhancement counseling, Freeborn et al. (2000) randomly assigned 514 patients to a brief motivational enhancement counseling session plus clinician advice in contrast to usual care. The patients were considered to be "hazardous drinkers," referring to people whose quantity and frequency of drinking is causing or likely to cause problems, but who still do not fit the criteria for alcohol dependence per se. Alcohol consumption and utilization patterns of health care were the pertinent outcome measures. There were no differences between the two groups, indicating that the intervention did not seem to have an effect.

In a look at more specialized modalities, Epstein and McCrady (1998) reported on the research literature supporting the efficacy of alcohol behavioral couples therapy (ABCT), grounded in social learning theory and family systems models. The authors reported on the cost-effectiveness/cost-benefit literature and indicated that ABCT is more effective than ABCT combined with relapse prevention. They concluded that ABCT is a well-articulated theoretical model that links addictive behaviors with relationship functioning. They cited substantial empirical support for the model and drew the following conclusions: 1) randomized clinical trials suggest the different types of spouse-involved therapy generally, and in ABCT in particular, appear to be more effective than treatments that do not include the spouse; 2) using the spouse to apply positive contingencies for sobriety-related behavior leads to more positive outcomes; 3) unilateral formats of ABCT are associated with increased probability that the drinker will become involved with treatment; 4) evidence does not exist to support the long-term superiority of behavioral over other interactional models of couples therapy for alcoholism; 5) studies suggest that a specific focus on relationship function may enhance long-term drinking outcomes and clearly enhances long-term marital stability and satisfaction; 6) evidence is equivocal about the necessary length and intensity of treatment, with one study suggesting that brief and extended interventions yield comparable results; and 7) cost studies suggest a positive benefit-to-cost ratio for ABCT.

Israel et al. (1996), in a complex study measuring the impact of screening and CBT counseling versus advice, revealed that the screening was effective in identifying 62% to 85% of the expected number of problem drinkers in a population of over 15,000 patients attending the private practices of 42 different primary care physicians. They also found that the CBT counseling was substantially superior to the advice-only condition. Others have been critical of this literature. Drummond (1997) took the rather pessimistic view that the research literature that extols the value of brief treatment, particularly in the hands of primary health care, is overstated and was critical of the meta-analyses done in this area. Howard (1993) took Holder et al. (1991) to task for their overly optimistic assessment of the cost-effectiveness of alcohol treatments. He objected to the generalizations brought forward and the selection of acceptable studies and interpretation of findings.

However, more recent work continues to demonstrate the success of relatively brief interventions. Murgraff et al. (2007), in the treatment of risky drinking on Friday among women, found a moderate response with a brief intervention in terms of follow-up. White et al. (2006) found that mandated students reduced their consumption of alcohol, as well as cigarette and marijuana use, with a relatively brief intervention. The issue of intensity of services is addressed by Bischof et al. (2008), who found in a proactive study in two Northern German cities that a stepped-care approach seemed to be the most cost-effective strategy of a brief intervention for individuals at risk for drinking. Doran et al. (2004) reviewed the literature in an effort to determine a level of GP detection of at-risk behavior for their patients, the rates at which they offered intervention, and the effectiveness of these interventions. They also wanted to develop a model based on this literature. They discovered that increasing rates of GP intervention achieves the greatest benefit and return on resources used. For instance, for every 5% increase in the rate of GP intervention, an additional 26,754 at-risk drinkers modify their behavior at a cost of $232 per patient. This compares with the cost per patient modifying drinking behavior of $233 and $208 for every 5% increase in the rates of detection and effectiveness, respectively.

Carroll and Rounsaville (1995) quoted Onken and Blaine (1990) to the effect that psychotherapy and counseling widely available in the United States is the backbone of treatment. Twelve-step programs are equally ubiquitous. McCrady and Langenbucher (1996), in their discussion of Holder et al.'s (1991) findings, pointed out that many of the studies in Holder et al.'s study were conducted with middle-class, socially stable patients without secondary psychiatric diagnosis and thus did not speak to the issue of the need for residential placements for patients who are dually diagnosed or who have eroded their social supports. Landry (1996) suggested that long-term residential placements are both effective and cost-effective in a number of cases of advanced addiction in which social and family supports are eroded. Minimalist therapeutic positions seem to disregard disastrous personal and social consequences of untreated substance abuse, the large numbers unsuccessfully treated by even the best brief interventions, and the data supporting improved yield through a flexible, intense approach guided by the needs of the individual patient. There are strong data from studies of alcohol, cocaine, and heroin abuse that it is cost-effective to address psychiatric comorbidity.

Many of these more recent approaches specifically address the issue of cost-effectiveness. French et al. (2008) studied 120 adolescents living with their families and attempted a cost-effectiveness analysis of four different interventions, including family based, individual, and group cognitive-behavioral approaches. Their results indicated that treatment results varied substantially across the four; however, family therapy showed significantly better substance use outcome compared to group treatment. However, after 7 months, group therapy caught up, both in terms of the delinquency outcome and the substance abuse outcome. Another cost-effectiveness study by Alessi et al. (2007) examined a low-cost contingency management (CM) approach compared with standard treatment and found that rates of substance use were lower in the CM participants at month 9 but not at month 6. This study suggested that it was feasible to deliver incentives for attendance at group, but further research is needed to understand the modest effects. Davidson et al. (2007) questioned whether behavioral broad spectrum treatment (BST) is more effective than motivational enhancement therapy for alcohol-dependent patients being treated with naltrexone. The authors completed a 3-month randomized control trial and determined that BST had a significantly higher percentage of days abstinent from alcohol, suggesting that the advantage of BST is worth the additional cost for patients whose psychosocial networks are supportive for continued drinking.

The use of the Internet and computer-based tools has also come into consideration. Hester and Miller (2006) reviewed the issues involving various Internet programs and noted those that have developed effectiveness as an intervention, particularly in terms of increasing patient motivation and reducing alcohol-associated harm through skill building. Mundt (2006) reported on a randomized control study of the Trial for Early Alcohol Treatment (TrEAT) project in determining the impact of computer and Internet-based approaches on reducing medical care expenses and clinic and hospital costs and concluded that Project TrEAT led to a reduction in alcohol consumption by high-risk drinkers, and a corresponding reduction in medical and societal costs. Mundt supported the cost-effectiveness of Project TrEAT, concluding that its costs were outweighed by its benefits.

Psychotherapy combined with medication has attracted attention. In a study of 1,383 alcohol-dependent patients, Doggrell (2006) examined the differential effectiveness of naltrexone, acomprosate, and behavioral intervention and found that there was no substantial difference among the three. Zarkin et al. (2005) presented a cost-analysis review of the COMBINE, a randomized controlled trial (RCT) comparing pharmacotherapies and behavioral interventions for outpatient treatment of alcohol dependence. The authors presented the estimated costs of 15 intake assessments plus the medical management and combined behavioral interventions for 9 of the 11 COMBINE sites. They concluded that labor costs are the main component of most interventions. The UKATT Research Team (2005; see also UKATT Research Team 2008) presented a study of cost-effectiveness and determined, based on a study of 742 patients with alcohol problems, that the therapies being investigated provided about five times as much savings in expenditures in health, social, and criminal justice services than the direct cost of the intervention.

Along the lines of cost-effectiveness considerations, Mortimer and Segal (2005) evaluated interventions in three clusters of mutually exclusive groups: 1) brief interventions for problem drinking; 2) psychotherapy for mild to moderate dependence; and 3) drug therapy adjunctive to counseling for detoxified patients with a history of severe physical dependence. The cost per QALY estimates for each of the interventions fell below any putative funding threshold for developed countries. Interventions for problem drinkers appeared to offer a better value than the interventions targeted at those with a history of severe physical dependence.

Barrett et al. (2006) studied 599 adults identified as hazardous drinkers who were randomly assigned either to an alcohol health worker, who delivered a brief intervention, or to an information-only control group. The outcomes were total cost, including health and social services, criminal justice, and productivity costs, and measures of alcohol consumption. At the 6-month follow-up, the levels of drinking were statistically significantly lower for those referred to an alcohol health worker than those who were given information only, and at the 12-month follow-up time they were observably lower. Costs were not significantly different at either follow-up time. The authors concluded that referral to an alcohol health worker and an alcohol education program produces favorable clinical outcomes and does not generate a significant increase in cost. However, the results are less robust than others have found.

Lash et al. (2005) studied the effect of a contracting intervention added to a 20-day residential treatment program for substance abuse disorder. Patients were randomly assigned to either standard treatment or standard treatment plus attendance contracting and prompting. The patients in the experimental approach showed fewer subsequent hospitalization days, lower costs, greater improvement in alcohol problem scores, and lower legal target problems in a 3-month follow-up than did the standard treatment group. In other measures, the two groups did not differ; however, the differences seem to support a cost-effectiveness difference.

Kunz et al. (2004) studied the cost-effectiveness of a brief intervention delivered to problem drinkers in an inner-city hospital. Over 1,000 patients were screened for problem drinking during a visit to the emergency department. The intervention was a brief counseling session and health information packet. The control group only received the packet. Outcomes at 3 months included looking at alcohol use, number of drinks, heavy drinking, and other factors. The average economic cost for the brief intervention was $632 per subject; intervention subjects had better 3-month outcomes than controls, but the difference was not always statistically significant. Cost-effectiveness ratios were relatively small for all outcomes. The authors concluded that this type of intervention has the potential to be cost-effective with further development. Kraemer (2007) performed a review of the cost-effectiveness of screening and brief intervention (SBI) for unhealthy alcohol use in medical settings and concluded that the reviewed studies strongly support SBI in medical settings as a reasonable deployment of health care resources and thereby illustrate the usefulness of an economic evaluation for assessing alcohol prevention.

Babor et al. (2007), following up on the idea of SBI, concluded that the studies yield short-term improvements in individual health, but the long-term effects are not yet clear despite promising simulation model results. Saitz (2007) also discussed the efficacy of SBI and stated that it can lead to substantial decreased consumption of primary care resources when used in the primary care setting. The author also concluded that further research is needed to determine the integration of SBI for alcohol and drugs in the real-world circumstances of primary care settings.

In summary, the cost-effectiveness literature is generally positive; however, there is much work to be done to clarify the complexity and the relationship between specific treatment approaches and characteristics of patients. The overwhelming cost and disabling consequences of addiction to alcohol are clear enough. Almost any treatment that can reduce the disabling consequences of alcohol abuse and addiction will be cost-effective.

# Nonlegal Drugs Use and Abuse: Marijuana, Cocaine, and Opiates

Kessler et al. (2001), in a survey of populations in different areas including Ontario, Canada, and the United States generally, as well as local samples in Fresno, California, and Mexico City, Mexico, recruited over 16,000 respondents. The significant findings were that most patients (50% in Ontario and 85% in Fresno) with substance abuse disorders sought treatment, but the lag between onset and treatment seeking averaged a decade or more. Predictors of treatment seeking included late onset of disorder versus early age, recentness of cohort (the most recent being the most likely to seek treatment), and specific symptoms of dependence, which include using large amounts, unsuccessful attempts to cut down, tolerance and withdrawal symptoms, and use of cocaine and heroin. The World Health Organization's (1998) Technical Report Series 873 is an excellent overview of drug treatment, including a conceptual section on economic considerations, as well as psychosocial interventions.

Miller et al. (1998) provided a description of an integrated addiction treatment system that consists of components of evaluation, intervention, detoxification, rehabilitation, and continuing care and discussed the cost-effectiveness of such a system. This article gives the sense of magnitude of patients in various treatments. The discussion of a cost-benefit analysis is crude, although they reference the CALDATA study (see below) (Gerstein et al. 1994).

Crits-Christoph and Siqueland (1996) conducted a meta-analysis of outcome studies for marijuana, cocaine, and opiate treatments. They reviewed controlled studies with objective outcome measures, which also attempted to define the treatment through provision of a treatment manual. Too few studies existed for a true meta-analysis. The authors cited difficulties with most studies, including small numbers of patients studied, highly varied populations, the scarcity of replication, very high dropout rates, no measure or control for therapist training and experience, and the scarcity of multisite studies. Despite these difficulties, the authors found definite trends emerging from their data. Intensive treatment (more than once a week) improved outcome on measures of substance abuse, legal involvement, and job and family stability. Treatment lengths greater than 6 months conferred added benefit that persisted at follow-up beyond 1 year. A broader range of treatment (e.g., drug counseling, job counseling, skill building in interpersonal problem solving, family therapy, and cognitive therapy for relapse prevention) provided added benefits that were sustained beyond 1 year. No estimates of cost of treatment were made. The authors concluded from the very high levels of legal and medical cost of opioid and crack addiction that any treatments that were effective would also be cost-effective.

In a study addressing the matching of patients to tailored treatments, Avants et al. (1998) hypothesized that methadone-maintained patients with high social anxiety would do better in a treatment that was low intensity and emphasized coping skills rather than a setting of high-intensity, socially demanding day treatment. Their randomized study of these two different intensities of psychosocial care found that when patients enrolled in a lower intensity psychosocial approach were compared with those enrolled in a higher intensity psychosocial approach, the socially anxious patients were drug free longer during treatment (patients who were not socially anxious did slightly better in the high-intensity intervention), were more likely to be abstinent at the termination of treatment, and were more likely to be compliant with HIV risk reduction behaviors if they were assigned to the lower intensity intervention in comparison with the higher intensity treatment. The low intervention treatment was provided at one-third of the cost of the higher intensity treatment.

The issue of combining psychosocial treatments with medications was also taken up in a study of methadone maintenance by Shaffer et al. (1997). Sixty-one patients were randomly assigned to methadone maintenance enhanced by traditional group psychotherapy or an alternative methadone maintenance treatment program involving Hatha yoga therapy. The results revealed no significant differences for drug use and criminal activities; however, both were effective in reducing these outcome measures. Patients with psychiatric symptoms and opiate dependence enrolled in a methadone maintenance program were studied in a random design study (Woody et al. 1995). Eighty-four subjects were randomly assigned into one of two different treatment approaches: 1) methadone maintenance for 24 weeks plus supplemental counseling, or 2) drug counseling plus supportive expressive psychotherapy and methadone maintenance. At the conclusion of the study, patients were not significantly different in the two groups in terms of opi-ate-positive urine samples, but the patients receiving supportive expressive psychotherapy had fewer cocaine-positive urine samples and required lower doses of methadone. Follow-up at 1 month revealed that both groups had made gains, but there were not significant differences between them. At 6-month follow-up, many of the gains made by the drug counseling had di-minished, whereas most of the gains made by the patients receiving sup-portive expressive psychotherapy remained. The significant differences that emerged between the two at the later follow-up were all in favor of support-ive expressive psychotherapy.

In a follow-up study of a randomized clinical trial of 100 methadone-maintained opiate users, Kraft et al. (1997) found at the 6-month follow-up time that the annual cost per abstinent patient for the methadone-maintained patients who had been treated in the methadone-only arm was $16,485; for the medium-intensity arm of methadone maintenance plus psychosocial counseling was $9,804; and for the intense-arm, methadone maintenance plus psychosocial counseling and medical and other psycho-social services was $11,818. The authors concluded that some psychosocial services were cost-effective; however, there was an asymptotic relationship between cost and effectiveness so that increasing intensity did not yield a proportionate increase in cost-effectiveness beyond a certain point.

In a study combining the effectiveness of psychosocial treatments with naltrexone for opiate dependence, Carroll et al. (2001) carried out a ran-domized study of 127 recently detoxified opiate-dependent individuals randomized into one of three conditions: 1) standard naltrexone treatment given three times a week; 2) naltrexone treatment plus CM, a form of vouchers contingent on drug-free urine and naltrexone compliance; or 3) naltrex-one treatment, CM, and involvement of a significant other whereby a family member participates in up to six family therapy sessions. The results re-vealed a significant main effect of CM in terms of improving treatment re-tention and reduction in opioid use. There was no significant effect of other involvement.

Carroll et al. (1994a) report a four-armed randomized study attempting to determine the effectiveness of psychotherapy and pharmacotherapy alone and in combination for cocaine addiction. These studies reveal the difficulty in measuring outcomes because of the heterogeneity of patients who use cocaine. They used a 2×2 design of cognitive-behavioral relapse prevention plus desipramine, clinical management plus desipramine, cog-nitive-behavioral relapse prevention plus placebo, and clinical management plus placebo. In their initial assessment at 12 weeks, they found no significant differences among the four groups. In the initial report they discovered that high-severity patients had significantly better outcome when treated with relapse prevention and clinical management, whereas desipramine was associated with improved abstinence initiation among lower severity patients. In the follow-up study of the same sample (Carroll et al. 1994b), investigators found at 1-year follow-up of the 121 subjects remaining in the study that abstinence during treatment was strongly associated with less cocaine use during follow-up and that there was a significant psychotherapy by time effect, suggesting a delayed improvement during follow-up for patients who receive the cognitive-behavioral relapse prevention compared with supportive clinical management.

In another approach, Brooner et al. (2007) performed a randomized clinical trial of 236 patients and found that the comparison between adaptive stepped-care and monetary-based voucher interventions for opiate dependence revealed that both were effective when compared with routine care in reducing opiate drug use among dependent patients. They offered no cost-effective data, however. Moore et al. (2007) performed a review applying a sensitivity analysis, using Australian data, looking at three different policy options for reducing heroin dependency and concluded that the relative costs were $5,000 (Australian) for pharmacotherapy maintenance; $11,000 (Australian) per year for residential rehabilitation; and $52,000 (Australian) per year for prison, leaving no doubt about the cost-effectiveness comparisons among these approaches. Gross et al. (2006) performed a study on 60 cocaine- and heroin-using patients, comparing medication contingencies with medication in combination with behavioral therapy, and found that the use of medication-based contingencies in combination with behavioral therapy may have feasibility but were not able to offer any cost-effectiveness data.

The interest in contingency-based programs for cocaine addiction/use has been widespread. Sigmon and Stitzer (2005) studied 102 patients enrolled in methadone maintenance treatment to examine the effect of attending group counseling. They found that adding a contingency reward for attending the counseling sessions increased attendance. The authors concluded that the data support effectiveness of low-cost incentive programs for participation in treatment. Vandrey et al. (2007) conducted a 16-week study comparing the effects of a goods-based versus cash-based program and found that the higher magnitude cash-based incentives produced greater cocaine abstinence compared with the control condition. The effect magnitude was not seen on the goods-based incentive vouchers. The efficacy and safety data revealed that giving cash to cocaine addicts did not increase their use of cocaine; on the contrary, when patients were tied to a contingency program, it had the effect of increasing their participation in the program. Other contingency approaches have been demonstrated by Petry et al. (2005), who treated 77 cocaine-dependent methadone patients in a random control design in which patients were assigned to standard treatment or standard treatment with CM. Patients with CM were more negative in urine samples for cocaine than those who were not, and they attended more groups than the patients in standard treatment.

Avants et al. (2004) evaluated 224 patients entering a methadone maintenance program who were randomly assigned to receive either standard care or counseling oriented toward risk reduction. The results showed that the patients receiving the harm reduction were more likely to be abstinent from cocaine and reported fewer unsafe sexual practices. The authors concluded that a weekly harm reduction group was somewhat more expensive than simply methadone maintenance but could bring about positive changes in behaviors and attitudes, particularly those associated with transmission of HIV.

Of two studies that examined psychotherapeutic treatments for marijuana abuses, the first by Dennis et al. (2004) measured in two randomized trials the effectiveness and cost-effectiveness of five short-term outpatient interventions for adolescents with cannabis use disorders. Trial 1 compared 5 sessions of motivational enhancement therapy plus CBT (MET/CBT5) with a 12-session regimen of MET and CBT (MET/CBT12) and family support network (FSN) that included family education and therapy components. Trial 2 compared MET/CBT5 with the adolescent community reinforcement approach (ACRA) and multidimensional family therapy (MDFT). Methodologically, it would have been preferable to have a no-treatment control group, but this was considered ethically impossible. Six hundred white male cannabis users ages 15–16 were randomly assigned. The days of abstinence and the percentage of adolescents in recovery (no drug use or abuse/dependence and living in the community) were measured during the 12 months after treatment. Two economic outcomes were measured: 1) the cost per day of abstinence over the 12-month follow-up, and 2) the cost per person in recovery at the end of the study. The costs estimates do not reflect other potential costs to society, such as subsequent treatment, missing school, health and other service utilization, arrests, and days in detention. Clinical outcomes were very similar for all treatments studied; however, cost-effectiveness differences were moderate to large in that the most cost-effective interventions were MET/CBT5 and MET/CBT12 in trial 1 and ACRA and MET/CBT5 in trial 2. Despite the greater efficacy of all treatment approaches for one-third of all subjects, two-thirds of subjects were still reporting substance use or related problems at the 12-month follow-up assessment.

In the second study, Olmstead et al. (2007) examined the cost-effectiveness of MET/CBT and CM to treat young adults with marijuana dependence. CM involved participants receiving vouchers redeemable for goods or services for attending counseling sessions or submitting marijuana-free urine specimens. One hundred and thirty-six marijuana-dependent young adults referred by the criminal justice system were randomized to one of four treatment conditions: 1) MET/CBT with CM; 2) MET/CBT without CM; 3) drug counseling (DC) with CM; and 4) DC without CM. Outcome measures included the longest duration of confirmed marijuana abstinence during treatment and the total number of marijuana-free urine specimens. Costs measured included the costs of therapy, patient drug testing, and those associated with the incentives component. Outcomes included incremental cost-effectiveness ratios that define the range of values over which each intervention would be considered cost-effective for improving each of the two patients outcomes measured during treatment. For example, the most effective treatment, MET/CBT with CM, was the most cost-effective at the highest threshold values, whereas the least effective treatment, DC, was the most effective at the lowest values. The threshold value indicates what society is willing to spend for a specific outcome. Specifically, in this study, the most effective treatment was also the most expensive because it added incremental costs. Given that marijuana is considered to be a gateway drug, if decision makers believe that improving treatment outcomes in young adults with marijuana dependence affects long-term substance abuse significantly, then they may be willing to invest in a more effective but expensive treatment for better long-term outcomes.

Abuse of stimulants has also been given attention. Stimulants are frequently used in conjunction with other drugs, and Peirce et al. (2006) reported on a random assignment of usual care with incentives trial on stimulant abstinence in patients on methadone maintenance treatment. They found that enrollees were much more likely to submit negative stimulant and alcohol samples of urine if they were given an incentive. Donovan and Wells (2007), in a study examining the potential role of the twelve-step program involvement in the treatment of methamphetamine addiction, performed a review of the literature to determine the possible extent in which involvement in twelve-step mutual self-help groups could play a role in the recovery process. And in doing so, they provided a thoughtful and useful summary.

# Dual Diagnosis

Psychoactive substance abuse, like alcohol abuse, is known to be a comorbid condition in a number of psychiatric illnesses. The likelihood of finding psychiatric illness in a substance-abusing as compared with a non-substance-abusing American is substantial (Regier et al. 1990). A substance-abusing American is 15.6 times more likely to be diagnosed with an antisocial personality disorder than an American who does not abuse substances. Similarly, a substance abuser is 10.9 times more likely to have an additional substance abuse problem, 7.4 times more likely to be schizophrenic, 5.8 times more likely to have an affective disorder, and five times more likely to suffer from an anxiety disorder than a non-substance abuser. Khantzian (1985) emphasized the manner in which psychiatric illness lowers affect tolerance and impulse control leading patients to "self-medicate." Vaillant (1980) noted that therapeutic traditions such as AA emphasized the way in which drugs induce psychosis, affective disturbance, or personality disorder in those with a normal premorbid personality. There is evidence (Khantzian 1985; Schuckit 1994) supporting both positions.

The significance of dual diagnosis from the perspective of the cost-effectiveness of treatment is that dually diagnosed patients are more likely to seek treatment for their substance abuse (Carroll and Rounsaville 1992) but are more difficult to treat (Luborsky et al. 1993; McLellan et al. 1983; Rounsaville et al. 1986). Nunes et al. (1991), Mason and Kocsis (1991), and Woody et al. (1985) all found that any Axis II disorder (but particularly antisocial personality disorder) is associated with a poorer prognosis. The severity of associated psychiatric symptoms worsens the prognosis of substance abuse treatment. Rounsaville et al. (1986), Kosten et al. (1989), and Woody et al. (1985) reported on the one exception to the previous point. Patients with antisocial personality disorder who are also depressed have a better prognosis than antisocial patients without depression. Woody et al. (1983, 1985, 1995) and Kadden et al. (1989) found that the prognosis for dually diagnosed patients improves with longer, more intensive treatment geared to address the addictive, intrapsychic, familial, social, and occupational aspects of their problems.

Maynard et al. (1999) found, in a before and after comparison of 534 patients with dual diagnosis of mental illness and substance abuse who were treated in a residential program, that there was improvement on almost all dimensions of outcome, especially before and after utilization of services. Furthermore, those who completed the program did better than those who did not complete the program in terms of utilization of counseling and medical services. The major weakness of this report is the absence of a random design and a comparison group. Nevertheless, the authors pointed out some interesting possibilities in making this comparison. For instance, they suggested the cost-offset effect of treating dually diagnosed or mentally ill and chemically abusing patients might be a significant aspect in assessing the cost-effectiveness of their treatment.

Chen et al. (2006) treated a group of 230 patients with dual substance use and psychiatric disorder. Participants received low- or high-service-intensity care in 1 of 14 residential programs and were followed for a year. High-severity patients treated in high-intensity programs had better alcohol, drug, and psychiatric outcomes at follow-up, as well as higher health care utilization and costs during the year between intake and follow-up, than those in the lower intensity program. For moderate-severity patients, high-intensity care improved the effectiveness of treatment in only one domain—drug abuse—and increased costs in the index stay but did not increase health care costs accumulated over the study year. Moderate-severity patients generally had similar outcomes in health care costs whether they were matched to low-intensity treatment or not. Matching high-severity patients to higher-service intensity improved the effectiveness of treatment, as well as increased health care costs.

Strong Kinnaman et al. (2007) used CM to treat a group of 59 dually diagnosed patients with illicit substance abuse. Their effort was to determine whether there was a difference in diagnosis and how CM was managed. They found that patients with diagnoses of schizophrenia and current substance abuse, as well as comorbid alcohol dependence, did respond to payment receipt. Tracy et al. (2007) carried out a study of applying CM to reduce substance abuse in individuals who were homeless and also had co-occurring psychiatric conditions. Overall retention in the study was high; participants assigned to CM reduced their cocaine and alcohol more than those in assessment only. The feasibility study suggests that application of low-cost CM procedures is reasonable and may reduce substance abuse.

# Survey Studies

A series of studies have surveyed alcohol and drug abusers who have made use of community treatment services in an effort to measure the impact of such treatment on the course of the illness. The purpose of these studies is to assess the effects of the broad range of substance abuse treatments as they are provided in a community on social costs associated with addiction. Mecca (1997) reviewed the California Drug and Alcohol Treatment Assessment (CALDATA) study. In this study the researchers interviewed 1,900 participants in California treatment programs 15–24 months after treatment. They found that participation in crime went from 74% of the population before treatment to 20% after treatment. Use of force or weapons was down 74.5%. Health care costs were also substantially lessened. Hospitalizations declined by 38% and hospital days by 25%. Emergency room admissions were reduced by 33%. Visits to the doctor declined 15%. Use of drugs declined 40%. The calculated cost-benefit ratio (70% of which came from reductions in crime) were as follows:

| | |
|---|---|
| Residential treatment: | $4.8 savings for every $1 treatment cost |
| Social model treatment: | $4.3 savings for every $1 treatment cost |
| Outpatient treatment: | $11.0 savings for every $1 treatment cost |
| Methadone (after discharge): | $12.6 savings for every $1 treatment cost |
| Methadone (continuing): | $4.8 savings for every $1 treatment cost |

Schildhaus et al. (1998) presented findings from the Services Research Outcomes Study (SROS). In this study the researchers interviewed 1,799 former clients from 99 drug treatment facilities to obtain a representative sample of the nearly 1 million people discharged from drug treatment across the United States in 1990. They used a survey technique to assess changes from the 5 years prior to treatment to the 5 years after treatment. They found substance abuse dropped 21% (ranging from 14% for heroin to 45% for crack). Different self-reported income-producing criminal activity (theft, burglary, dealing drugs, fraud, forgery, or prostitution) dropped after treatment in a range from 25% to 38% depending on the category of criminal activity. Drunk driving offenses dropped 25%. Measures of life stability improved after treatment. Compared with the period before treatment, there was a 40% decrease in time spent on the street, a 20% decrease in those who were victims of assault, a 30% decrease in loss of child custody, and a 43% decrease in suicide attempts.

Of course, there are serious methodological difficulties in patient self-report surveys such as SROS and CALDATA. Some difficulties, such as the reliability of substance abusers' self-report on such things as their own criminal and substance-abusing activity, were addressed by the authors of the studies. Other difficulties, such as the effect of age on criminal activity and substance abuse (the effect of the natural course of the illness on the outcome variables), are highly significant in considering efficacy and cost benefit and were not addressed by the authors. Anglin and Hser (1990) suggested that although each of the many studies are limited by methodological considerations, the studies when taken together offer support of the efficacy of treatment. Others suggest that a series of unreliable invalid measures cannot be mathematically manipulated into a reliable and valid result. The SROS survey found, for instance, that teenagers, unlike any other group, actually increased their cocaine use after treatment. This certainly leaves open the possibility that some of the "therapeutic effect" measured by SROS may be a measure of the effects of the passage of time on the illness and not the effects of treatment.

# Conclusion

The medical consequences of abusing a substance may be absent, mild, chronically disabling, or immediately life threatening. Illness can result from direct exposure to the psychoactive substance, physical neglect secondary to the addiction, trauma while intoxicated, or exposure to pathogens attendant to the lifestyle or route of administration of the drug. The psychological and social consequences of substance use vary considerably depending on the type of drug, the genetic and psychological vulnerabilities of the individual, the age at which the abuse began, and the family, local, and wider cultural response to the abuser's conduct. On each of these axes an individual may be found anywhere on a continuum from safe to imminent danger.

The multiaxial complexity of substance abuse makes generalizing from studies risky. However, certain facts are sufficiently established to guide us in our clinical work and policy recommendations (Carroll and Rounsaville 1992; Carroll et al. 1994a, 1994b, 1994c, 1998). Diagnostic and educational activities by primary medical practitioners have a high cost benefit and are underutilized. They represent a highly cost-effective form of supportive counseling. Empathy, respect, and concern are essential in any treatment. Behavioral aversive strategies help some patients, but therapies that seek to stimulate shame and guilt are counterproductive. Cognitive-behavioral psychotherapeutic strategies for building motivation to quit, arranging the circumstances of quitting, and handling relapse have proved beneficial. Specific forms of family psychotherapy (family strategies) that improve communication and reduce recrimination also have proven benefit and can assist in keeping some in treatment who would otherwise drop out. Motivational interviewing is used in a variety of addictions to address the issue of enhancing motivation. Despite substantial studies that have demonstrated the external validity quite well (namely, the degree to which the results of a study can be generalized or extended to settings or populations other than those in the particular experiment), the internal validity (the ability of the research design to rule out alternative explanations for the results) studies have been variable and weak. Investigators have not been able to identify cost-effectiveness studies for motivational interviewing directly; however, the treatment is relatively straightforward to learn, and the application of it, in most circumstances, is very low intensity and not time consuming. Any effectiveness of motivational interviewing is likely to be cost-effective (Burke et al. 2002).

Establishment of reinforcement schedules in the community can be highly useful. Treatments to help patients regulate painful affect, including Rogerian therapy, family therapy directed toward lowering levels of conflict within the family, and appropriate psychotherapy, are useful. Those who are dually diagnosed obtain significant benefit from appropriate treatment of their accompanying psychiatric disorder, which may of course include psychotherapy. While not reviewed systematically in this chapter, it is clear that use of appropriate medication to treat a comorbid psychiatric condition or to block the psychoactive effects of various substances potentiates the effects of many forms of psychotherapy by alleviating symptoms that interfere with treatment and by permitting patients to remain in the treatment setting long enough for treatment to work (Carroll et al. 1994a, 1994b; Irvin et al. 1999).

The survey literature (in what is probably its most reliable data) finds that most people seeking substance abuse treatment in the United States are dually diagnosed, use multiple substances, and are in rather advanced stages of addiction with multiple intrapsychic, occupational, medical, family, legal, and other social problems. Common sense along with what scientific data are available suggests that addressing these different problems with modalities of treatment appropriate to the problem improves outcome on a number of measures. However, we face a number of challenges. We need better treatments for those who do not respond well to current treatment. We must further our skill in matching treatment to patient. A particularly challenging area of investigation is the examination of interventions that can help reestablish a firm supportive cultural structure in those communities where both personal ties and social mores have been shattered. The dispossessed substance-abusing children of the world await this research. The development of expertise in rebuilding cultural structures has implications far beyond the control of substance abuse.

# References

Alessi SM, Hanson T, Wieners M, et al: Low-cost contingency management in community clinics: delivering incentives partially in group therapy. Exp Clin Psychopharmacol 15:293–300, 2007

Alterman AI, Gariti P, Mulvaney F: Short- and long-term smoking cessation for three levels of intensity of behavioral treatment. Psychol Addict Behav 15:261–264, 2001

Anglin MD, Hser Y: Treatment of drug abuse, in Crime and Justice: An Annual Review of Research, Vol 13. Edited by Tonry M, Wilson JO. Chicago, IL, Chicago University Press, 1990, pp 393–460

Anthony JC, Eaton WW, Mandell W: Psychoactive drug dependence and abuse: more common in some occupations than others? Journal of Employee Assistance Research 1:148–186, 1992

Anthony JC, Warner LA, Kessler RC: Comparative epidemiology of dependence on tobacco, alcohol, controlled substances, and inhalants: basic findings from the national comorbidity survey. Exp Clin Psychopharmacol 2:244–268, 1994

Anthony JC, Arria AM, Johnson EO: Epidemiological and public health issues for tobacco, alcohol, and other drugs. Review of Psychiatry 14:15–49, 1996

Avants SK, Margolin A, Kosten TR, et al: When is less treatment better? The role of social anxiety in matching methadone patients to psychosocial treatments. J Consult Clin Psychol 66:924–931, 1998

Avants SK, Margolin A, Usubiaga MH, et al: Targeting HIV-related outcomes with intravenous drug users maintained on methadone: a randomized clinical trial of a harm reduction group therapy. J Subst Abuse Treat 26:67–78, 2004

Babor TF, McRee BG, Kassebaum PA, et al: Screening, Brief Intervention, and Referral to Treatment (SBIRT): toward a public health approach to the management of substance abuse. Subst Abus 28:7–30, 2007

Barrett B, Byford S, Crawford MJ, et al: Cost-effectiveness of screening and referral to an alcohol health worker in alcohol misusing patients attending an accident and emergency department: a decision-making approach. Drug Alcohol Depend 81:47–54, 2006

Bischof G, Grothues JM, Reinhardt S, et al: Evaluation of a telephone-based stepped care intervention for alcohol-related disorders: a randomized controlled trial. Drug Alcohol Depend 93:244–251, 2008

Brandon TH: Behavioral tobacco cessation treatments: yesterday's news or tomorrow's headlines? J Clin Oncol 19 (suppl 18):64S–68S, 2001

Breslau N, Johnson EO, Hiripi E, et al: Nicotine dependence in the United States: prevalence, trends, and smoking persistence. Arch Gen Psychiatry 58:810–816, 2001

Brooner RK, Kidorf MS, King VL, et al: Comparing adaptive stepped care and monetary-based voucher interventions for opioid dependence. Drug Alcohol Depend 88 (suppl 2):S14–S23, 2007

Burke BL, Arkowitz H, Dunn C: Efficacy of Motivational Interviewing: Adaptations, what we know so far, in Motivational Interviewing: Preparing People for Change, 2nd Edition. Edited by Miller WR, Rollnick S. New York, Guilford, 2002, pp 217–250

Carroll KM, Rounsaville BJ: Contrast of treatment-seeking and untreated cocaine abusers. Arch Gen Psychiatry 49:464–471, 1992

Carroll KM, Rounsaville BJ: Psychosocial treatments for substance dependence, in The American Psychiatric Press Review of Psychiatry, Vol 14. Edited by Oldham JM, Riba MB. Washington, DC, American Psychiatric Press, 1995, pp 127–149

Carroll KM, Rounsaville BJ, Gordon LT, et al: Psychotherapy and pharmacotherapy for ambulatory cocaine abusers. Arch Gen Psychiatry 51:177–187, 1994a

Carroll KM, Rounsaville BJ, Nich C, et al: One-year follow-up of psychotherapy and pharmacotherapy for cocaine dependence. Delayed emergence of psychotherapy effects. Arch Gen Psychiatry 51:989–997, 1994b

Carroll KM, Nich C, Ball SA, et al: Treatment of cocaine and alcohol dependence with psychotherapy and disulfiram. Addiction 93:713–727, 1998

Carroll KM, Ball SA, Nich C, et al: Targeting behavioral therapies to enhance naltrexone treatment of opioid dependence: efficacy of contingency management and significant other involvement. Arch Gen Psychiatry 58:755–761, 2001

Centers for Disease Control and Prevention: Cigarette smoking-attributable mortality and years of potential life lost—United States, 1990. JAMA 270:1408, 1410, 1413, 1993

Centers for Disease Control and Prevention: Medical-care expenditures attributable to cigarette smoking—United States, 1993. JAMA 272:428–429, 1994

Chen S, Barnett PG, Sempel JM, et al: Outcomes and costs of matching the intensity of dual-diagnosis treatment to patients' symptom severity. J Subst Abuse Treat 31:95–105, 2006

Cisler R, Holder HD, Longabaugh R, et al: Actual and estimated replication costs for alcohol treatment modalities: case study from Project MATCH. J Stud Alcohol 59:503–512, 1998

Cloninger C: Genetics of substance abuse, in The American Psychiatric Publishing Textbook of Substance Abuse Treatment, 2nd Edition. Galanter M, Kleber HD. Washington, DC, American Psychiatric Press, 1999, pp 59–66

Committee on Treatment of Alcohol Problems, Institute of Medicine: Broadening the Base of Treatment for Alcohol Problems. Washington, DC, National Academy Press, 1990

Compton WM, Thomas YF, Stinson FS, et al: Prevalence, correlates, disability, and comorbidity of DSM-IV drug abuse and dependence in the United States: results from the national epidemiologic survey on alcohol and related conditions. Arch Gen Psychiatry 64:566–576, 2007

Crits-Christoph P, Siqueland L: Psychosocial treatment for drug abuse. Selected review and recommendations for national health care. Arch Gen Psychiatry 53:749–756, 1996

Davidson D, Gulliver SB, Longabaugh R, et al: Building better cognitive-behavioral therapy: is broad-spectrum treatment more effective than motivational-enhancement therapy for alcohol-dependent patients treated with naltrexone? J Stud Alcohol Drugs 68:238–247, 2007

Dennis M, Godley SH, Diamond G, et al: The Cannabis Youth Treatment (CYT) Study: main findings from two randomized trials. J Subst Abuse Treat 27:197–213, 2004

Doggrell SA: Which treatment for alcohol dependence: naltrexone, acamprosate and/or behavioural intervention? Expert Opin Pharmacother 7:2169–2173, 2006

Donovan DM, Wells EA: "Tweaking 12-Step": the potential role of 12-Step self-help group involvement in methamphetamine recovery. Addiction 102 (suppl 1):121–129, 2007

Doran CM, Shakeshaft AP, Fawcett JE: General practitioners' role in preventive medicine: scenario analysis using alcohol as a case study. Drug Alcohol Rev 23:399–404, 2004

Drummond DC: Alcohol interventions: do the best things come in small packages? Addiction 92:375–379, 1997

Epstein EE, McCrady BS: Behavioral couples treatment of alcohol and drug use disorders: current status and innovations. Clin Psychol Rev 18:689–711, 1998

Freeborn DK, Polen MR, Hollis JF, et al: Screening and brief intervention for hazardous drinking in an HMO: effects on medical care utilization. J Behav Health Serv Res 27:446–453, 2000

French MT, Zavala SK, McCollister KE, et al: Cost-effectiveness analysis of four interventions for adolescents with a substance use disorder. J Subst Abuse Treat 34:272–281, 2008

Gelernter J: Genetic factors in alcoholism: evidence and implications, in The Psychopharmacology of Alcohol Abuse. Edited by Kranzler H. New York, Springer-Verlag, 1995, pp 297–313

Gerstein DR, Johnson RA, Harwood HJ: Evaluating Recovery Services: The California Drug and Alcohol Treatment Assessment (CALDATA). Sacramento, CA, California Department of Alcohol and Drug Programs, 1994

Gordon L, Graves N, Hawkes A, et al: A review of the cost-effectiveness of face-to-face behavioural interventions for smoking, physical activity, diet and alcohol. Chronic Illn 3:101–129, 2007

Gross A, Marsch LA, Badger GJ, et al: A comparison between low-magnitude voucher and buprenorphine medication contingencies in promoting abstinence from opioids and cocaine. Exp Clin Psychopharmacol 14:148–156, 2006

Hall SM, Reus VI, Munoz RF, et al: Nortriptyline and cognitive-behavioral therapy in the treatment of cigarette smoking. Arch Gen Psychiatry 55:683–690, 1998

Halpin HA, McMenamin SB, Rideout J, et al: The costs and effectiveness of different benefit designs for treating tobacco dependence: results from a randomized trial. Inquiry 43:54–65, 2006

Harrison PA, Hoffmann NG: CATOR Report: Adult Inpatient Completers One Year Later. St. Paul, MN, Ramsey Clinic, 1989

Hester RK, Miller JH: Computer-based tools for diagnosis and treatment of alcohol problems. Alcohol Res Health 29:36–40, 2006

Holder H, Longabaugh R, Miller WR, et al: The cost effectiveness of treatment for alcoholism: a first approximation. J Stud Alcohol 52:517–540, 1991

Howard MO: Assessing the comparative cost-effectiveness of alcoholism treatments: a comment on Holder, Longabaugh, Miller and Rubonis. J Stud Alcohol 54:667–675, 1993

Irvin JE, Bowers CA, Dunn ME, et al: Efficacy of relapse prevention: a meta-analytic review. J Consult Clin Psychol 67:563–570, 1999

Israel Y, Hollander O, Sanchez-Craig M, et al: Screening for problem drinking and counseling by the primary care physician-nurse team. Alcohol Clin Exp Res 20:1443–1450, 1996

Kadden RM, Cooney NL, Getter H, et al: Matching alcoholics to coping skills or interactional therapies: posttreatment results. J Consult Clin Psychol 57:698–704, 1989

Kendler KS: Twin studies of psychiatric illness: an update. Arch Gen Psychiatry 58:1005–1014, 2001

Kessler RC, Aguilar-Gaxiola S, Berglund PA, et al: Patterns and predictors of treatment seeking after onset of a substance use disorder. Arch Gen Psychiatry 58:1065–1071, 2001

Kessler RC, Berglund P, Demler O, et al: Lifetime prevalence and age-of-onset distributions of DSM-IV disorders in the National Comorbidity Survey Replication. Arch Gen Psychiatry 62:593–602, 2005a

Kessler RC, Chiu WT, Demler O, et al: Prevalence, severity, and comorbidity of 12-month DSM-IV disorders in the National Comorbidity Survey Replication. Arch Gen Psychiatry 62:617–627, 2005b

Khantzian EJ: The self-medication hypothesis of addictive disorders: focus on heroin and cocaine dependence. Am J Psychiatry 142:1259–1264, 1985

Klesges RC, Haddock CK, Lando H, et al: Efficacy of forced smoking cessation and an adjunctive behavioral treatment on long-term smoking rates. J Consult Clin Psychol 67:952–958, 1999

Kosten TA, Kosten TR, Rounsaville BJ: Personality disorders in opiate addicts show prognostic specificity. J Subst Abuse Treat 6:163–168, 1989

Kraemer KL: The cost-effectiveness and cost-benefit of screening and brief intervention for unhealthy alcohol use in medical settings. Subst Abus 28:67–77, 2007

Kraft MK, Rothbard AB, Hadley TR, et al: Are supplementary services provided during methadone maintenance really cost-effective? Am J Psychiatry 154:1214–1219, 1997

Kunz FM Jr, French MT, Bazargan-Hejazi S: Cost-effectiveness analysis of a brief intervention delivered to problem drinkers presenting at an inner-city hospital emergency department. J Stud Alcohol 65:363–370, 2004

Landry MJ: Overview of addiction treatment effectiveness (DHHS Publ No SMA-96-3081). Rockville, MD, Substance Abuse and Mental Health Services Administration, Office of Applied Studies, 1996

Lash SJ, Gilmore JD, Burden JL, et al: The impact of contracting and prompting substance abuse treatment entry: a pilot trial. Addict Behav 30:415–422, 2005

Law M, Tang JL: An analysis of the effectiveness of interventions intended to help people stop smoking. Arch Intern Med 155:1933–1341, 1995

Lichtenstein E, Hollis JF, Severson HH, et al: Tobacco cessation interventions in health care settings: rationale, model, outcomes. Addict Behav 21:709–720, 1996

Luborsky L, Diguer L, Luborsky E, et al: Psychological health-sickness (PHS) as a predictor of outcomes in dynamic and other psychotherapies. J Consult Clin Psychol 61:542–548, 1993

Mason BJ, Kocsis JH: Desipramine treatment of alcoholism. Psychopharmacol Bull 27:155–161, 1991

Mattson ME: Matching patients to alcoholism treatment, in The Encyclopedia of Psychotherapy. Edited by Hersen M, Sledge W. New York, Academic Press, 2002, pp 123–130

Maynard C, Cox GB, Krupski A, et al: Utilization of services for mentally ill chemically abusing patients discharged from residential treatment. J Behav Health Serv Res 26:219–228, 1999

McCrady BS, Langenbucher JW: Alcohol treatment and health care system reform. Arch Gen Psychiatry 53:737–746, 1996

McLellan AT, Luborsky L, Woody GE, et al: Predicting response to alcohol and drug abuse treatments. Role of psychiatric severity. Arch Gen Psychiatry 40:620–625, 1983

Mead M: New Lives for Old: Cultural Transformation—Manus, 1928-1952. New York, Harper Collins, 1956

Mecca AM: Blending policy and research: the California outcomes study. J Psychoactive Drugs 29:161–163, 1997

Miller NS, Swift RM, Gold MS: Health care economics for integrated addiction treatment in clinical settings. Psychiatr Ann 28:682–689, 1998

Miller WR, Brown JM, Simpson T, et al: What works? A methodological analysis of the alcohol treatment outcome literature, in Handbook of Alcoholism Treatment Approaches: Effective Alternatives, 2nd Edition. Edited by Hester RK, Miller WR. Needham Heights, MA, Allyn & Bacon, 1995, pp 12–44

Moher M, Hey K, Lancaster T: Workplace interventions for smoking cessation. Cochrane Database Syst Rev 2:CD003440, 2005

Moore TJ, Ritter A, Caulkins JP: The costs and consequences of three policy options for reducing heroin dependency. Drug Alcohol Rev 26:369–378, 2007

Mortimer D, Segal L: Economic evaluation of interventions for problem drinking and alcohol dependence: cost per QALY estimates. Alcohol Alcohol 40:549–555, 2005

Mundt MP: Analyzing the costs and benefits of brief intervention. Alcohol Res Health 29:34–36, 2006

Murgraff V, Abraham C, McDermott M: Reducing Friday alcohol consumption among moderate, women drinkers: evaluation of a brief evidence-based intervention. Alcohol Alcohol 42:37–41, 2007

Nunes EV, Quitkin FM, Brady R, et al: Imipramine treatment of methadone maintenance patients with affective disorder and illicit drug use. Am J Psychiatry 148:667–669, 1991

Olivier D, Lubman DI, Fraser R: Tobacco smoking within psychiatric inpatient settings: biopsychosocial perspective. Aust N Z J Psychiatry 41:572–580, 2007

Olmstead TA, Sindelar JL, Easton CJ, et al: The cost-effectiveness of four treatments for marijuana dependence. Addiction 102:1443–1453, 2007

Onken L, Blaine J: Psychotherapy and counseling research in drug abuse treatment: questions, problems, and solutions, in Psychotherapy and Counseling in the Treatment of Drug Abuse (NIDA Res Monogr 104). Rockville, MD, National Institute of Drug Abuse, 1990, pp 1–5

Peirce JM, Petry NM, Stitzer ML, et al: Effects of lower-cost incentives on stimulant abstinence in methadone maintenance treatment: a National Drug Abuse Treatment Clinical Trials Network study. Arch Gen Psychiatry 63:201–208, 2006

Petry NM, Martin B, Simcic F Jr: Prize reinforcement contingency management for cocaine dependence: integration with group therapy in a methadone clinic. J Consult Clin Psychol 73:354–359, 2005

Powell BJ, Penick EC, Read MR, et al: Comparison of three outpatient treatment interventions: a twelve-month follow-up of men alcoholics. J Stud Alcohol 46:309–312, 1985

Regier DA, Farmer ME, Rae DS, et al: Comorbidity of mental disorders with alcohol and other drug abuse. Results from the Epidemiologic Catchment Area (ECA) Study. JAMA 264:2511–2518, 1990

Regier DA, Narrow WE, Rae DS, et al: The de facto US mental and addictive disorders service system. Epidemiologic catchment area prospective 1-year prevalence rates of disorders and services. Arch Gen Psychiatry 50:85–94, 1993

Rice D, Kelman S, Miller L, et al: The economic costs of alcohol and drug abuse and mental illness (DHHS Publ No ADM-90-1694). Rockville, MD, Alcohol, Drug Abuse, and Mental Health Administration, 1990

Rigotti NA, Pasternak RC: Cigarette smoking and coronary heart disease: risks and management. Cardiol Clin 14:51–68, 1996

Ross HE, Glaser FB, Germanson T: The prevalence of psychiatric disorders in patients with alcohol and other drug problems. Arch Gen Psychiatry 45:1023–1031, 1988

Rounsaville BJ, Kosten TR, Weissman MM, et al: Prognostic significance of psychopathology in treated opiate addicts. A 2.5-year follow-up study. Arch Gen Psychiatry 43:739–745, 1986

Saitz R: Screening and brief intervention enter their 5th decade. Subst Abus 28:3–6, 2007

Schildhaus S, Gerstein DR, Brittingham A, et al: Services Research Outcomes Study. Rockville, MD, Substance Abuse and Mental Health Services Administration, Office of Applied Statistics, 1998

Schuckit M: The relationship between alcohol problems, substance abuse, and psychiatric syndromes, in DSM-IV Sourcebook. Edited by Widiger T, Frances A, Pincus H. Washington, DC, American Psychiatric Association Press, 1994, pp 45–66

Shaffer HJ, LaSalvia TA, Stein JP: Comparing Hatha yoga with dynamic group psychotherapy for enhancing methadone maintenance treatment: a randomized clinical trial. Altern Ther Health Med 3:57–66, 1997

Sigmon SC, Stitzer ML: Use of a low-cost incentive intervention to improve counseling attendance among methadone-maintained patients. J Subst Abuse Treat 29:253–258, 2005

Stead LF, Lancaster T: Group behaviour therapy programmes for smoking cessation. Cochrane Database Syst Rev 2:CD001007, 2005

Strong Kinnaman JE, Slade E, Bennett ME, et al: Examination of contingency payments to dually diagnosed patients in a multi-faceted behavioral treatment. Addict Behav 32:1480–1485, 2007

Tracy K, Babuscio T, Nich C, et al: Contingency management to reduce substance use in individuals who are homeless with co-occurring psychiatric disorders. Am J Drug Alcohol Abuse 33:253–258, 2007

Treno AJ, Holder HD: Measurement of alcohol-involved injury in community prevention: the search for a surrogate III. Alcohol Clin Exp Res 21:1695–1703, 1997

UKATT Research Team: Cost effectiveness of treatment for alcohol problems: findings of the randomised UK alcohol treatment trial (UKATT). BMJ 331:544, 2005

UKATT Research Team: UK Alcohol Treatment Trial: client-treatment matching effects. Addiction 103:228–238, 2008

U.S. Department of Health and Human Services: Smoking cessation: clinical practice guideline No 18 (AHCPR Publ No 96-0692). Rockville, MD, U.S. Department of Health and Human Services, 1996

Vaillant GE: Natural history of male psychological health: VIII. Antecedents of alcoholism and "orality." Am J Psychiatry 137:181–186, 1980

Vandrey R, Bigelow GE, Stitzer ML: Contingency management in cocaine abusers: a dose-effect comparison of goods-based versus cash-based incentives. Exp Clin Psychopharmacol 15:338–343, 2007

West R, McNeill A, Raw M: Smoking cessation guidelines for health professionals: an update. Health Education Authority. Thorax 55:987–999, 2000

West R, McNeill A, Raw M: Smokeless tobacco cessation guidelines for health professionals in England. Br Dent J 196:611–618, 2004

Westmaas JL, Nath V, Brandon TH: Contemporary smoking cessation. Cancer Control 7:56–62, 2000

White HR, Morgan TJ, Pugh LA, et al: Evaluating two brief substance-use interventions for mandated college students. J Stud Alcohol 67:309–317, 2006

Wolfenden L, Wiggers J, Knight J, et al: Increasing smoking cessation care in a preoperative clinic: a randomized controlled trial. Prev Med 41:284–290, 2005

Woody GE, Luborsky L, McLellan AT, et al: Psychotherapy for opiate addicts. Does it help? Arch Gen Psychiatry 40:639–645, 1983

Woody GE, McLellan AT, Luborsky L, et al: Sociopathy and psychotherapy outcome. Arch Gen Psychiatry 42:1081–1086, 1985

Woody GE, McLellan AT, Luborsky L, et al: Psychotherapy in community methadone programs: a validation study. Am J Psychiatry 152:1302–1308, 1995

World Health Organization: WHO Expert Committee on Drug Dependence: 30th Report (WHO Technical Report Series No 873). Geneva, World Health Organization, 1998

Zarkin GA, Bray JW, Mitra D, et al: Cost methodology of COMBINE. J Stud Alcohol Suppl:50–55; discussion 33, 2005

## Summary of studies addressing cost-effectiveness in the treatment of substance abuse

| Articles | Subjects | Treatment | Outcome |
|---|---|---|---|
| **Treatment of tobacco addiction** | | | |
| Centers for Disease Control and Prevention 1993 | Review. | NA | Report that details the mortality and years of potential life lost attributable to cigarette smoking in the United States based on data from 1990. |
| Centers for Disease Control and Prevention 1994 | Review. | NA | Report that details the medical care expenditures attributable to cigarette smoking in the United States based on data from 1993. |
| Alterman et al. 2001 | 240 one-pack-a-day smokers: assigned to one of three different interventions with 80 in each treatment cell. | 1. A low-intensity (LI) group that received 8 weeks of nicotine replacement therapy (NRT) and one advice and education (A&E) session with a nurse practitioner (NP). 2. A moderate-intensity (MI) group with NRT and four A&E sessions with an NP. 3. A high-intensity (HI) group that received NRT, four A&E sessions, and 12 weeks of individualized cognitive-behavioral therapy (CBT). | Biochemically confirmed abstinence rates at 9, 26, and 52 weeks posttreatment initiation were highest for the HI (45%, 37%, 35%) group, followed by the LI (35%, 30%, and 27%) and MI (27%, 12%, 12%) groups. Group differences approached statistical significance at 9 weeks and were statistically significant at both 26 and 52 weeks. |

## Summary of studies addressing cost-effectiveness in the treatment of substance abuse *(continued)*

| Articles | Subjects | Treatment | Outcome |
|---|---|---|---|
| **Treatment of tobacco addiction *(continued)*** | | | |
| Moher et al. 2005 | Review. | Various. | Workplace interventions aimed at helping individuals to stop smoking included 10 studies of group therapy (GT), 7 studies of individual counseling (IC), 9 studies of self-help materials (SH), and 5 studies of NRT. The results were consistent with those found in other settings. GT, IC, and NRT increased cessation rates in comparison with no treatment or minimal intervention controls. SH were less effective. Workplace interventions aimed at the workforce as a whole included 14 studies of tobacco bans, 2 studies of social support, 4 studies of environmental support, 5 studies of incentives, and 8 studies of comprehensive (multi-component) programs. Tobacco bans decreased cigarette consumption during the working day, but their effect on total consumption was less certain. There was a lack of evidence that comprehensive programs reduced the prevalence of smoking. Competitions and incentives increased attempts to stop smoking, but there was less evidence that they increased the rate of quitting. |

**Summary of studies addressing cost-effectiveness in the treatment of substance abuse *(continued)***

| Articles | Subjects | Treatment | Outcome |
|---|---|---|---|
| **Treatment of tobacco addiction *(continued)*** | | | |
| Stead and Lancaster 2005 | Review. | Various group approaches. | There was an increase in cessation with the use of a group program ($N$=4,395, odds ratio [OR] 2.04, 95% confidence interval [CI] 1.60 to 2.60). Group programs were more effective than no-intervention controls (seven trials, $N$=815, OR 2.17, 95% CI 1.37 to 3.45). There was no evidence that group therapy was more effective than a similar intensity of individual counseling. There was limited evidence that the addition of group therapy to other forms of treatment, such as advice from a health professional or nicotine replacement, produced extra benefit. |
| Halpin et al. 2006 | 393 adult smokers enrolled in a California preferred provider organization. | Random assignment to one of three different benefit designs for treating tobacco dependence: drugs only (NRT patch, nasal spray, inhaler, and Zyban); drugs and counseling (drugs and proactive telephone counseling); and drugs if counseling (drugs conditional on enrollment in counseling). | After 8 months, there were no significant increases in quit attempts or quit rates in the groups with covered drugs and counseling compared with the group with drug coverage only. Therefore, costs rose with no increase in quit rates when proactive telephone counseling was added to coverage of pharmacotherapy, regardless of benefit design. |

## Summary of studies addressing cost-effectiveness in the treatment of substance abuse *(continued)*

| Articles | Subjects | Treatment | Outcome |
|---|---|---|---|
| **Treatment of tobacco addiction** *(continued)* | | | |
| Gordon et al. 2007 | Review. | Various behavioral approaches. | There was considerable variation among the studies by target populations, intervention components, primary outcomes, and economic methods, but the reported incremental cost-effectiveness ratios were consistently low (e.g., <14,000 euros per quality-adjusted life-year [QALY] gained for smoking-cessation programs in 2006 euros) as compared with preventive pharmaceutical and invasive interventions. Interventions targeting high-risk-population subgroups were relatively better value for money as compared with those targeting general populations. |
| **Alcohol addiction and psychotherapy** | | | |
| Holder et al. 1991 | An analysis of cost-effectiveness of alcoholism treatment modalities based on 1) findings from clinical trials, 2) costs for treatment in settings and/or by providers, and 3) recommendations from treatment experts. | Various. | The results of this first effort to establish initial cost/effectiveness considerations are intended to stimulate researchers to conduct the types of clinical studies where both cost and effectiveness are carefully measured to increase the scientific basis for future cost/effect policy considerations. The authors expect future clinical studies will revise the results of this initial effort. |

## Summary of studies addressing cost-effectiveness in the treatment of substance abuse *(continued)*

| Articles | Subjects | Treatment | Outcome |
|---|---|---|---|
| **Alcohol addiction and psychotherapy** *(continued)* | | | |
| Cisler et al. 1998 | Examines the relative costs of three manual-guided, individually delivered treatments and the costs of replicating them in nonresearch settings. | Various individual treatments. | For Project MATCH, motivational enhancement therapy (MET) cost twice as much or more per patient contact hour (mean=$498) than CBT (mean=$198) and twelve-step facilitation treatment (TSF) (mean=$253) but was less costly per research participant (mean=$1,700) than both CBT (mean=$1,901) and TSF (mean=$1,969). For clinical replication, high-end per-patient costs ranged from $512 for MET to $750 for TSF to $788 for CBT: a cost savings for MET of $238 (32%) over TSF and $276 (35%) over CBT. |
| Doran et al. 2004 | Review intended to determine 1) level of general practitioner (GP) detection of at-risk drinking, 2) rates at which intervention is offered, and 3) effectiveness of interventions. | Secondary intentions were to develop a model based on these findings that can be used in conjunction with scenario analysis and to consider the cost implications of current efforts and various scenarios. This study deals specifically with Australian general practice. | The results suggest that increasing rates of GP intervention achieves greatest benefit and return on resource use. For every 5% point increase in the rate of GP intervention, an additional 26,754 at-risk drinkers modify their drinking behavior at a cost of $231.45 (Australian) per patient. This compares with a cost per patient modifying drinking behavior of $232.60 and $208.31 (Australian) for every 5% point increase in the rates of detection and effectiveness, respectively. |

**Summary of studies addressing cost-effectiveness in the treatment of substance abuse** *(continued)*

| Articles | Subjects | Treatment | Outcome |
|---|---|---|---|
| **Alcohol addiction and psychotherapy** *(continued)* | | | |
| Kunz et al. 2004 | 1,036 subjects were screened for problem drinking during their visit to an emergency department. Eligible participants (*N*=294) were randomly assigned to either a brief intervention group or a control group. As the result of attrition, a final sample of 194 (90 brief intervention; 104 control) participants remained at follow-up. | The intervention consisted of a brief counseling session and a health information packet. The control group received only the packet. Intervention cost data were collected and analyzed using the Drug Abuse Treatment Cost Analysis Program. | The average economic cost of the brief intervention was $632 per subject, of which screening ($497) was the largest component. In all cases, intervention subjects had better 3-month outcomes than control subjects, but the differences were not always statistically significant. Cost-effectiveness ratios were relatively small for all three outcomes, suggesting this type of intervention has the potential to be cost-effective under full implementation. |
| Lash et al. 2005 | 102 individuals scheduled to begin a 28-day substance use disorder residential treatment program. | Random assignment to either standard treatment (STX) or STX plus attendance contracting and prompting (CP). | CP participants showed fewer subsequent hospitalization days, lower hospitalization costs, greater improvement in alcohol problem scores, and lower legal problem scores at a 3-month follow-up than the STX group. The two groups did not differ on treatment entry rate, time in treatment, or drug use problem scores. |

## Summary of studies addressing cost-effectiveness in the treatment of substance abuse *(continued)*

| Articles | Subjects | Treatment | Outcome |
|---|---|---|---|
| **Alcohol addiction and psychotherapy *(continued)*** | | | |
| Mortimer and Segal 2005 | Review. | The evaluated interventions were divided into mutually exclusive programs: 1) brief interventions, 2) psychotherapy for mild to moderate dependence, and 3) drug-therapy adjuvant to counseling for detoxified patients with a history of severe dependence. | Cost per QALY estimates for each of the interventions fall below any putative funding threshold for developed economies. Interventions for problem drinkers appear to offer better value than interventions targeted at those with a history of severe physical dependence. |
| UKATT Research Team 2005 | 742 clients with alcohol problems; 617 (83.2%) were interviewed at 12 months and full economic data were obtained on 608 (98.5% of 617). | Main economic measures: QALYs, costs of trial treatments, and consequences for public sector resources (health care, other alcohol treatment, social services, and criminal justice services). | Both therapies saved about five times as much in expenditure on health, social, and criminal justice services as they cost. Neither net savings nor cost-effectiveness differed significantly between the therapies, despite the average cost of social behavior and network therapy (221 pounds sterling; $385; 320 euros) being significantly more than that of motivational enhancement therapy (129 pounds sterling). If a QALY were worth 30,000 pounds sterling, then the motivational therapy would have a 58% chance of being more cost-effective than the social therapy, and the social therapy would have a 42% chance of being more cost-effective than the motivational therapy. |

## Summary of studies addressing cost-effectiveness in the treatment of substance abuse *(continued)*

| Articles | Subjects | Treatment | Outcome |
| --- | --- | --- | --- |
| **Alcohol addiction and psychotherapy *(continued)*** | | | |
| Zarkin et al. 2005 | Review. | Cost-analysis review of the treatments used in the COMBINE study. | The authors present the estimated cost per activity for 15 intake assessments plus the medical management (MM) and combined behavioral intervention (CBI) sessions for 9 of the 11 COMBINE sites. Labor costs represent the bulk of the total cost for all activities. The CBI session is more expensive than the MM session. |
| Barrett et al. 2006 | 599 adults identified as drinking hazardously according to the Paddington Alcohol Test. | Random assignment to referral to an alcohol health worker (AHW) who delivered a brief intervention (*n*=287) or to an information-only control (*n*=312). Total societal costs and clinical measures of alcohol consumption were measured. | Levels of drinking were observably lower in those referred to an AHW at 12 months follow-up and statistically significantly lower at 6 months follow-up. Total costs were not significantly different at either follow-up. Referral to AHWs in an accident and emergency department (AED) produces favorable clinical outcomes and does not generate a significant increase in cost. A decision-making approach revealed that there is at least a 65% probability that referral to an AHW is more cost-effective than the information-only control in reducing alcohol consumption among AED attendees with a hazardous level of drinking. |

**Summary of studies addressing cost-effectiveness in the treatment of substance abuse *(continued)***

| Articles | Subjects | Treatment | Outcome |
|---|---|---|---|
| **Alcohol addiction and psychotherapy** *(continued)* | | | |
| Mundt 2006 | 392 intervention and 382 control subjects. | Randomized controlled trial of screening and brief intervention (SBI) in primary care clinics. | This study revealed that Project TrEAT led to a reduction in alcohol consumption by high-risk drinkers and a corresponding reduction in medical and societal costs. Overall, this study supported the cost-effectiveness of Project TrEAT, concluding that its costs were outweighed by its benefits. |
| Babor et al. 2007 | Review. | SBIRT | With the accumulation of positive evidence, implementation research on alcohol SBI was begun in the 1990s, followed by trials of similar methods for other substances (e.g., illicit drugs, tobacco, prescription drugs) and by national demonstration programs in the United States and other countries. That SBIRT yields short-term improvements in individuals' health is irrefutable; long-term effects on population health have not yet been demonstrated, but simulation models suggest that the benefits could be substantial. |
| Kraemer 2007 | Review. | SBI | Overall, the reviewed studies support alcohol SBI in medical settings as a wise use of health care resources and illustrate the usefulness of economic evaluation for assessing alcohol prevention and treatment programs. |

**Summary of studies addressing cost-effectiveness in the treatment of substance abuse *(continued)***

| Articles | Subjects | Treatment | Outcome |
|---|---|---|---|
| **Alcohol addiction and psychotherapy *(continued)*** | | | |
| French et al. 2008 | 120 adolescents (96 boys and 24 girls) and their families. | The present study attempted a cost-effectiveness analysis of four interventions, including family based, individual, and group cognitive–behavioral approaches, for adolescents with a substance use disorder. | Results indicated that treatment costs varied substantially across the four interventions. Moreover, family therapy showed significantly better substance use outcome compared with group treatment at the 4-month assessment, but group treatment was similar to the other interventions for substance use outcome at the 7-month assessment and for delinquency outcome at both the 4- and 7-month assessments. These findings over a relatively short follow-up period suggest that the least expensive intervention (group) was the most cost-effective. |
| **Nonlegal drugs—use and abuse: marijuana, cocaine, and opiates** | | | |
| Kraft et al. 1997 | 100 methadone-maintained opiate users randomly assigned to three treatment groups with different levels of support services over a 24-week trial. | One group received methadone treatment with a minimum of counseling, the second received methadone plus more intensive counseling, and the third received methadone plus enhanced counseling, medical, and psychosocial services. | The follow-up analysis reaffirmed the preliminary findings that the methadone plus counseling level provided the most cost-effective implementation of the treatment program. At 12 months, the annual cost per abstinent client was $16,485, $9,804, and $11,818 for the low, intermediate, and high levels of support, respectively. Abstinence rates were highest, but modestly so, for the group receiving the high-intensity, high-cost methadone with enhanced services intervention. |

## Summary of studies addressing cost-effectiveness in the treatment of substance abuse *(continued)*

| Articles | Subjects | Treatment | Outcome |
|---|---|---|---|
| Nonlegal drugs—use and abuse: marijuana, cocaine, and opiates *(continued)* | | | |
| Dennis et al. 2004 | 600 cannabis users were predominantly white males, ages 15–16 years. | Trial 1 compared 5 sessions of motivational enhancement therapy plus CBT (MET/CBT5) with a 12-session regimen of MET and CBT (MET/CBT12) and another that included family education and therapy components (family support network [FSN]). Trial 2 compared MET/CBT5 with the adolescent community reinforcement approach (ACRA) and multidimensional family therapy. | The clinical outcomes were very similar across sites and conditions; however, after controlling for initial severity, the most cost-effective interventions were MET/CBT5 and MET/CBT12 in trial 1 and ACRA and MET/CBT5 in trial 2. |

**Summary of studies addressing cost-effectiveness in the treatment of substance abuse *(continued)***

| Articles | Subjects | Treatment | Outcome |
|---|---|---|---|
| Nonlegal drugs—use and abuse: marijuana, cocaine, and opiates *(continued)* | | | |
| Moore et al. 2007 | Review. | Sensitivity analyses using Australian data, including varying the magnitude and duration of treatment effects, and ascribing positive outcomes only to treatment completers. | If the postprogram abstinence rates are sustained for 2 years, then for an average heroin user the cost of averting a year of heroin use is approximately $5,000 (Australian) for pharmacotherapy maintenance, $11,000 (Australian) for residential rehabilitation, and $52,000 (Australian) for prison. Varying the parameters does not change the ranking of the programs. If the completion rate in pharmacotherapy maintenance was raised above 95% (by the threat of prison for noncompleters), the combined model of treatment plus prison may become the most cost-effective option. |

**Summary of studies addressing cost-effectiveness in the treatment of substance abuse *(continued)***

| Articles | Subjects | Treatment | Outcome |
|---|---|---|---|
| Nonlegal drugs—use and abuse: marijuana, cocaine, and opiates *(continued)* | | | |
| Olmstead et al. 2007 | A total of 136 marijuana-dependent young adults, all referred by the criminal justice system. | Random assignment to one of four treatment conditions: MET/CBT with contingency management (CM), MET/CBT without CM, drug counseling (DC) with CM, and DC without CM. Patient outcome measures include the longest duration of confirmed marijuana abstinence during treatment and the total number of marijuana-free urine specimens provided during treatment. | Given the relatively small and specialized nature of the study sample, and the fact that the authors examined a CM procedure with a single reinforcement schedule, additional studies are warranted to determine the reliability and generalizability of the results both to alternative marijuana-using populations and to CM procedures with alternative incentive parameters. Nevertheless, the relative durability of effects of MET/CBT compared with DC through the 6-month follow-up, and its cost-effectiveness over a comparatively wide range of threshold values, underscores the promise of this approach. |

## Summary of studies addressing cost-effectiveness in the treatment of substance abuse *(continued)*

| Articles | Subjects | Treatment | Outcome |
| --- | --- | --- | --- |
| **Dual diagnosis** | | | |
| Kosten et al. 1989 | 150 treated opioid addicts. | Rates of depression and alcoholism as well as assessments of specific problems were measured in a 2.5-year follow-up. | Using DSM-III criteria, the authors found that borderline personality disorder predicted more depressive disorders and alcoholism at follow-up; yet greater recovery from these disorders was seen. Borderline patients had more severe psychiatric problems as measured by the Addiction Severity Index (ASI). Other ASI outcomes differed by personality disorder; antisocial addicts had more legal problems, and narcissistic addicts had more medical problems. These results suggest that treatment for opiate addicts be tailored to the specific needs of the patients, which can be predicted, in part, by their comorbid personality disorder diagnosis. |

## Summary of studies addressing cost-effectiveness in the treatment of substance abuse *(continued)*

| Articles | Subjects | Treatment | Outcome |
|---|---|---|---|
| **Dual diagnosis** *(continued)* | | | |
| Chen et al. 2006 | 230 patients with dual substance use and psychiatric disorders. | Participants received low or high service-intensity acute care in 1 of 14 residential programs and were followed up for 1 year (80%) using the ASI. Patients' health care utilization was assessed from charts, Department of Veterans Affairs (VA) databases, and health care diaries; costs were assigned using methods established by the VA Health Economics Resource Center. | High-severity patients treated in high-intensity programs had better alcohol, drug, and psychiatric outcomes at follow-up, as well as higher health care utilization and costs during the year between intake and follow-up than did those in low-intensity programs. For moderate-severity patients, high service intensity improved the effectiveness of treatment in only a single domain (drug abuse) and increased costs of the index stay but did not increase health care costs accumulated over the study year. Moderate-severity patients generally had similar outcomes and health care costs whether they were matched to low-intensity treatment or not. For high-severity patients, matching to higher service intensity improved the effectiveness of treatment as well as increased health care costs. |
| **General topics** | | | |
| Luborsky et al. 1993 | Systematic review of quantitative studies on Sigmund Freud's proposition that the poorer the psychological health, the more limited are the benefits from treatment. | This article reviews 1) main methods of measurement, 2) the record of predictive success, 3) validity studies, 4) the relation to psychiatric diagnosis, 5) prediction in forms of treatment other than psychotherapy, and 6) theories of why psychological health predicts outcomes of psychotherapy. | The majority of the studies show significant prediction of outcomes of psychotherapy, with correlations between .2 and .35. |

## Summary of studies addressing cost-effectiveness in the treatment of substance abuse *(continued)*

| Articles | Subjects | Treatment | Outcome |
|---|---|---|---|
| **General topics** *(continued)* | | | |
| Regier et al. 1993 | 20,291 adults in the National Institute of Mental Health Epidemiologic Catchment Area Program. | Interviews. | An annual prevalence rate of 28.1% for addictive disorders was found, composed of a 1-month point prevalence of 15.7% (at wave 1) and a 1-year incidence of new or recurrent disorders identified in 12.3% of the population at wave 2. During the 1-year follow-up period, 6.6% of the total sample developed one or more new disorders after being assessed as having no previous lifetime diagnosis at wave 1. An additional 5.7% of the population, with a history of some previous disorder at wave 1, had an acute relapse or suffered from a new disorder in 1 year. Irrespective of diagnosis, 14.7% of the U.S. population in 1 year reported use of services in one or more component sectors of the de facto U.S. mental and addictive service system. Persons with specific disorders varied in the proportion who used services, from a high of more than 60% for somatization, schizophrenia, and bipolar disorders to a low of less than 25% for addictive disorders and severe cognitive impairment. |

## Summary of studies addressing cost-effectiveness in the treatment of substance abuse *(continued)*

| Articles | Subjects | Treatment | Outcome |
|---|---|---|---|
| **General topics *(continued)*** | | | |
| Gerstein et al. 1994 | Participants were selected at random from treatment or discharge lists from four types of programs, including both residential and community-based programs. The sample of approximately 3,000 individuals represented the nearly 150,000 individuals in treatment. | Standard drug treatment vs. none. | Results revealed treatment costs of $209 million and savings of $1.5 billion during treatment and in the 1st year afterward. The savings resulted mostly from reductions in crime. The cost-benefit ratios for society ranged from 2:1 to more than 4:1, depending on the treatment type; however, methadone treatment that ended in discharge resulted in net losses, mainly from participants' earnings losses. Benefits persisted for participants followed as long as 2 years. Results also revealed that treatment resulted in reductions in crime, alcohol and drug use, and health care. The analysis concluded that drug treatment programs were a good investment. |
| Miller et al. 1998 | Commentary. | — | The authors provide an explanation of the current addiction treatment system and how it continues to evolve in clinical practice. |

# 8 | Psychotherapy for Patients With Medical Conditions

William H. Sledge, M.D.
Joel Gold, M.D.

**H**ealth is an important issue for society in general as well as for the individuals in a society. Every person will at one time or another become medically ill themselves or become involved in the care of family or friends who require medical attention. Illness poses special dilemmas for those who are sick as well as for their loved ones and others who depend on them. While there is a broad range of seriousness among illnesses and all illnesses are not fatal or disabling, the ambiguity of medical symptoms, particularly at their initial manifestation, poses threats to the function and perhaps life of the individual. It is a narcissistic injury in most cases to discover that one is ill, however fleeting and limited. It means, at the least, a temporary diminution of function and vitality and may be accompanied by pain, suffering, and disfigurement. Because illness may also herald a permanently disabling or life-threatening condition, being ill is frequently associated with a heightened emotional state of fear, anxiety, and need.

Furthermore, the requirements of the sick role are such that the ill person must seek competent medical care. The sick person must depend on the competence of medical caregivers without a good means of assessing that

competency himself or herself. The ill person must submit to the invasion of
body and privacy that such care entails, telling his or her story to someone
who may be a stranger and allowing that person access to his or her body,
secrets, and fears. Therefore, the ill person not only is in a heightened state
of fear and anxiety but also is dependent on others (who may be strangers)
for diagnosis and treatment. The ill person must trust that these caregivers
will be benignly motivated and highly skilled. It is no wonder that patients
may "regress" under these circumstances and that there can be tragic fail-
ures of communication.

The personal demands for the physician are also great and require substantial discipline and adaptation to negotiate the professionalization of this
intimate relationship. Parsons (1951) wrote about how the profession of
medicine is structured to ensure access to health care according to the needs
of society and the application of technical knowledge within the circum-
stance of this highly charged relationship. Sometimes this relationship does
not function well and patients do not receive the care that they need or desire (Sledge and Feinstein 1997).

# Emotional Disorders in
# Medically Ill Patients

Psychological and physical health have long been recognized as being inti-
mately connected. Indeed, the mind-body dualism of Western intellectual
tradition has not served the integrated care of ill people well. We do not
intend a comprehensive treatment of this topic; clearly the radical reduc-
tionism of a strictly biological approach has allowed great advances in the
understanding of the biological basis of diseases, but this approach has not,
to date, been able to accommodate a comprehensive understanding of the
social and psychological dimensions of illness and the care of ill people
(Engel 1977). It is a truism and established common sense that one's mental
state can affect one's physical well-being. There is also a wealth of scientifi-
cally collected evidence to support this idea. While this mutually influencing
boundary of mind and body has been recognized for many eons, recently
more compelling concrete evidence indicating the details of this direct relationship between the two has begun to emerge. It is important to stress
the bidirectional influences between the domains of physical and mental (Ader
et al. 1990; Kiecolt-Glaser and Glaser 1992). Psychological distress contributes to physical illnesses and vice versa. While it is not always clear as to which
comes first, the studies cited below clearly point to this interconnectedness
of psyche and soma and to the importance of attending to them both in the
effort to care for the ill.

An often-cited groundbreaking study of this bidirectionality in terms of psychotherapy (Baxter et al. 1992) found that patients with obsessive-compulsive disorder treated with behavioral therapy had the same changes in brain metabolism as did those treated with pharmacotherapy. As research progresses in fields such as psychoneuroendocrinology (Ader et al. 1990; Kennedy et al. 1988; Kiecolt-Glaser and Glaser 1992), more evidence that the effect one's mental state has on one's physical health will come to light. In the meantime, however, we can look to clinical studies that show that medically ill people who receive some form of psychotherapy feel better and live longer than those who do not. More important, perhaps, those receiving psychological support experience a better understanding of themselves, their relationship to their illness, and a greater sense of well-being (House et al. 1988).

# Emotional Distress, Psychopathology, and Medical Conditions

Emotional distress is associated with disease and disability that, in and of themselves, are experienced as emotionally stressful and may exacerbate underlying psychiatric and medical disorders, or even produce new ones. Consequently, the coexistence of emotional distress rising to the level of diagnosable psychopathology is relatively common. Katon (1987) reported a 6%–10% prevalence of depression among primary care populations. Furthermore, Katon and Russo (1989) found that patients with major depression had significantly higher positive somatic symptoms than those without a psychiatric disorder. Katon and Roy-Byrne (1989) described physical symptoms mimicking medical illness among patients with panic disorder, leading to higher medical utilization and patient suffering.

Patients who have high levels of stress are subject to greater rates of mortality and have weakened immune functioning. House et al. (1988) described an increased risk of death among people with poor social relationships, noting that this risk is as great as smoking or high serum cholesterol. Zubenko et al. (1997) studied 809 elderly patients with DSM-III-R (American Psychiatric Association 1987) diagnoses of organic mental, mood, or psychotic disorders, following acute admission for these disorders over a period of 5 years 9 months. They reported that these patients had mortality ratios that were 1.5 to 2.5 times that of the age-matched general population. Spiegel and Kato (1996) reviewed 19 articles and concluded that social isolation increases mortality risk from cancer.

Various studies implicate psychological stress as damaging to one's immune system (Ader et al. 1990; Kennedy et al. 1988). Kennedy et al. (1988)

observed changes in herpes virus latency, decreases in the percentage of t-helper lymphocytes, and decreases in the number of natural killer cells in subjects exposed to acute or chronic psychological stressors. These changes were correlated with loneliness and depression. Moreover, positive impacts on immune functioning have been effected through various cognitive-behavioral strategies (Kiecolt-Glaser and Glaser 1992), as well as brief group psychotherapy (Fawzy et al. 1990b, 1993).

# Psychotherapy

Although we have defined psychotherapy as an attempt to relieve suffering and restore or increase capacity and function through disciplined talking and listening, for the purposes of this chapter, we review interventions that are formally psychotherapy as well as other psychological approaches. We have both practical and conceptual reasons for taking this broad, liberal definition of psychotherapy. Practically, there are very few studies of formal psychotherapy for the care of medical conditions with or without recognized psychopathology. Even fewer address cost-effectiveness. Our conceptual reason that may explain the practical issue is that care is not organized and delivered in such a way for psychotherapy to be the main focus of such care and in many instances even to be a part of care. In the face of diagnosable medical pathology, the medical care dominates the provision of services, as well it should. Furthermore, even when there are recognized and acknowledged mental pain and suffering and psychopathology, most doubly-diagnosed patients prefer to focus on their medical care. And there is the issue of the relative blindness to psychological issues that is characteristic of American and even Western medical approaches.

But there is a psychological dimension to all medical care. All events in the encounter of patient and caregiver (Sledge and Feinstein 1997) are important to one or both parties in the exchange even though we may not explicitly recognize these interventions in how we organize and pay for these encounters. Perhaps the most salient psychological "service" is that of the relationship between patient and physician. And indeed, there is a vast literature that suggests the importance of this critical relationship, but there is remarkably very little empirical research on what are the critical, curative features in such a relationship.

Here for the purposes of this review, we will not include studies of the generic, nonspecific features of the doctor-patient relationship unless they address some specific intervention. However, we will include other psychological interventions designed to be helpful and that are psychotherapy-like in their deployment, for example, such services as consultations, liaison activities, psychoeducation, and clinical case management (Sledge et al. 1995);

furthermore, dedicated self-help and support groups will be included in our review. This approach is justified in that it resembles how care is delivered and organized, and it provides data to begin to make reasonable inferences in the face of the absence of definitive data. The table at the end of this chapter summarizes the salient studies with a specific cost-effectiveness dimension. The criteria for including studies in the table are the use of a random design methodology in assigning patients, the presence of a clear, well-defined psychological intervention, and outcome measured clinically as well as utilization and/or cost. We also included salient reviews.

# Role of Psychological Approaches

Given the ubiquity of psychological and social issues, it would be reasonable to suppose that psychological approaches may have a role in the treatment of medical conditions through reducing pain and suffering, promoting recovery, and enhancing compliance and thereby hastening recovery from medical illnesses. Indeed, the available evidence suggests that this is so. Whether such approaches are cost-effective has been frequently difficult to determine, even when there is clear evidence that the interventions are clinically effective. Most studies are not designed to test the idea that psychotherapeutic approaches are cost-effective for the emotional distress and overall outcome of the treatment of medical conditions. Cost-effective studies are complex and expensive to implement, largely because the estimation of costs takes considerable effort and unusual access to business records and in part because a consensus about a proper outcome metric is only now emerging (Wolff et al. 1997). For outcome measurement to be truly comprehensive, the study must include a subjective measure of pain and suffering, the state of function, quality of life (best measured in terms of quality-adjusted life years), morbidity and mortality, utilization of services, and the costs of those services. As Wells and Sturm (1995, p. 85) put it in their review of the care for depression, "If we want to spend our…dollars efficiently, an important criterion should be the health improvement realized for each additional dollar spent. Cost-effective does not necessarily mean cheap but instead means high-value; quality improvement may be cost-effective even if it increases direct treatment costs."

## Clinical Vignette

In the September 8, 1997, issue of *The New Yorker*, Dr. Jerome Groopman, an oncologist at Beth Israel Deaconess Hospital in Boston, eloquently described his treatment of Kirk Bains (the name had been changed), a wealthy, 54-year-old, venture capitalist who had renal cell carcinoma. The cancer had spread to his bones, liver, and lungs; his abdomen was swollen with ascites; and he was jaundiced. He had been told by other eminent oncologists that he had only weeks to live. Mr. Bains presented himself as a go-for-it-all risk-taker who refused to give up. He implored Dr. Groopman to treat him with whatever experimental therapy he could design. Though skeptical at first, Dr. Groopman was taken with Mr. Bains's positive outlook and consented to treat him. After warning the patient of the terrible side effects to come, Dr. Groopman prescribed a never-before attempted combination of interleukin-2, vinblastin, and progesterone.

Although the predicted side effects did come, they did not kill the patient, and he soon began to respond to the therapy. Both doctor and patient considered the remission of the cancer close to miraculous. However, in the wake of his recovery, Mr. Bains appeared to lose his positive outlook. His wife stated that while he used to read three newspapers per day, Mr. Bains no longer read any. Dr. Groopman became concerned that the patient might have become depressed, but Mr. Bains assured him he was not depressed; he had no problems with sleep, concentration, or appetite—he only felt that the information in the newspapers no longer seemed important to him.

Several months later, the cancer recurred. Dr. Groopman expected Mr. Bains once again to mount a strong fight against the disease, but instead found him resigned to death. The doctor found out that the remission forced the patient to look back and assess his life. Mr. Bains came to realize that he had wasted his life pursuing money instead of cultivating relationships. He decided that he had been self-absorbed and uncaring. He stated that "the remission meant nothing, because it was too late to relive my life." Mr. Bains died shortly thereafter, and Dr. Groopman realized that the patient's cancer had not been his only problem.

In an insightful letter to *The New Yorker*, on October 6, 1997, Dr. Jacqueline Persons, an associate clinical professor of psychiatry at the University of California, San Francisco, commented that "if [the patient] had received psychological care comparable to the outstanding and aggressive care he received for his cancer, he might have been able to bring his [last months] to a more dignified, peaceful conclusion." Had Mr. Bains received some form of psychotherapy, he may have had the desire and energy to once again fight the cancer. He may have lived longer. But the real message of this case is not about extending life. When faced with the end of his life, the patient examined it and came away with many regrets. If Mr. Bains had seen a mental health professional while his cancer was being treated, he might have been able to meet life's greatest challenge, death, with greater understanding and acceptance, rather than with despair and regret.

# Search Methodology

Below, selected studies supporting the use of psychotherapy in the medically ill are described. They are grouped according to medical illnesses for which the psychotherapy was used. These studies were found by doing a MEDLINE search from January 1984 to December 2007 and used the keyword "psychotherapy" cross-referenced with the keywords "cancer," "HIV," "diabetes," "cardiac," "pain," and "medical illness." All studies were screened for cost-sensitive outcomes of psychotherapy. In addition, for appropriate background, studies regarding cost of illness and efficacy of psychotherapy for medical-surgical patients were included. The review table at the end of this chapter summarizes selected studies that used a random assignment design to compare a psychological treatment with a standardized treatment along outcome measures of cost and/or utilization as well as clinical improvement.

# Effect of Psychopathology on Medical Expenditures

Levenson et al. (1990) screened a group of 455 medical inpatients and found that 27.9% were "very depressed" and 27.5% were "very anxious." These patients with significant psychopathology or pain had a 40% longer median length of hospital stay, 35% greater mean hospital costs, and more procedures performed than those with little psychopathology or pain. Browne et al. (1990) found that in patients with chronic illness the strongest correlate of total health services consumed was psychosocial adjustment, as defined by completing a series of inventories, with a total annual cost per poorly adjusted patient of $23,883, as compared with only $9,791 if well adjusted. Verbosky et al. (1993) compared 24 medical/surgical inpatients for whom psychiatric consultation was requested for depression or dysthymia with 24 inpatients with matched medical diagnoses who did not require psychiatric consultation. They found that the depressed group had a mean length of stay that was twice that of the nondepressed group (20 days vs. 10 days).

A number of studies suggest that medically ill patients with concomitant psychiatric illness do not respond as well to somatic therapies if their psychiatric illnesses are left untreated (Cohen et al. 1997; Gavard et al. 1993; Hellman et al. 1990; Jacobson 1996a, 1996b; Katon 1987; Levenson et al. 1990; Meyer et al. 1981; Smith et al. 1986, 1995; Spiegel 1996; Verbosky et al. 1993). By extension, the cost of medical care rises for patients with ongoing mental disorders (Druss et al. 2000). If their psychiatric symptoms are treated along with their other medical illnesses, the overall cost to society of care may be lowered (Rosenheck et al. 1999).

Psychotherapeutic interventions with families of medically ill patients may also lower health care expenditures. In a study by Mittelman et al. (1996), caregivers of patients with Alzheimer's disease who received six sessions of individual and family counseling within 4 months of enrollment in the study were only two-thirds as likely to place the patient in a nursing home at any given point in time as were the control caregivers. Also, the median time from baseline to nursing home placement was 329 days longer in the treatment group than in the control group.

# Psychotherapy With Somatization Disorder Patients

Smith et al. (1986) found that the per capita cost of health care for patients with somatization disorder is up to nine times the average. In a randomized controlled trial, they found that psychiatric consultation lowered the cost of health care in these patients by 53%. The same research team (Kashner et al. 1995) also found that group therapy, in addition to psychiatric consultation, over a 1-year period following the therapy yielded a 52% net savings in health care charges compared with controls who received standard medical care. The more group sessions the patients attended, the greater their improvement in general and mental health. In a related study, Smith et al. (1995) randomly selected physicians who were treating patients with somatization syndrome, that is, patients who sought help for 6–12 unexplained physical symptoms but did not meet criteria for somatization disorder. The physicians in the experimental group received psychiatric consultation letters recommending a management approach to these patients. The control group did not receive the letter until 1 year into the study. Patients of the physicians who received the letter early reported increased physical functioning, and the intervention reduced annual medical charges by 32.9%.

# Impact of Psychological Services on Patients With Co-occurring Psychiatric and Medical Diagnoses and Utilization of Care/Cost Offset

In a review of 13 controlled studies of hospitalized surgical or heart attack patients, Mumford et al. (1982) found that modest psychological interventions reduced hospital stay approximately 2 days below the 9.92 day average. These studies focused on short, inpatient psychiatric interventions and not on longer term psychotherapy. In another careful meta-analysis of 58 controlled studies and analyses of Blue Cross and Blue Shield Federal Employees Plan, Mumford et al. (1984) provided evidence that outpatient psychiatric services effectively reduce the cost of other medical care. They found that 85% of the studies showed a reduction in utilization, primarily through reduced inpatient stays.

Meyer et al. (1981) investigated general medical outpatients with comparable medical and emotional problems, defined by a series of rating scales, who were randomly assigned to one of two groups: 72 patients were treated only by internists, whereas 62 others also received 10 weekly psychotherapeutic visits. Significantly more patients who had undergone psychotherapy remained improved at 1-year follow-up. Hellman et al. (1990) performed a randomized prospective study, in which primary care patients with physical symptoms with a psychosomatic component (e.g., palpitations, headache, gastrointestinal upset) were put in one of two behavioral medicine groups. One group focused on the mind-body relationship, relaxation training, and cognitive restructuring, whereas the other group focused only on information about stress management. Patients in the first group showed significantly greater reductions in health maintenance organization visits, as well as subjective diminution in symptoms, compared with those in the group receiving only information.

Using an episode of care analysis, Kessler et al. (1982) found that cost-offset effects are most pronounced for characteristics related to the psychiatric care and that there is a peaking of medical expenditures before the mental health care and that the offset is relatively short term. Luborsky et al. (2004) reviewed the evidence of the relation of having a period of psychotherapy and comparing it with a measure of improved health care. Three interrelated types of studies were identified and examined: 1) reduction in physical illness through psychotherapy, especially for the patients' survival time during the interval between diagnosis and endpoint; 2) reduction in pain in relation to receiving psychotherapy; and 3) reduction in cost and medical treatment in relation to receiving psychotherapy. An average effect size under each type revealed that survival time was not affected by psychotherapy for severely ill patients but was possibly effective for low-severity patients, and for reduction in pain, physical illness, and cost, there was clearly an effect of psychosocial treatment.

# Psychotherapy in Patients With Cancer

The diseases for which the effectiveness of psychotherapy has been extensively studied are the cancers (Spiegel 1996). For generations, the very word "cancer," usually spoken in a whisper, was tantamount to a death sentence. Although the ability to treat effectively and even to cure cancers has improved dramatically, the fear associated with such a diagnosis has not abated proportionally. As such, many who are faced with a fight against malignancy can become despairing and withdrawn. If these patients are allowed to feel defeated and unsupported, the chance of survival may be hampered. The psychological distress associated with cancer is substantial. Derogatis et al. (1983) reported that 47% of 215 cancer patients screened had a DSM-III diagnosis (American Psychiatric Association 1980).

Many studies address the issue of whether psychotherapy increases survival, and this area has had some controversy. Spiegel et al. (1989) studied the effect of psychosocial intervention on survival time in 86 patients with breast cancer. They found that mean survival time almost doubled, from 18.9 months in the control group to 36.6 months in the group treated for 1 year with weekly supportive therapy and self-hypnosis for pain. Of particular interest is the fact that divergence in survival time began at 20 months after entry, supporting the notion that continued psychotherapy, as opposed to very brief intervention, is necessary for the positive effect to become manifest.

However, Linn et al. (1982) in a similar test of counseling with metastatic lung cancer patients found that patients felt better but did not have increased survival rates. Andersen (1992) offered a possible explanation for the fact that Linn et al. did not find a similar survival advantage using psychotherapy with metastatic lung cancer patients by postulating that Spiegel et al.'s experimental intervention was of considerably longer duration and contributed to the survival benefit of breast cancer patients in a dose-response relationship. In another study, Gellert et al. (1993) found that a similar support program, but lacking psychotherapy, conferred no survival advantage. After finding that the decreased anxiety and depression of malignant melanoma patients treated with six structured support group sessions was maintained 6 months out, Fawzy and colleagues (Fawzy et al. 1990a, 1990b; Fawzy et al. 1993) looked at the same patients 5–6 years later. They found that the experimental group had greater disease-free intervals, fewer recurrences, and an overall longer survival than did the control group, with 13 recurrences and 10 deaths in the control group of 34, as compared with 7 recurrences and 3 deaths in the experimental group of the same size. These findings were statistically significant. In addition, Richardson et al. (1990) reported that a group of patients with leukemia and lymphoma who participated in educational and supportive programs experienced enhanced survival. These programs were specifically geared to increasing compliance, which they did, and yet had an effect on survival beyond the effect of the compliance.

Kuchler et al. (2007) also investigated the impact of psychotherapy support on survival for patients with gastrointestinal cancers undergoing surgery. A randomized control trial was conducted enrolling 271 patients with primary cancer diagnoses of esophagus, stomach, liver/gallbladder, pancreas, or colon/rectum. They were stratified by gender and randomly assigned to a control group that received standard care as provided on the surgical settings or to an experimental group that received formal psychotherapeutic support in addition to routine care. A Kaplan-Meier survival curve demonstrated statistically significantly better survival for the experimental group than the control group, and the unadjusted significance level was quite high for 10 years. Secondary analysis found that the differences in favor of the experimental group occurred in patients with stomach, pancreatic, primary liver, or colorectal cancer. The authors concluded that patients with these disorders benefit from a formal program of psychotherapy support, which actually increases survival times.

The issue of whether psychotherapy has an impact on quality of life in cancer is much better established than the issue of whether psychosocial/ psychotherapy has an impact on survival. Cheung et al. (2003) evaluated the effects of progressive muscle relaxation training (PMRT) on anxiety and quality of life in colorectal cancer patients after they had undergone stoma surgery. A random control design method was used with repeated measures over 10 weeks postsurgery. There were 59 participants randomly assigned to a control condition receiving routine care (*n*=30) or an experimental group receiving routine care and PMRT (*n*=29). The outcome measure was the State-Trait Anxiety Inventory and two quality-of-life scales. PMRT significantly decreased state anxiety and improved generic quality of life in the experimental group, manifested as statistically significant results in the domains of physical health, psychological health, social concerns, and environment. In both groups, measures of social relationships were decreased. The authors suggest that PMRT should be incorporated in the long-term care of colorectal cancer patients and is "probably" cost-effective. Kissane et al. (2007) studied 485 women with advanced breast cancer who were randomly assigned to supportive-expressive group therapy (SEGT) plus three classes of relaxation therapy or to the control condition, receiving three classes of relaxation therapy. The primary outcome was survival; psychosocial well-being was appraised only secondarily. The results revealed that SEGT did not prolong survival but did increase quality of life and offered protection from depression. In another study of group therapy for metastatic breast cancer patients, Lemieux et al. (2006) examined the impact of group psychosocial support on health care costs. A total of 235 women with metastatic breast cancer from seven Canadian centers took part in the study in a randomized controlled trial evaluating the effect of weekly group therapy plus standard care versus standard care alone on survival and pain, psychosocial functioning, and health-related quality of life. The economic analysis was based on a subset of patients from the three largest trial sites that had the most reliable prospective reporting of health care utilization. While the results in this study showed no significant difference between the intervention arm and the control arm in survival, the patients who received the group therapy had better mood and pain control. The difference in total health care costs between the two groups was not statistically significant. In fact, although the group therapy patients' treatment was more expensive, it was also more cost-effective by virtue of the significantly superior impact on mood and pain control.

Many studies also stress the improved quality of life that psychotherapy confers. Trijsburg et al. (1992) reviewed 22 controlled studies of psychosocial interventions in patients with cancer. They noted positive physical or psychological benefits conferred on patients in 19 of the 22 studies. Cain et al. (1986) described decreased depression and anxiety, better relationships with caregivers, fewer sexual dysfunctions, and greater participation in leisure activities in a group of women with gynecological cancers who underwent eight support group counseling sessions; this improvement was observed 6 months later. Forester et al. (1985) examined the effects of psychotherapy in patients undergoing radiation therapy for cancer. They found that these patients, who received weekly psychotherapy for 10 sessions, had statistically significant declines in both emotional and physical manifestations of distress.

Sometimes, beneficial studies were surprising in how the benefit was realized. Jacobsen et al. (2002) studied the effect of a form of stress management training on quality-of-life assessments in patients undergoing chemotherapy for cancer; 411 patients were randomly assigned to receive usual care, which included a professionally administered form of stress management training or a patient self-administered form of self-management training. Follow-up tests revealed that the patients who received the self-administered intervention reported statistically significantly better physical functioning, greater vitality, fewer role limitations because of emotional problems, and better mental health. Patients who received the professionally administered intervention fared no better in terms of quality of life than patients receiving usual care only. Costs of the self-administered intervention were estimated to be 66% from the perspective of the payer to 68% from the societal perspective, less than the average cost of professionally administered psychosocial interventions. This study demonstrates that under the proper conditions, self-administered stress management can supersede and displace professionally administered access to psychosocial care and be equally or more effective.

Linn and Linn (1981) reported improvement in quality of life as measured by depression, life satisfaction, and self-esteem in terminally ill cancer patients who received counseling. Spiegel et al. (1981) also found less mood disturbance and less phobic behavior among women with metastatic breast cancer who participated in supportive group psychotherapy. Spiegel (1994, 1995) concluded that psychosocial treatments in cancer patients decrease depression and anxiety, improve quality of life, and enhance the ability of the medically ill to cope with the illness. And, as noted above, this group of investigators also found significantly improved survival time.

# Psychotherapy in Patients With Cardiac and Cardiovascular Diseases

Links between psychological health and cardiac disease have been found in numerous studies. For example, individuals who have hostile, controlling, and socially dominant (type A) personalities have been shown to be at greater risk for coronary heart disease (Houston et al. 1992). Mittleman et al. (1995) described episodes of anger precipitating acute myocardial infarction (MI). Based on interviews with 1,623 patients following an MI, the authors reported that those who experienced an episode of anger had increased their risk of having an MI within the following 2 hours, by 2.3 times. Furthermore, caregivers who are stressed due to caring for family members with Alzheimer's disease but who have high social supports have shown typical age-related decreases in heart-rate reactivity. In contrast, those with low social supports have shown increased reactivity, as well as increased systolic blood pressure (Uchino et al. 1992). Their findings suggest that chronic stress can contribute to harmful cardiac changes, which can be moderated through social support. Ironson et al. (1992) examined the effect of psychological stress on myocardial ischemia and found that, in both healthy controls and in cardiac patients, anger significantly reduced left ventricular ejection fraction.

The phenomenon of the "cardiac cripple" has also been described. Patients with heart disease, even when doing well, may become so frightened of the prospect of another MI that they stop doing the things that they enjoy. This kind of behavior can be associated with a decline in enthusiasm for living and subsequent depression. Ironically, this pattern may worsen a cardiac patient's prognosis. These patients need support and encouragement in order for them to make the most of their lives, despite their cardiac conditions. Also, a variation on this theme are patients with chest pain, no evidence of cardiovascular disease, but continued worry and concern that they are severely ill with a cardiac disorder. Mayou et al. (1997) studied such a group in a randomized comparison of cognitive-behavioral therapy (CBT) against usual care and found that there were significant differences at 3 months in terms of mood and activity. At 6 months significant differences remained but were not as dramatic.

Blumenthal and Wei (1993), in a review of behavioral and psychological therapies in the rehabilitation of patients with cardiac disease, concluded that these therapies showed promise in improving both quantity and quality of life. Linden et al. (1996) performed a meta-analysis of the use of psychosocial interventions in cardiac rehabilitation. In comparing 2,024 patients who received psychosocial treatment with 1,156 control patients, they found reductions in psychological distress, systolic blood pressure, heart rate, cholesterol levels, cardiac recurrence rates, and mortality in the treated patients.

Gould et al. (1995) randomly selected patients with coronary artery disease, documented by positron-emission tomography (PET) scans and arteriography, either for usual care by their physicians or for an experimental intervention consisting of very low-fat vegetarian diet, smoking cessation, mild to moderate exercise, stress management, and group therapy. After 5 years, the 20 patients in the experimental group showed improvement in ventricular perfusion seen arteriographically and on PET images, whereas stenosis worsened in the 15 patients in the control group.

Johannesson et al. (1995) actually carried out cost-effectiveness analysis of a multiple risk factor reduction program that consisted of advice rendered in individual and group settings based on nutritional and behavioral treatment principles as well as drugs to achieve the goals of the program of smoking cessation, serum cholesterol reduction, and diastolic blood pressure "normalization." The study used an open randomized allocation of parallel treatments to the experimental program or usual care (drugs alone) with a 3-year follow-up for 508 patients. The cost-effectiveness analysis used a societal perspective with the measure of cost-effectiveness being measured as the cost per life year gained (in Swedish 1991 crowns, SEK). Interventions with SEK 100,000 per life year ratios or less are considered to be highly cost-effective. This study revealed a cost-effectiveness ratio of SEK 4,000 largely because of the reduction in coronary heart disease by 11% and stroke by 70%.

In another cost-effectiveness study, Davidson et al. (2007) evaluated hospitalization cost offset of hostility management group therapy for patients with coronary artery disease; 26 male patients with MI or unstable angina were randomly assigned to either 2 months of cognitive-behavioral group therapy or an informational or control session. Results revealed that therapy patients had a significantly shorter length of stay, 0.38 days versus 2.15 days, $t(15.2)=-2.29$, $P=0.04$. The average hospitalizations were significantly lower for therapy patients (average $245 vs. $1,333) than for the controls, $t=-2.27$, $P=0.04$. Cost-offset ratio was calculated by dividing the $1,088 of hospital savings by the $560 of therapy expense, revealing a ratio of 1:1.94. This meant that for every dollar spent on therapy, there is an approximate savings of $1.94 in hospitalization cost in the following 6 months. The authors concluded that these findings strongly support the hospitalization cost offset of hostility reduction in coronary artery disease patients. Along similar lines, Moore et al. (2007), who developed a novel outpatient cognitive-behavioral chronic disease management program (CB-CDMP), found that their program improved angina status and quality of life. They took 271 patients with chronic refractory angina and reduced their hospital admissions from 2.4 per year to 1.78 per year ($P<0.001$). The authors believe that the CB-CDMP approach was a low-cost alternative to palliative revascularization.

And in another study examining a therapeutic addition to a stressful surgical procedure, Lewin et al. (2009) attempted to assess the clinical effectiveness and cost-effectiveness of a brief, home-based cognitive-behavioral rehabilitation program for patients who were undergoing an implantation of a cardiac defibrillator. This was a random control design study in which the control group received usual care and advice from an experienced health care professional. The authors concluded that the therapy plan improved health-related quality of life, reduced the incidence of clinically significant psychological distress, and significantly reduced unplanned readmissions and that this was a cost-effective and easily implemented method for delivering rehabilitation and psychological care to patients undergoing implantation of a cardiac defibrillator.

# Psychotherapy in Patients With Diabetes

The prevalence of depression is greater in adults with insulin-dependent diabetes mellitus (IDDM) than in the general population (Gavard et al. 1993; Popkin et al. 1988). Moreover, patients with poorly controlled diabetes mellitus have higher incidences of psychiatric illnesses, including depression and eating disorders, than do those with tighter glycemic control (Lustman et al. 1986; Polonsky et al. 1994). They are also more likely to live in families with high levels of conflict (Anderson et al. 1981). In addition, diabetic patients who are depressed are more likely to have serious retinopathy, often a sequela of diabetes, than those without depression (Cohen et al. 1997). Patients who develop severe complications, such as renal failure or loss of vision, often experience periods of mourning their loss of function (Jacobson 1996a, 1996b; Jacobson et al. 1994). Kent et al. (1994) found that patients with severely unstable diabetes had higher mortality rates, more serious medical complications, lower quality-of-life scores, and more frequent psychosocial disruptions. Patients with IDDM may have greater prevalence of anxiety disorders than the general population, which can be confusing, as anxiety can mimic symptoms of abnormal glycemia (Jacobson 1996a, 1996b).

Studies in which psychotherapy is a treatment for patients with IDDM demonstrate a positive effect of psychological treatment on course of illness and outcome. Moran et al. (1991) compared two groups of poorly controlled diabetic children. While the control group received only inpatient medical care, the experimental group also received psychoanalytic psychotherapy three to four times a week for 15 weeks. The treatment group had improved glycemic control 1 year after discharge, whereas the comparison group returned to poor metabolic control within 3 months. Similarly, glycemic control was improved in a study of insulin-dependent diabetics who underwent cognitive analytic therapy (Fosbury et al. 1997). Bernbaum et al. (1989) studied 29 subjects with IDDM and non-IDDM subjects who were visually impaired. They entered a 12-week program that included education and group support. Indices of glycemic control and psychosocial functioning improved, as did exercise tolerance. Padgett et al. (1988) performed a meta-analysis of 93 studies of 7,451 patients who received psychosocial interventions in the management of their diabetes mellitus. All subtypes of intervention, including education, learning/behavior modification, and counseling, yielded moderate but significant gains in physical outcome and psychological status.

Hampson et al. (2001), in a review of 62 studies in the literature, found that roughly 40% were randomized controlled trials. The studies took place in a variety of settings and used different interventions. The mean pooled effect size for the psychotherapy interventions was found to be 0.37 for psychosocial outcomes and 0.33 for glycated hemoglobin. That included outliers; without outliers, the effectiveness was 0.08, indicating that the interventions had small to medium beneficial effect on diabetes management outcomes in general but big effects on patients with severe control problems over time. They noted that all studies reported beneficial effects and concluded from this review that educational and psychosocial interventions have small to medium beneficial effects on various diabetes management outcomes and that well-designed trials continue to be needed in different cultural and political climates.

In a study to monitor costs and to assess cost-effectiveness, Katon et al. (2006) examined 418 patients with diabetes and depression from 18 primary care clinics from 8 health care organizations in five states. Patients with diabetes and depression were randomly assigned to usual care or to the IMPACT intervention, which included a behavioral activation intervention (such as structured positive activities) and a choice of either problem-solving treatment (a six- to eight-session manualized psychotherapy program) or enhanced treatment with antidepressant medication. Initial medication treatment was augmented with problem-solving therapy based on partial response or nonresponse and vice versa. The primary dependent cost variable was total outpatient costs (including both mental health and non-mental health costs). Total mental health costs were $1,019 higher in IMPACT versus usual-care patients. However, over a 24-month period, non-mental health medication costs were $271 lower and other outpatient costs $722 lower in IMPACT patients, suggesting a considerable medical cost offset in non-mental health ambulatory care costs. Total outpatient services were thus only $25 higher in IMPACT versus usual-care patients, yielding an incremental cost-effectiveness ratio of 25 cents per depression-free day. Over 2 years, the grand total of health care costs (inpatient and outpatient) was $896 lower in IMPACT compared with usual-care patients. In addition, over a 24-month period, the IMPACT patients experienced 115 more depression-free days compared with the usual-care patients. This particular study reveals both cost-effectiveness and cost-offset effect for the intervention studied.

In another examination of incremental cost and cost-effectiveness for a depression treatment program for diabetic outpatients, a randomized controlled trial involving 329 depressed diabetic patients compared systematic depression treatment with care as usual (Simon et al. 2007). The intervention, systematic depression treatment, began with either a 12-month problem-solving psychotherapy or an antidepressant pharmacotherapy program, depending on each patient's preference. Subsequent treatment (combining psychotherapy and medication, adjustments to medication, and specialty referral) was adjusted according to the clinical response. Depressive symptoms were assessed at 3, 5, 12, and 24 months as were health service costs. The interventions followed a stepped-care model with the step 1 treatment being either antidepressant medication or psychotherapy. Step 2 included the addition of a second treatment modality, adding medication for those beginning with psychotherapy and/or medication adjustment. Effectiveness was defined as the number of depression-free days during follow-up. Patients in the intervention group experienced approximately 20 more depression-free days in the first year compared with patients given usual care; in the 2nd year, intervention patients experienced an additional increment of 33 days. Outpatient depression treatment costs were $700 higher in the intervention group during the 1st year, and general medical outpatient costs were somewhat lower so that total outpatient costs in the two groups were approximately equal. During the 2nd year of follow-up, outpatient depression treatment costs were approximately $100 higher in the intervention group, but total outpatient costs were approximately $1,400 lower. Over the 2-year follow-up period, the authors estimated that the intervention reduced outpatient health service cost by approximately $300 in that $800 of additional depression treatment costs was offset by a decrease of approximately $1,100 in costs of general medical care. The overall economic value of this intervention also included both cost savings and clinical benefits. The gain in depression-free days in year 2 was 1.5 times as large as in year 1, even though all intervention treatment ended at 12 months. Thus, the clinical benefits of systematic depression treatment persisted long after the end of the formal intervention, and it was noted that the positive effects of the intervention on the use of health services may not appear for 12 months or more.

# Psychotherapy in Patients With Musculoskeletal Disease

Two quasi-experimental studies suggest that consultation and/or psychiatric liaison services substantially reduce health services utilization (and costs) for elderly patients with hip fractures. Levitan and Kornfeld (1981) reported that the length of hospitalization for postoperative elderly patients who received consultation from a liaison psychiatrist was 12 days shorter than for those who did not. In addition, twice as many of the group receiving consultation returned home, rather than to a nursing home, compared with control patients. Strain et al. (1991) reported 56% and 60% prevalence of DSM-III disorders in two groups of elderly patients admitted for hip fractures. Psychiatric consultation for all patients admitted in a year shortened their length of stay and saved $166,926 and $97,361, respectively, at the two sites studied. This was in comparison with the previous year, when psychiatric consultation was only used in the traditional manner, that is, in cases where psychiatric illness was suspected because of overt signs and symptoms.

As one might expect, there are studies addressing the treatment of low back pain that have interesting results. Johnson et al. (2007) reported a random control trial to determine whether, among patients with persistent, disabling low back pain, a group program of exercise and education that uses a CBT approach reduces pain and disability over 12 months, the cost-effectiveness of the intervention, and whether patient preference for type of treatment influences outcome. The authors discovered that the intervention program produced only modest effects in reducing low back pain and disability over a 1-year period. There was some ambiguity as to whether the patient preference for treatment influences the outcome, and this clearly warrants further investigation.

In a review of 12 years of studies on carpal tunnel syndrome, Feuerstein et al. (1999) found that CBT yields significant reductions in associated pain, anxiety, and depression. Addressing disability, Schweikert et al. (2006) attempted to investigate whether the cost-effectiveness and the return to work were better with CBT added to standard therapy compared with simply a 3-week inpatient rehabilitation program for patients with low back pain. A sophisticated economic evaluation alongside an effectiveness trial was performed; 409 patients were studied who were admitted over a 3-week inpatient rehabilitation. The cost of the CBT for the treatment arm was approximately 127 euros; however, there was significant improvement in quality-adjusted life year. The authors concluded that adding a cognitive-behavioral component to standard therapy could reduce work days lost and increase indirect cost savings. From a societal perspective, the cost of the psychological treatment was compensated by lower indirect costs.

# Psychological Intervention for HIV

In a carefully constructed economic evaluation using cost-utility analysis, Johnson-Masotti et al. (2000) compared three related CBT interventions to assess cost-effectiveness in the reduction of HIV risk behaviors in adults with severe mental illness. These treatment approaches were single session, dyadic, multisession, and advocacy training. The results were different for men and women. For women only the single session was cost-effective, and for men all three were cost-effective but the advocacy intervention, which was the most expensive, was also the most cost-effective.

# Psychotherapy in Patients With Pain

Somatic pain and psychic pain have long been associated. Walker et al. (1988) interviewed 25 women with chronic pelvic pain and compared them with a control group of 30 women with specific gynecological conditions. Both groups underwent diagnostic laparoscopy. The women with chronic pelvic pain had significantly higher prevalence of major depression, substance abuse, adult sexual dysfunction, somatization, and histories of childhood and adult sexual abuse than did women in the control group. Rosenthal (1993) also concluded that chronic pelvic pain is often a somatic expression of depression in women with histories of sexual or physical abuse. Lim (1994) reminded clinicians to bear in mind the psychogenic causes of pain and to refer such cases to a mental health professional early, in order to avoid undue suffering and inefficient use of health care resources. However, the mental health provider may not be so essential. In a meta-analysis of home-based treatment programs (self-study, tapes, books, educational materials), Haddock et al. (1997) found that home-based programs are equal in effectiveness to clinic-based approaches and that their cost-effectiveness scores were up to five times more effective than clinic-based therapies.

Investigators have conducted studies regarding the efficacy of psychotherapy in treating a variety of pain disorders. Peters et al. (2000) found that a cognitive-behavioral pain management program in a military hospital setting resulted in an improvement in all outcome measures (pain ratings, relaxation skills, quality of life, satisfaction ratings, and medical utilization). There was an 87% reduction in outpatient medical visits in the first 3 months of the program with a projected annual savings of $78,960 for the care of these 61 patients. Cognitive-behavioral therapy has been shown to aid in the management of both rheumatoid and osteoarthritis (Keefe and Caldwell 1997), as well as chronic back pain (Linton 1994). Turner and Jensen (1993) randomly assigned 102 outpatients with chronic low back pain to cognitive therapy/relaxation training groups or to a waiting-list control group. Pain intensity decreased significantly in treatment groups but not in the control group. These improvements were present at 6 and 12 months. In a similar study, forty-four 7- to-14-year-olds with recurrent abdominal pain were randomly selected for either cognitive behavioral family intervention (CBFI) or standard pediatric care. The group who received CBFI had a higher rate of complete elimination of pain, lower levels of relapse at 6 and 12 months, and lower levels of interference with activities as a result of pain (Sanders et al. 1994).

Cognitive-behavioral therapy has also been used in the treatment of pain for patients with advanced cancer (Loscalzo 1996). Arathuzik (1994) studied 24 women with metastatic breast cancer who were experiencing pain. Women who were enrolled in CBT had significantly greater ability to decrease pain than did women who were not. Spiegel and Bloom (1983) found that women with metastatic breast cancer who were offered weekly group therapy demonstrated significantly less self-rated pain and suffering than women in the control group. Changes in pain measures were significantly correlated with changes in self-rated total mood disturbance.

# Psychotherapy in Patients With Gastrointestinal Disorders

Investigators have long recognized the strong link between psychological variables and gastrointestinal illness. Even many without disease can recognize in themselves the relationship between mental state and gastrointestinal functioning. Anxious and depressed people commonly report suffering from symptoms including constipation, diarrhea, and abdominal cramping. Drossman et al. (1990) found that a high frequency of women (44% of 206) who were referred for gastrointestinal disorders reported past physical and sexual abuse.

Guthrie et al. (1993) randomly selected 102 subjects with chronic, refractory irritable bowel syndrome (IBS) for either psychotherapy or supportive listening. After 12 weeks, the women in psychotherapy showed physical and psychological improvements that were significantly greater than those found in the supportive listening group. There was a similar trend with men, but the difference did not reach the level of statistical significance. At the end of this trial, the supportive listening subjects were offered psychotherapy. Those who accepted showed marked improvements. One year later, patients who had received psychotherapy remained well, those who had dropped out had severe symptoms, and most control patients who had refused psychotherapy had relapsed. Van Dulmen et al. (1996) studied the efficacy of CBT in the treatment of IBS. The 25 patients who received CBT (eight 2-hour sessions over 3 months) had significantly greater improvement in their abdominal complaints than did the 20 control patients. These improvements persisted in follow-up.

In their study of 257 patients with severe IBS, Creed et al. (2003) randomly assigned patients to 1) eight sessions of individual psychotherapy, 2) 20 mg daily of paroxetine, or 3) routine care by a gastroenterologist or general practitioner. Outcomes were rated according to severity of abdominal pain, physical-health-related quality of life, and mental-health-related quality of life. Because IBS is the major cause of referrals to gastroenterology clinics in the Western world, costing $8 billion a year in the United States, with severe IBS leading to a threefold increase in work absenteeism and physician visits and to significantly impaired health-related quality of life, cost-effective treatments are enormously valuable in this condition. In addition, pharmacologic treatments aimed at intestinal symptoms have been disappointing in this group of patients. In this study, direct health care costs were measured as well as direct non-health care costs, including patient expenditures as a result of the illness, nonprescription medication, and days lost from work. The results demonstrated that the severity and frequency of abdominal pain had improved for all three groups without significant differences. For the mental component of health-related quality of life, both the psychotherapy and paroxetine groups showed improvement compared with treatment as usual. However at 1-year follow-up, there was no significant difference among the three groups. For the physical component of the health-related quality of life, both the psychotherapy and paroxetine groups showed a small improvement after 3 months. At 1-year follow-up, however, both treatment groups had a statistically significant improvement over treatment as usual. With regard to costs, the direct health care costs were significantly greater for psychotherapy (but not for paroxetine) compared with treatment as usual. However, during the 1-year follow-up, direct health care costs were significantly lower for psychotherapy (but not for paroxetine) compared with treatment as usual. The difference was created by a reduction in gastroenterologist and other medical visits, a high proportion of direct health care costs in all groups. The costs of days lost from work remained similar in all groups. However, psychotherapy, but not paroxetine, was associated with a small reduction in the number of patients claiming disability benefits. Overall, the magnitude of improvement in the physical component of health-related quality of life from either psychotherapy or paroxetine was noted to be remarkable at no additional cost.

# Psychotherapy and Transplantation

Recipients of kidney transplant may develop emotional problems, including medical noncompliance, compromised quality of life, and difficulty integrating the newly acquired organ into the sense of self. Baines et al. (2004) attempted to determine the effectiveness of group versus individual psychotherapy on the expression of depression in a group of recipients of a cadaver kidney transplant. A random controlled design was used, with the two comparison groups being those who received either group or individual therapy. The Beck Depression Inventory was the main outcome measure. Forty-nine patients were in individual therapy and 40 were in group therapy, and of these 89 patients, 82 completed 12 weeks of therapy. The results revealed that both individual and group therapy were beneficial; however, individual therapy was found to lower Beck Depression Inventory scores greater than group therapy at the end of the treatment time.

# Miscellaneous Illnesses

O'Dowd et al. (2006) intended to test the idea that group CBT could produce an effective and cost-effective management strategy for patients in primary care with chronic fatigue syndrome/myalgic encephalopathy. The authors performed a double-blind randomized control trial with three arms. Outcomes were assessed at 6 and 12 months. The authors found that with the 153 patients recruited into the trial, group CBT did not achieve the expected change in the primary outcome measures, as a significant number did not achieve scores within the normal range postintervention. The treatment did not return a significant number of subjects to within the normal range on this domain; however, improvements were evident in some areas, and CBT was effective in treating symptoms of fatigue, mood, and physical fitness in chronic fatigue syndrome.

# Conclusion

Psychiatric disorders can place patients at increased risk for physical ailments, and medical illness is often accompanied by psychological distress. Psychotherapeutic interventions can and should be used, in conjunction with standard medical treatments, when working with the medically ill who have concomitant psychiatric illness and/or distress. Furthermore, in many medical illnesses in which there is no overt psychopathology or unusual psychological distress, psychologically oriented treatments when deployed with appropriate biologically based treatments have been shown to reduce suffering, reduce costs, improve overall cost-effectiveness, increase quality of life, and, in some cases, extend life.

# References

Ader R, Felten D, Cohen N: Interactions between the brain and the immune system. Annu Rev Pharmacol Toxicol 30:561–602, 1990

American Psychiatric Association: Diagnostic and Statistical Manual of Mental Disorders, 3rd Edition. Washington, DC, American Psychiatric Association, 1980

American Psychiatric Association: Diagnostic and Statistical Manual of Mental Disorders, 3rd Edition, Revised. Washington, DC, American Psychiatric Association, 1987

Andersen BL: Psychological interventions for cancer patients to enhance the quality of life. J Consult Clin Psychol 60:552–568, 1992

Anderson BJ, Miller JP, Auslander WF, et al: Family characteristics of diabetic adolescents: relationship to metabolic control. Diabetes Care 4:586–594, 1981

Arathuzik D: Effects of cognitive-behavioral strategies on pain in cancer patients. Cancer Nurs 17:207–214, 1994

Baines LS, Joseph JT, Jindal RM: Prospective randomized study of individual and group psychotherapy versus controls in recipients of renal transplants. Kidney Int 65:1937–1942, 2004

Baxter LR, Schwartz JM, Bergman KS, et al: Caudate glucose metabolic rate changes with both drug and behavior therapy for obsessive-compulsive disorder. Arch Gen Psychiatry 49:681–689, 1992

Bernbaum M, Albert SG, Brusca SR, et al: A model clinical program for patients with diabetes and vision impairment. Diabetes Educ 15:325–330, 1989

Blumenthal JA, Wei J: Psychobehavioral treatment in cardiac rehabilitation. Cardiol Clin 11:323–331, 1993

Browne GB, Arpin K, Corey P, et al: Individual correlates of health service utilization and the cost of poor adjustment to chronic illness. Med Care 28:43–58, 1990

Cain EN, Kohorn EI, Quinlan DM, et al: Psychosocial benefits of a cancer support group. Cancer 57:183–189, 1986

Cheung YL, Molassiotis A, Chang AM: The effect of progressive muscle relaxation training on anxiety and quality of life after stoma surgery in colorectal cancer patients. Psychooncology 12:254–266, 2003

Cohen ST, Welch G, Jacobson AM, et al: The association of lifetime psychiatric illness and increased retinopathy in patients with type I diabetes mellitus. Psychosomatics 38:98–108, 1997

Creed F, Fernandes L, Guthrie E, et al: The cost-effectiveness of psychotherapy and paroxetine for severe irritable bowel syndrome. Gastroenterology 124:303–317, 2003

Davidson KW, Gidron Y, Mostofsky E, et al: Hospitalization cost offset of a hostility intervention for coronary heart disease patients. J Consult Clin Psychol 75:657–662, 2007

Derogatis LR, Morrow GR, Fetting J, et al: The prevalence of psychiatric disorders among cancer patients. JAMA 249:751–757, 1983

Drossman DA, Leserman J, Nachman G, et al: Sexual and physical abuse in women with functional or organic gastrointestinal disorders. Ann Intern Med 113:828–833, 1990

Druss BG, Rosenheck RA, Sledge WH: Health and disability costs of depressive illness in a major U.S. corporation. Am J Psychiatry 157:1274–1278, 2000

Engel GL: The need for a new medical model: a challenge for biomedicine. Science 196:129–136, 1977

Fawzy FI, Cousins N, Fawzy NW, et al: A structured psychiatric intervention for cancer patients. I. Changes over time in methods of coping and affective disturbance. Arch Gen Psychiatry 47:720–725, 1990a

Fawzy FI, Kemeny ME, Fawzy NW, et al: A structured psychiatric intervention for cancer patients. II. Changes over time in immunological measures. Arch Gen Psychiatry 47:729–735, 1990b

Fawzy FI, Fawzy NW, Hyun CS, et al: Malignant melanoma. Effects of an early structured psychiatric intervention, coping, and affective state on recurrence and survival 6 years later. Arch Gen Psychiatry 50:681–689, 1993

Feuerstein M, Burrell LM, Miller VI, et al: Clinical management of carpal tunnel syndrome: a 12-year review of outcomes. Am J Ind Med 35:232–245, 1999

Forester B, Kornfeld DS, Fleiss JL: Psychotherapy during radiotherapy: effects on emotional and physical distress. Am J Psychiatry 142:22–27, 1985

Fosbury JA, Bosley CM, Ryle A, et al: A trial of cognitive analytic therapy in poorly controlled type I patients. Diabetes Care 20:959–964, 1997

Gavard JA, Lustman PJ, Clouse RE: Prevalence of depression in adults with diabetes. An epidemiological evaluation. Diabetes Care 16:1167–1178, 1993

Gellert GA, Maxwell RM, Siegel BS: Survival of breast cancer patients receiving adjunctive psychosocial support therapy: a 10-year follow-up study. J Clin Oncol 11:66–69, 1993

Gould KL, Ornish D, Scherwitz L, et al: Changes in myocardial perfusion abnormalities by positron emission tomography after long-term, intense risk factor modification. JAMA 274:894–901, 1995

Guthrie E, Creed F, Dawson D, et al: A randomised controlled trial of psychotherapy in patients with refractory irritable bowel syndrome. Br J Psychiatry 163:315–321, 1993

Haddock CK, Rowan AB, Andrasik F, et al: Home-based behavioral treatments for chronic benign headache: a meta-analysis of controlled trials. Cephalalgia 17:113–118, 1997

Hampson SE, Skinner TC, Hart J, et al: Effects of educational and psychosocial interventions for adolescents with diabetes mellitus: a systematic review. Health Technol Assess 5:1–79, 2001

Hellman CJ, Budd M, Borysenko J, et al: A study of the effectiveness of two group behavioral medicine interventions for patients with psychosomatic complaints. Behav Med 16:165–173, 1990

House JS, Landis KR, Umberson D: Social relationships and health. Science 241:540–545, 1988

Houston BK, Chesney MA, Black GW, et al: Behavioral clusters and coronary heart disease risk. Psychosom Med 54:447–461, 1992

Ironson G, Taylor CB, Boltwood M, et al: Effects of anger on left ventricular ejection fraction in coronary artery disease. Am J Cardiol 70:281–285, 1992

Jacobsen PB, Meade CD, Stein KD, et al: Efficacy and costs of two forms of stress management training for cancer patients undergoing chemotherapy. J Clin Oncol 20:2851–2862, 2002

Jacobson AM: The psychological care of patients with insulin-dependent diabetes mellitus. N Engl J Med 334:1249–1253, 1996a

Jacobson AM: Psychological perspectives in the care of patients with diabetes mellitus, in Psychiatric Secrets. Edited by Jacobson J, Jacobson A. Philadelphia, PA, Hanley & Belfus, 1996b, pp 443–450

Jacobson AM, de Groot M, Samson JA: The evaluation of two measures of quality of life in patients with type I and type II diabetes. Diabetes Care 17:267–274, 1994

Johannesson M, Agewall S, Hartford M, et al: The cost-effectiveness of a cardiovascular multiple-risk-factor intervention programme in treated hypertensive men. J Intern Med 237:19–26, 1995

Johnson RE, Jones GT, Wiles NJ, et al: Active exercise, education, and cognitive behavioral therapy for persistent disabling low back pain: a randomized controlled trial. Spine 32:1578–1585, 2007

Johnson-Masotti AP, Pinkerton SD, et al: Cost-effectiveness of an HIV risk reduction intervention for adults with severe mental illness. AIDS Care 12:321–332, 2000

Kashner TM, Rost K, Cohen B, et al: Enhancing the health of somatization disorder patients. Effectiveness of short-term group therapy. Psychosomatics 36:462–470, 1995

Katon W: The epidemiology of depression in medical care. Int J Psychiatry Med 17:93–112, 1987

Katon W, Roy-Byrne PP: Panic disorder in the medically ill. J Clin Psychiatry 50:299–302, 1989

Katon W, Russo J: Somatic symptoms and depression. J Fam Pract 29:65–69, 1989

Katon W, Unutzer J, Fan MY, et al: Cost-effectiveness and net benefit of enhanced treatment of depression for older adults with diabetes and depression. Diabetes Care 29:265–270, 2006

Keefe FJ, Caldwell DS: Cognitive behavioral control of arthritis pain. Med Clin North Am 81:277–290, 1997

Kennedy S, Kiecolt-Glaser JK, Glaser R: Immunological consequences of acute and chronic stressors: mediating role of interpersonal relationships. Br J Med Psychol 61 (part 1):77–85, 1988

Kent LA, Gill GV, Williams G: Mortality and outcome of patients with brittle diabetes and recurrent ketoacidosis. Lancet 344:778–781, 1994

Kessler LG, Steinwachs DM, Hankin JR: Episodes of psychiatric care and medical utilization. Med Care 20:1209–1221, 1982

Kiecolt-Glaser JK, Glaser R: Psychoneuroimmunology: can psychological interventions modulate immunity? J Consult Clin Psychol 60:569–575, 1992

Kissane DW, Grabsch B, Clarke DM, et al: Supportive-expressive group therapy for women with metastatic breast cancer: survival and psychosocial outcome from a randomized controlled trial. Psychooncology 16:277–286, 2007

Kuchler T, Bestmann B, Rappat S, et al: Impact of psychotherapeutic support for patients with gastrointestinal cancer undergoing surgery: 10-year survival results of a randomized trial. J Clin Oncol 25:2702–2708, 2007

Lemieux J, Topp A, Chappell H, et al: Economic analysis of psychosocial group therapy in women with metastatic breast cancer. Breast Cancer Res Treat 100:183–190, 2006

Levenson JL, Hamer RM, Rossiter LF: Relation of psychopathology in general medical inpatients to use and cost of services. Am J Psychiatry 147:1498–1503, 1990

Levitan SJ, Kornfeld DS: Clinical and cost benefits of liaison psychiatry. Am J Psychiatry 138:790–793, 1981

Lewin RJ, Coulton S, Frizelle DJ, et al: A brief cognitive behavioural preimplantation and rehabilitation programme for patients receiving an implantable cardioverter-defibrillator improves physical health and reduces psychological morbidity and unplanned readmissions. Heart 95:63–69, 2009

Lim LE: Psychogenic pain. Singapore Med J 35:519–522, 1994

Linden W, Stossel C, Maurice J: Psychosocial interventions for patients with coronary artery disease: a meta-analysis. Arch Intern Med 156:745–752, 1996

Linn BS, Linn MW: Late stage cancer patients: age differences in their psychophysical status and response to counseling. J Gerontol 36:689–692, 1981

Linn MW, Linn BS, Harris R: Effects of counseling for late stage cancer patients. Cancer 49:1048–1055, 1982

Linton SJ: Chronic back pain: integrating psychological and physical therapy—an overview. Behav Med 20:101–104, 1994

Loscalzo M: Psychological approaches to the management of pain in patients with advanced cancer. Hematol Oncol Clin North Am 10:139–155, 1996

Luborsky L, German RE, Diguer L, et al: Is psychotherapy good for your health? Am J Psychother 58:386–405, 2004

Lustman PJ, Griffith LS, Clouse RE, et al: Psychiatric illness in diabetes mellitus. Relationship to symptoms and glucose control. J Nerv Ment Dis 174:736–742, 1986

Mayou RA, Bryant BM, Sanders D, et al: A controlled trial of cognitive behavioural therapy for non-cardiac chest pain. Psychol Med 27:1021–1031, 1997

Meyer E 3rd, Derogatis LR, Miller MJ, et al: Addition of time-limited psychotherapy to medical treatment in a general medical clinic. Results at one-year follow-up. J Nerv Ment Dis 169:780–790, 1981

Mittleman MA, Maclure M, Sherwood JB, et al: Triggering of acute myocardial infarction onset by episodes of anger. Determinants of Myocardial Infarction Onset Study Investigators. Circulation 92:1720–1725, 1995

Mittelman MS, Ferris SH, Shulman E, et al: A family intervention to delay nursing home placement of patients with Alzheimer disease. A randomized controlled trial. JAMA 276:1725–1731, 1996

Moore RK, Groves DG, Bridson JD, et al: A brief cognitive-behavioral intervention reduces hospital admissions in refractory angina patients. J Pain Symptom Manage 33:310–316, 2007

Moran G, Fonagy P, Kurtz A, et al: A controlled study of psychoanalytic treatment of brittle diabetes. J Am Acad Child Adolesc Psychiatry 30:926–935, 1991

Mumford E, Schlesinger HJ, Glass GV: The effect of psychological intervention on recovery from surgery and heart attacks: an analysis of the literature. Am J Public Health 72:141–151, 1982

Mumford E, Schlesinger HJ, Glass GV, et al: A new look at evidence about reduced cost of medical utilization following mental health treatment. Am J Psychiatry 141:1145–1158, 1984

O'Dowd H, Gladwell P, Rogers CA, et al: Cognitive behavioural therapy in chronic fatigue syndrome: a randomised controlled trial of an outpatient group programme. Health Technol Assess 10:iii–iv, ix–x, 1–121, 2006

Padgett D, Mumford E, Hynes M, et al: Meta-analysis of the effects of educational and psychosocial interventions on management of diabetes mellitus. J Clin Epidemiol 41:1007–1030, 1988

Parsons T: Social structure and dynamic process: the case of modern medical practice, in The Social System. Toronto, Free Press, 1951

Peters L, Simon EP, Folen RA, et al: The COPE program: treatment efficacy and medical utilization outcome of a chronic pain management program at a major military hospital. Mil Med 165:954–960, 2000

Polonsky WH, Anderson BJ, Lohrer PA, et al: Insulin omission in women with IDDM. Diabetes Care 17:1178–1185, 1994

Popkin MK, Callies AL, Lentz RD, et al: Prevalence of major depression, simple phobia, and other psychiatric disorders in patients with long-standing type I diabetes mellitus. Arch Gen Psychiatry 45:64–68, 1988

Richardson JL, Shelton DR, Krailo M, et al: The effect of compliance with treatment on survival among patients with hematologic malignancies. J Clin Oncol 8:356–364, 1990

Rosenheck RA, Druss B, Stolar M, et al: Effect of declining mental health service use on employees of a large corporation. Health Aff (Millwood) 18:193–203, 1999

Rosenthal RH: Psychology of chronic pelvic pain. Obstet Gynecol Clin North Am 20:627–642, 1993

Sanders MR, Shepherd RW, Cleghorn G, et al: The treatment of recurrent abdominal pain in children: a controlled comparison of cognitive-behavioral family intervention and standard pediatric care. J Consult Clin Psychol 62:306–314, 1994

Schweikert B, Jacobi E, Seitz R, et al: Effectiveness and cost-effectiveness of adding a cognitive behavioral treatment to the rehabilitation of chronic low back pain. J Rheumatol 33:2519–2526, 2006

Simon GE, Katon WJ, Lin EH, et al: Cost-effectiveness of systematic depression treatment among people with diabetes mellitus. Arch Gen Psychiatry 64:65–72, 2007

Sledge WH, Feinstein AR: A clinimetric approach to the components of the patient-physician relationship. JAMA 278:2043–2048, 1997

Sledge WH, Astrachan B, Thompson K, et al: Case management in psychiatry: an analysis of tasks. Am J Psychiatry 152:1259–1265, 1995

Smith GR Jr, Monson RA, Ray DC: Psychiatric consultation in somatization disorder. A randomized controlled study. N Engl J Med 314:1407–1413, 1986

Smith GR Jr, Rost K, Kashner TM: A trial of the effect of a standardized psychiatric consultation on health outcomes and costs in somatizing patients. Arch Gen Psychiatry 52:238–243, 1995

Spiegel D: Health caring. Psychosocial support for patients with cancer. Cancer 74 (suppl 4):1453–1457, 1994

Spiegel D: Essentials of psychotherapeutic intervention for cancer patients. Support Care Cancer 3:252–256, 1995

Spiegel D: Cancer and depression. Br J Psychiatry Suppl:109–116, 1996

Spiegel D, Bloom JR: Group therapy and hypnosis reduce metastatic breast carcinoma pain. Psychosom Med 45:333–339, 1983

Spiegel D, Kato PM: Psychosocial influences on cancer incidence and progression. Harv Rev Psychiatry 4:10–26, 1996

Spiegel D, Bloom JR, Yalom I: Group support for patients with metastatic cancer. A randomized outcome study. Arch Gen Psychiatry 38:527–533, 1981

Spiegel D, Bloom JR, Kraemer HC, et al: Effect of psychosocial treatment on survival of patients with metastatic breast cancer. Lancet 2:888–891, 1989

Strain JJ, Lyons JS, Hammer JS, et al: Cost offset from a psychiatric consultation-liaison intervention with elderly hip fracture patients. Am J Psychiatry 148:1044–1049, 1991

Trijsburg RW, van Knippenberg FC, Rijpma SE: Effects of psychological treatment on cancer patients: a critical review. Psychosom Med 54:489–517, 1992

Turner JA, Jensen MP: Efficacy of cognitive therapy for chronic low back pain. Pain 52:169–177, 1993

Uchino BN, Kiecolt-Glaser JK, Cacioppo JT: Age-related changes in cardiovascular response as a function of a chronic stressor and social support. J Pers Soc Psychol 63:839–846, 1992

van Dulmen AM, Fennis JF, Bleijenberg G: Cognitive-behavioral group therapy for irritable bowel syndrome: effects and long-term follow-up. Psychosom Med 58:508–514, 1996

Verbosky LA, Franco KN, Zrull JP: The relationship between depression and length of stay in the general hospital patient. J Clin Psychiatry 54:177–181, 1993

Walker E, Katon W, Harrop-Griffiths J, et al: Relationship of chronic pelvic pain to psychiatric diagnoses and childhood sexual abuse. Am J Psychiatry 145:75–80, 1988

Wells KB, Sturm R: Care for depression in a changing environment. Health Aff (Millwood) 14:78–89, 1995

Wolff N, Helminiak TW, Tebes JK: Getting the cost right in cost-effectiveness analyses. Am J Psychiatry 154:736–743, 1997

Zubenko GS, Mulsant BH, Sweet RA, et al: Mortality of elderly patients with psychiatric disorders. Am J Psychiatry 154:1360–1368, 1997

## Summary of studies addressing the cost-effectiveness of psychotherapy of patients with medical conditions

| Articles | Patients | Treatment | Outcome |
|---|---|---|---|
| **Psychotherapy in patients with cancer** | | | |
| Jacobsen et al. 2002 | 411 patients about to start chemotherapy. | Participants were randomly assigned to receive usual psychosocial care only, a professionally administered form of stress management training, or a patient self-administered form of stress management training. Quality-of-life assessments were conducted before randomization and before the 2nd, 3rd, and 4th treatment cycles. Intervention costs were estimated from both payer and societal perspectives. | Compared with patients who received usual care only, patients receiving the self-administered intervention reported significantly ($P \leq 0.05$) better physical functioning, greater vitality, fewer role limitations because of emotional problems, and better mental health. In contrast, patients who received the professionally administered intervention fared no better in terms of quality of life than patients receiving usual care only. Costs of the self-administered intervention were estimated to be 66% (from a payer perspective) to 68% (from a societal perspective) less than the average costs of professionally administered psychosocial interventions for patients starting chemotherapy. |

## Summary of studies addressing the cost-effectiveness of psychotherapy of patients with medical conditions *(continued)*

| Articles | Patients | Treatment | Outcome |
|---|---|---|---|
| **Psychotherapy in patients with cancer *(continued)*** | | | |
| Cheung et al. 2003 | 59 patients. | Participants were randomly assigned to a control group receiving routine care ($n=30$) and an experimental group receiving routine care and progressive muscle relaxation training (PMRT) through two teaching sessions and practice at home for the first 10 weeks. The State–Trait Anxiety Inventory and two Quality of Life Scales were used to collect the data of interest in three occasions, namely during hospitalization, at week 5, and at week 10 postsurgery. | Use of PMRT significantly decreased state anxiety and improved quality of life in the experimental group ($P<0.05$). Social relationships decreased in both groups. In relation to the disease-specific quality-of-life measure, differences were observed only in the 10-week assessment, with the experimental group reporting better quality of life at 10 weeks but not over time as compared with the control group. PMRT should be incorporated in the long-term care of colorectal cancer patients, as it can improve their psychological health and quality of life. This may be a cost-effective intervention that needs minimal training. |

**Summary of studies addressing the cost-effectiveness of psychotherapy of patients with medical conditions** *(continued)*

| Articles | Patients | Treatment | Outcome |
|---|---|---|---|
| **Psychotherapy in patients with cancer** *(continued)* | | | |
| Kissane et al. 2007 | 485 women with advanced breast cancer recruited between 1996 and 2002; 227 women (47%) consented. | Participants were randomly assigned within an average 10 months of cancer recurrence in a 2:1 ratio to intervention with 1 year or more of weekly supportive-expressive group therapy (SEGT) plus three classes of relaxation therapy (147 women) or to control receiving three classes of relaxation therapy (80 women). | SEGT did not prolong survival: median survival 24.0 months in SEGT and 18.3 in controls; univariate hazard ratio for death, 0.92 (95% confidence interval [CI] 0.69, 1.26); multivariate hazard ratio, 1.06 (95% CI 0.74, 1.51). Significant predictors of survival were treatment with chemotherapy and hormone therapy ($P<0.001$), visceral metastases ($P<0.001$), and advanced disease at first diagnosis ($P<0.05$). SEGT ameliorated and prevented new DSM-IV depressive disorders ($P=0.002$), reduced hopelessness-helplessness ($P=0.004$), trauma symptoms ($P=0.04$), and improved social functioning ($P=0.03$). |

## Summary of studies addressing the cost-effectiveness of psychotherapy of patients with medical conditions *(continued)*

| Articles | Patients | Treatment | Outcome |
|---|---|---|---|
| **Psychotherapy in patients with cancer *(continued)*** | | | |
| Kuchler et al. 2007 | Consenting patients (*N*=271) with a preliminary diagnosis of cancer of the esophagus, stomach, liver/ gallbladder, pancreas, or colon/ rectum. | Participants were stratified by gender and randomly assigned to a control group that received standard care as provided on the surgical wards or to an experimental group that received formal psychotherapeutic support in addition to routine care during the hospital stay. Survival status for all patients was determined from records and from three external sources. | Kaplan–Meier survival curves demonstrated better survival for the experimental group than the control group. The unadjusted significance level for group differences was *P*=0.0006 for survival to 10 years. Cox regression models that took TNM (tumor, node, metastasis) staging or the residual tumor classification and tumor site into account also found significant differences at 10 years. Secondary analyses found that differences in favor of the experimental group occurred in patients with stomach, pancreatic, primary liver, or colorectal cancer. |

**Summary of studies addressing the cost-effectiveness of psychotherapy of patients with medical conditions _(continued)_**

| Articles | Patients | Treatment | Outcome |
|---|---|---|---|
| **Psychotherapy in patients with cardiac and cardiovascular diseases** | | | |
| Davidson et al. 2007 | 26 male patients with myocardial infarction or unstable angina. | Patients were randomly assigned to either 2 months of cognitive-behavioral group therapy or an information (control) session. | Therapy patients had a shorter average length of hospital stay ($N=13$, $M=0.38$ days, $SD=0.96$) than did control patients ($N=13$, $M=2.15$ days, $SD=2.6$), $t_{15,2}=-2.29$, $P=0.04$, over 6 months following therapy. The average hospitalization costs were significantly lower for therapy patients ($M=\$245$, $SD=\$627$) than for control patients ($M=\$1,333$, $SD=\$1,609$), $t_{15,6}=-2.27$, $P=0.04$. The cost-offset ratio is calculated by dividing the \$1,088 of hospitalization savings by the \$560 of therapy expense (\$1.00:\$1.94), indicating that for every \$1 spent on therapy, there is an approximate savings of \$2 in hospitalization costs in the following 6 months. These findings support the hospitalization cost offset of hostility reduction in coronary heart disease patients. |

**Summary of studies addressing the cost-effectiveness of psychotherapy of patients with medical conditions *(continued)***

| Articles | Patients | Treatment | Outcome |
|---|---|---|---|
| **Psychotherapy in patients with cardiac and cardiovascular diseases *(continued)*** | | | |
| Moore et al. 2007 | 430 outpatients were referred between January 1, 1997 and January 10, 2002, of whom 383 were diagnosed with chronic refractory angina (CRA). | CRA is an increasingly prevalent, complex chronic pain condition that results in frequent hospitalization for chest pain. It has previously been shown that a novel outpatient cognitive-behavioral chronic disease management program (CB-CDMP) improves angina status and quality of life in such patients. | In the present study of 271 CRA patients enrolled in the CB-CDMP, total hospital admissions were reduced from 2.40 admissions per patient per year to 1.78 admissions per patient per year ($P<0.001$). The rising trend of total hospital bed day occupancy prior to enrollment fell from 15.48 days per patient per year to a stable 10.34 days per patient per year ($P<0.001$). |
| Lewin et al. 2009 | Consecutive series of patients undergoing implantation with an implantable cardioverter-defibrillator (ICD). 192 patients were recruited to the study (71 intervention, 121 control). | The control group received usual care and advice from an experienced health care professional. The intervention group received usual care plus the ICD plan. | At 6 months after surgery, the intervention group had better physical health (37.83 vs. 34.24; $P<0.01$), fewer limitations in physical activity (34.02 vs. 31.72; $P=0.04$), a greater reduction in the proportion of patients with a borderline diagnosis of anxiety (21% vs. 13%; $P=0.60$) and depression (13% vs. 2%; $P=0.30$), more planned ECGs (89% vs. 66%; $P=0.04$), and 50% fewer unplanned admissions (11% vs. 22%; $P<0.01$). |

**Summary of studies addressing the cost-effectiveness of psychotherapy of patients with medical conditions *(continued)***

| Articles | Patients | Treatment | Outcome |
|---|---|---|---|
| **Psychotherapy in patients with diabetes** | | | |
| Hampson et al. 2001 | Review. | To examine the effectiveness of educational and psychosocial interventions for adolescents with type 1 diabetes designed to improve their diabetes management. Specifically, it addressed the following research questions:<br><br>1. Do educational and psychosocial interventions for adolescents with type 1 diabetes have beneficial effects on biological and psychosocial outcomes?<br>2. Are there types or features of interventions that have been shown to be more effective than others?<br>3. What evidence is there of the cost-effectiveness of interventions? | 25 randomized control trials were examined in more detail and three of the most effective were described in depth. Effect sizes could be calculated for 14 studies. The mean (pooled) effect size for psychosocial outcomes was 0.37 and 0.33 for glycated hemoglobin with outliers (0.08 without outliers), indicating that these interventions have small to medium beneficial effects on diabetes management outcomes. |

*Psychotherapy for Patients With Medical Conditions*        **263**

**Summary of studies addressing the cost-effectiveness of psychotherapy of patients with medical conditions** *(continued)*

| Articles | Patients | Treatment | Outcome |
|---|---|---|---|
| **Psychotherapy in patients with musculoskeletal disease** | | | |
| Schweikert et al. 2006 | 409 patients with chronic low back pain who were admitted to a 3-week inpatient rehabilitation. | Participants were randomly assigned to usual care or usual care plus cognitive-behavioral therapy (CBT). | Average incremental costs for psychological treatment during rehabilitation were 127 euros (95% CI 125.6, 130.9; $P<0.001$). Six months after rehabilitation, patients in the intervention group were absent from work an average of 5.4 (95% CI −1.4, 12.1; $P=0.12$) days less than patients receiving usual treatment. Between groups, there were no significant differences in quality-adjusted life years (QALYs) gained or in direct medical or nonmedical costs. The CBT showed lower indirect costs: 751 euros (95% CI −145, 1,641; $P=0.097$). |
| Johnson et al. 2007 | Patients ages 18–65 years consulting with low back pain (LBP) were recruited; those still reporting LBP 3 months after the initial consultation were randomly assigned between the two trial arms. A total of 196 subjects (84%) completed follow-up 12 months after the completion of the intervention. | Patients in the intervention arm received a program of eight 2-hour group exercise sessions over 6 weeks comprising active exercise and education delivered by physiotherapists using a CBT approach. Both arms received an educational booklet and audio-cassette. The primary outcome measures were pain (0–100 Visual Analogue Scale) and disability (Roland and Morris Disability Scale; score 0–24). | The intervention showed only a small and nonsignificant effect at reducing pain (−3.6 mm; 95% CI −8.5, 1.2 mm) and disability (−0.6 score; 95% CI −1.6, 0.4). The cost of the intervention was low with an incremental cost-effectiveness ratio of pound sterling 5,000 ($8,650) per QALY. In addition, patients allocated to the intervention who had expressed a preference for it had clinically important reductions in pain and disability. |

**Summary of studies addressing the cost-effectiveness of psychotherapy of patients with medical conditions** *(continued)*

| Articles | Patients | Treatment | Outcome |
|---|---|---|---|
| **Psychotherapy and transplantation** | | | |
| Baines et al. 2004 | The control arm was composed of 37 consecutive patients who had received a first cadaver kidney; 89 recipients of first cadaver kidney transplants into the study were randomly allocated into two study groups: 49 for individual therapy and 40 for group therapy. | Recipients of first cadaver kidney transplants were randomly assigned into two groups to receive a 12-week course of group or individual psychotherapy. The Beck Depression Inventory (BDI) was used as a measure of change in emotional state, pretherapy, and at 3, 6, 9, and 12 months. A higher score on BDI was suggestive of psychological dysfunction. | The mean score was $26.3 \pm 7.9$ before and $18.9 \pm 9.0$ after therapy in the individual treatment group ($P=0.001$). This was in comparison with a mean score of $30.2 \pm 3.8$ before and $26.0 \pm 4.2$ after therapy for the group therapy arm ($P=0.01$). Improvement appeared to be more significant in the individual therapy compared with group therapy ($P=0.01$). Lowering of scores was progressive and sustained ($P=0.01$). In the control arm, mean score was $9.4 \pm 5.4$ before and $20.5 \pm 5.5$ at the end of the first year ($P=0.005$), suggesting a significant worsening of BDI scores. Multivariate analysis of age, gender, employment status, duration of dialysis, etiology of kidney failure, diabetes mellitus, and psychotherapy received at any time before transplantation did not affect results. |

**Summary of studies addressing the cost-effectiveness of psychotherapy of patients with medical conditions *(continued)***

| Articles | Patients | Treatment | Outcome |
|---|---|---|---|
| **Miscellaneous illnesses** | | | |
| Luborsky et al. 2004 | Review. | A dedicated review of the evidence for the relation of having a period of psychotherapy and then comparing it with a measure of improved physical health. The authors attempted to make it the first intended-to-be-complete review of this type. Three interrelated types of studies were examined: Type 1: reduction in physical illnesses through psychotherapy, especially for the patient's survival time during the interval between diagnosis and an end point. Type 2: reduction in pain in relation to receiving psychotherapy. Type 3: reduction in costs of treatment in relation to receiving psychotherapy. To find the relevant studies on these topics, we performed a literature search using both PsycINFO and MEDLINE databases. | An average of the effect sizes under each type was taken to calculate the mean effect size along with its confidence interval. Results (Type 1) on survival time for the combined severe patients did not reach even the lowest significant level of effect size, although the low-severity patients seemed to fit the hypothesis better, but the other two reduction topics (Types 2 and 3) clearly did achieve it. |

**Summary of studies addressing the cost-effectiveness of psychotherapy of patients with medical conditions *(continued)***

| Articles | Patients | Treatment | Outcome |
|---|---|---|---|
| Miscellaneous illnesses *(continued)* | | | |
| O'Dowd et al. 2006 | Adults with a diagnosis of chronic fatigue syndrome/myalgic encephalopathy (CFS/ME) referred by their general practitioner. A total of 153 patients were recruited to the trial and 52 were randomly assigned to receive CBT, 50 to education and support group (EAS), and 51 to standard medical care (SMC). | A double-blind, randomized controlled trial was adopted with three arms. Outcomes were assessed at baseline and 6 and 12 months after first assessment and results were analyzed on an intention-to-treat basis. The three interventions were group CBT incorporating graded activity scheduling, EAS, and SMC. The primary outcome measure was the 36-item Short Form (SF-36) physical and mental health summary scales. Other outcome measures included the Chalder Fatigue Scale, Hospital Anxiety and Depression Scale, General Health Questionnaire, and measures of physical function. | Group CBT did not achieve the expected change in the primary outcome measure as a significant number did not achieve scores within the normal range postintervention. The treatment did not return a significant number of subjects to within the normal range on this domain; however, significant improvements were evident in some areas. Group CBT was effective in treating symptoms of fatigue, mood, and physical fitness in CFS/ME. It was found to be as effective as trials using individual therapy in these domains. However, it did not bring about improvement in cognitive function or quality of life. There was also evidence of improvement in the EAS group, which indicates that there is limited value in the nonspecific effects of therapy. |

# Psychotherapy for Children and Adolescents

Jules Bemporad, M.D.

**W**hile the cost-effectiveness of psychotherapy with children and adolescents has not been demonstrated in large-scale studies involving large samples, smaller, focused research reports have shown that psychotherapy does reduce the need for further treatment or is helpful in returning children who are receiving medication for a variety of disorders to appropriate functioning or prevents future intervention by social agencies or the juvenile justice system. In contrast, the efficacy of verbal therapies on everyday functioning has been substantiated in a sizable literature. Four meta-analytic reports, surveying hundreds of published studies, found that treated children did better than matched controls. These four studies reviewed research involving most forms of psychotherapy performed by a variety of mental health professionals for children with diverse problems. More focused studies have also demonstrated significant beneficial effect of psychotherapy as well as providing guidance in selecting appropriate types of therapy for different problems. Although a direct relationship between psychotherapy and reduced cost has not been established beyond a doubt, it may be assumed that children who are less encumbered by psychological problems, as a result of psychotherapeutic intervention, will require fewer psychiatric or medical services in the future.

To the degree that psychotherapy will reduce direct or indirect expenditures incurred by similarly impaired, but untreated, individuals, its cost-effectiveness with children and adolescents is difficult to determine with accuracy. However, a number of studies (cited below) show that psychotherapy with children ensures better control of chronic illness such as diabetes, reduces visits to a health maintenance organization (HMO) for medical visits, lessens the need for social services or institutionalization for youngsters with attention-deficit/hyperactivity disorder (ADHD), and helps to restore adequate social functioning in children with depression.

Nevertheless, estimates of cost-effectiveness of the psychotherapy with children presents certain complications that are usually absent in similar studies of the treatment of adults. Children are not employed, so that indirect costs, such as decreased productivity or days of work lost, cannot be calculated. Intangible costs, such as pain or suffering alleviated, are difficult to quantify into monetary units. There is often "cost shifting" whereby social agencies, special schools, and the juvenile justice system end up paying the cost of treatment. The actual expenditure or frequency of such services is unknown and so cannot be considered in estimating the cost-benefit of psychotherapy. Direct costs, the expense of the treatment itself, are also hard to calculate because children are seen in a variety of settings that vary enormously in terms of expenditure. At the low-cost end of the spectrum might be a resource room for a dozen children once a week in a public school where service is delivered by existing school personnel, and at the high-cost end might be a specialized inpatient unit for eating-disordered adolescents with highly trained staff involved in a carefully constructed ward milieu treatment and intensive psychotherapy. Perhaps the best that can be offered at our current level of knowledge is a statement on the effectiveness (rather that the cost-effectiveness) of psychotherapy for the pediatric population. It may be assumed that if such treatment is effective in ameliorating symptoms and in promoting healthier everyday functioning, such treatment should reduce the need for later treatment and indirect costs of decreased productivity of the working parent(s) and of involvement of ancillary agencies or personnel (i.e., school guidance counselors). A mentally healthier child or adolescent should be less of a drain on social or school agencies, as well as less of a burden on his or her family and less of a drain on society as an adult.

# Search Methodology

A MEDLINE search for publications on cost-effectiveness or cost offset for child or adolescent psychotherapy produces few appropriate citations. A similar search for simply effectiveness of psychotherapy for this population resulted in a multitude of citations that are reviewed and compared in the meta-analytic studies described below.

# Specific Characteristics of Patient Population

Any evaluation of the effectiveness of psychotherapy in children and adolescents should consider the particular developmental characteristics of this patient group. In contrast to adults, children and adolescents are in the process of rapid psychological change and usually have not consolidated a persistent mode of functioning. As such, their behavior, including some considered to be symptoms of psychopathology, may abate on its own as developmental challenges are met, mastered, and integrated. Among such transient and normal "developmental crises" (Group for the Advancement of Psychiatry 1966) may be included the so-called 8-month anxiety of the infant, the separation anxiety and phobias of the preschooler, the compulsive or ritualistic behavior of the school-age child, and the mood changes and behavioral fluctuations of the adolescent. These psychological alterations reflect the organism's attempt to complete successfully psychosocial tasks in the maturational process and can be of brief and limited duration. Therefore, some symptoms of younger individuals are a normal part of growing up and should, under expectable circumstances, disappear without treatment as development continues. As Anna Freud (1965) observed, "In fact, where pathology is not too severe, the child analyst will often query after the successful conclusion of a treatment how much of the improvement he can claim as outcome of his therapeutic measures and how much he must ascribe to maturation and to spontaneous developmental moves" (p. 28).

Another differential characteristic of the pediatric population is its material and psychological reliance on parents or other adults. This dependency means that children usually are identified as requiring intervention when their behavior becomes troublesome to others rather than only to themselves. Therefore, case finding and eventual treatment may be determined largely by the relative concern or indifference of family members or other adults, such as school personnel, who interact daily with the child or adolescent. Parents or guardians become highly instrumental in the compliance with therapeutic indications. It is they who decide whether the child will keep appointments or take medication, when indicated. It is not unusual for the parents of a child with ADHD, which is basically a neurodevelopmental condition requiring pharmacotherapy, to refuse to put their child on medication, forcing the clinician to utilize nonpharmacological treatment approaches that, while beneficial in conjunction with medication, are of limited utility by themselves (Abikoff 1991). On the positive side, parents may insist that a child continue treatment even when the child would prefer to engage in more pleasurable activities or when the therapy forces him or her to face unpleasant realities.

Another important aspect of the dependency of this age group is its selective greater reactivity to changes within the home situation rather than in the extrafamilial environment. Children and adolescents are greatly affected by the events occurring within the family setting, and their disorders have their origins in the vicissitudes of relationships with needed loved ones, such as divorce, abuse, or bereavement. Other childhood disorders such as depression, delinquency, or anxiety disorders may be the result of being raised in chronically dysfunctional families. In such cases, effective treatment should involve the entirety of the child's psychosocial experience, extending beyond individual care. For example, Puig-Antich et al. (1985b) recommended psychotherapy for depressed children to remedy the multiple social problems exhibited by such children. Medication alone was not sufficient to restore a child to healthy functioning in terms of relationships or self-esteem. Another study comparing children with ADHD, some of whom received only medication and some who received psychotherapy that often involved the family in addition to medication, revealed that, as adults, the medication-only group had a significantly higher rate of arrests and institutionalization than the multitreatment group (Satterfield et al. 1987). Therefore, effective treatment may involve family members and other influential individuals, as well as the child, in order to affect his or her level of functioning. Toward this end, Henggeler et al. (1994) reported that multisystemic therapy, which targets intervention with family, peers, school, and community, is more successful than one-dimensional therapies in treating severely disturbed, predominantly antisocial, adolescents.

The recognition of the power of the family, as well as other factors such as poverty, lack of social supports, and peer influence, to instigate or to perpetuate childhood disorders has obvious import for the effectiveness of therapeutic intervention. Outcome studies performed in community clinics that serve predominantly children who come from multiproblem families with social and economic disadvantages can be expected to show less effectiveness than studies carried out with children from affluent and relatively untroubled families.

This last influence relates to two other factors that should be taken into account when efficacy studies are evaluated. The first relates to the level of skill and training of the therapist. Community clinics and public sector service delivery centers are often, but not always, staffed with less-experienced, less-educated, and lower-paid practitioners than those who offer services in private practice or academic settings. Even when public sector providers possess the adequate skill and training, their caseloads may be so overwhelming that less-than-optimal care has to be delivered if all children in need are to be provided for.

A second relevant factor in assessing efficacy studies is the goal of treatment. Some studies focus on symptom suppression only or identify only one presenting symptom as the therapeutic target. Other studies may be more ambitious and aim at amelioration of the child's total psychological functioning as well as his or her immediate environment. The latter studies usually report less impressive results than those who select children with only one symptom (i.e., a healthier cohort) or who concentrate only on symptom removal (reduced expectations).

In summary, a variety of factors, beyond the identified child patient, may influence greatly the relative efficacy of psychotherapeutic intervention. The dysfunction of the child's everyday environment, the compliance of the parents with treatment recommendations, the developmental level of the child, the extent of the goals of treatment, and the setting and skill of the practitioner must all be considered in reviewing studies. Unfortunately, such information is all too lacking in published reports so that often the conclusions reached cannot be accepted with the desired certainty.

# Types of Outcome Studies

The literature on psychotherapy with children and adolescents can be divided into three major types. In the early years of child psychotherapy, most of the literature consisted of single case reports written by clinicians that described the (usually psychoanalytic) therapy of a child as elucidating a particular psychodynamic formulation. As the field became more established, clinical researchers reported small series of cases with similar disorders or difficulties, with or without a control group. These studies attempted to define diagnostic characteristics or personality functioning of the children in question as much as their responses to treatment. The well-known work of Johnson and her colleagues (Johnson et al. 1941) on school phobia can serve as an apt illustration of this type of contribution. Later clinical series have focused less on the description or causes of a specific disorder and more on the effect of treatment, particularly behavioral therapy of isolated symptoms. These studies draw their subjects from advertisements rather than random clinical samples presenting for help and usually include a matched control group.

Finally, the third type of study on the effects of therapy utilizes a recently developed statistical tool for meta-analysis. This technique typically consists of comparing pre- and posttreatment variables or comparing treated and matched control groups. The degree of difference found, for example in treated versus control subjects, on a relevant measure is calculated and divided by some measure of sample variability, usually the standard deviation of score in the control group, to yield an effect size. This resultant statistic can be summed for a number of studies to generate an average effect size representing the effects of treatment in a large number of pooled studies. Obviously, care must be taken to assure that outcome measures are clearly defined and that the research methodology is sound. Studies that lack scientific rigor are discarded from the final analysis. Assuming the inclusion of accurate research studies, effect size has been used increasingly to determine the impact of intervention as well as to measure the effectiveness of different treatments, on varying populations with diverse problems. The advantage of a meta-analysis study is the attempt to eliminate the subjectivity found in a narrative review of studies by supplying a numerical index of outcome.

The following selective review will not attempt to exhaust the literature on psychotherapy with the pediatric population. Only some studies with control groups and sound methodology will be included, as will be reviews of the field in general using meta-analytic techniques (see summary table at the end of this chapter).

## Meta-Analytic Studies

There have been four major meta-analytic studies performed assessing the effects of psychotherapy on children and adolescents. All have reported an appreciable effect size (ES), thereby demonstrating a significant beneficial effect. These studies are summarized briefly below; the reader desiring a more detailed exposition is referred to an excellent review by Weisz and Weiss (1993).

Casey and Berman (1985) surveyed outcome of psychotherapy of children up to and including age 12 (mean age=8–9 years). Their review included 64 studies published between 1952 and 1983. The type of presenting problem, sources of referral, and treatment methods varied considerably. Their results revealed an ES of 0.71, indicating that the treated children were functioning better than 76% of the control group children following therapeutic intervention.

Weisz et al. (1987) conducted a broad-based meta-analysis on the effects of psychotherapy on patients ages 4–18 years. They surveyed 105 studies (32 of which had been included in Casey and Berman's prior review) published between 1958 and 1984. Again the subjects varied widely (children with retardation or organic disabilities were excluded) as did the treatment methods and sources of referral. These authors found an ES score of 0.79 (across 163 treatment vs. control comparisons) indicating that the average treated child scored better than 79% of the control untreated group. Only 6% of the treatment control comparisons yielded a negative ES score, indicating that the control group was functioning better than the treatment groups.

Kazdin et al. (1990) conducted a third meta-analysis on the effects of psychotherapy. They utilized 105 studies on children ages 4–18 published between 1970 and 1988. (Thirteen percent of these also had been surveyed by Casey and Berman [1985] and 18% had been included in Weisz et al.'s [1987] study.) This study also revealed a sizable ES score, indicating beneficial effect of treatment (for treatment vs. no treatment, ES=0.88; for treatment vs. active control, ES=0.77).

A fourth meta-analytic study was conducted by Weisz and colleagues (J. R. Weisz, B. Weiss, T. Morton, D. Granger, and S. Han, "Meta-Analysis of Psychotherapy Outcome Research With Children and Adolescents," unpublished work, 1992, extensively described in Weisz and Weiss 1993). This investigation focused on studies not included in prior studies except for those reported by Kazdin et al. (1990) and published studies on general psychotherapy with patients of all ages that may have included children. These authors surveyed 110 studies on children between the ages of 1.5 and 17.6 years published between 1967 and 1991. Again, a broad range of children, referral sources, and treatment methods were included. The derived ES score was 0.71, indicating that the average treated child scored better than 76% of the nontreated children.

These four large-scale meta-analytic studies yielded remarkably similar results: children who received a variety of psychotherapeutic interventions improved more than roughly three-fourths of the control group children who did not receive treatment. This robust, repeated finding points to definite positive results from psychotherapy. Taking into account the stated limitations of the meta-analytic technique, these findings in over 200 separate studies surveyed make a strong argument for the effectiveness of psychotherapy.

## Focused Studies on Efficacy

As stated earlier, meta-analytic studies are able to yield information on general trends but cannot specify which treatment is best for which condition in detail. Studies that are surveyed may differ in patient problems, treatment methods, or outcome measures. A few studies summarized below are exemplary in choosing outcomes that can be measured accurately and describe their methodology in great detail.

Moran et al. (1991) randomly assigned children ages 6–18 years consecutively admitted for brittle diabetes to a control group receiving standard medical treatment or to an additional course of psychoanalytically oriented therapy three to five times a week during their hospital stay (5–28 weeks, mean 15 weeks). Treatment was unstructured but focused on age-appropriate concerns and adaptive strategies. Follow-up at 1 year past discharge showed the treatment group was in greater diabetic control (as measured by blood sugar levels) and functioning better in their everyday lives. The therapy group should require less frequent medical visits resulting in cost savings.

Heinicke and Ramsey-Klee (1986) assessed the effects of psychoanalytic-oriented therapy on children ages 7–10 years presenting with learning disorders and academic problems. Children were assigned to treatment once weekly or four times a week. Both frequencies of treatment were judged positively, but greater improvement was shown by the more frequent session group at 1-year follow-up. Outcome measures included self-esteem and relationships in addition to academic achievement and reading ability, reducing the need for intensive professional contact in the future.

Finney et al. (1991) looked at the effect of brief targeted therapy on later utilization of medical services by children enrolled in an HMO. The treatment group consisted of 93 children (ages 1–15, mean 6.4 years) who had been referred to the Behavioral Pediatrics Service for a variety of difficulties categorized as behavior, toileting, psychosomatic, and school problems. The control group consisted of 93 matched children in the HMO system who had not been so referred. Treatment consisted of one to six 50-minute sessions addressing the specific problems via behavior modification utilizing parent behavior management techniques. Planned telephone contact after treatment was used to ensure implementation of treatment recommendations. At outcome, 76% of parents reported that the referral problem has been resolved or improved, 20% reported the problem as unchanged, and 4% reported the problem as worse. Therapists' independent ratings agreed with 80% of parent ratings. HMO visits for the year preceding and following treatment were tabulated and compared. It was found that children with behavior problems and toileting problems had reduced HMO utilization significantly whereas those with psychosomatic and school problems did not. The control group showed no change in HMO visits. Therefore, this study indicated that brief focal intervention can be effective with some childhood problems but not with others. In addition, this study also demonstrates a cost-offset effect where there was a reduction in subsequent medical care.

Weiss and Hechtman (1986) reviewed follow-up studies of children with ADHD. They reported overwhelming evidence that children who received psychotherapy along with medication fared much better as adults than children who received medication alone. They specifically emphasized a difference in self-esteem and social functioning between the two groups. As mentioned earlier, Satterfield et al. (1987) found significant differences in arrests and institutionalization as well. Also, as stated earlier, Puig-Antich (1985b) found that medication alone was not sufficient in remitting the full spectrum of depressive disorders in children and recommended psychotherapy to achieve a full recovery.

In a unique study actually measuring the cost-effectiveness of treatments involving psychotherapy for children, Jensen et al. (2005) examined the major forms of ADHD treatments used in the National Institute of Mental Health's Multimodal Treatment Study of Children With ADHD. A total of 579 children with ADHD ages 7–9.9 years were assigned to 14 months of one of four interventions: 1) medication management, 2) intensive behavioral treatment (psychosocial therapy), 3) the combination of medication management and behavioral treatment, or 4) community care. Treatment costs varied fourfold, medication management alone being the least expensive, behavioral treatment the next least expensive, followed by combined treatment. The community care group had lower costs of medication as well as less intensive and less effective treatment. Medical management was both more effective and more costly than community care. Medical management was judged to be more cost-effective than combination treatment or behavioral treatment alone, although it was noted that medical management was less effective than the combination of medical management and the psychotherapeutic behavioral treatment. When making a judgment of relative cost-effectiveness, it is important to keep in mind that the assessment of cost-effectiveness includes judging the acceptability of increments of higher costs for increments of greater improvement. ADHD is the most prevalent behavioral disorder in children and a costly major public health problem. While the direct costs associated with providing each of the treatments were measured in this study, given the 14-month outcome analyses, the findings did not address the potential longer term cost-effectiveness of treatment or the broader societal costs incurred as a result of ADHD. These may include parental work absences and loss of income, the costs of special education and other social services, and the costs of the juvenile justice system, all costs stemming from the illness. The authors noted that children with ADHD incur medical costs similar to those of children with asthma. ADHD children have $1,000–$2,000 higher medical costs than healthy children and $3,000 higher costs for auto accidents as well as increased used of other expensive special education, juvenile justice, and social services. Given these considerations, the modest incremental costs for more effective versus less effective programs (the combination of medical management and behavioral treatment vs. the less costly medical management alone) should perhaps be considered.

The Treatment for Adolescents With Depression Study (TADS) compared the effectiveness of 36 weeks of randomized treatment for 327 adolescents ages 12–17 years with major depressive disorder to 1) fluoxetine hydrochloride, 2) cognitive-behavioral therapy (CBT), or 3) their combination. At week 12 the rates of response were 73% for combination therapy, 62% for fluoxetine, and 48% for CBT. At week 18 the rates were 85% combination therapy, 69% fluoxetine therapy, and 65% CBT. By week 24, the three treatment groups' response rates converged and remained so to 36 weeks, at which point the response rates were 86% for combination treatment and 81% for fluoxetine therapy and for CBT. A finding of great importance was that patients treated with fluoxetine alone were twice as likely as patients treated with combination therapy or CBT to experience a suicidal event, indicating that CBT seems to protect against suicidality in patients treated with fluoxetine. The authors concluded that the combination of fluoxetine and CBT is superior to either monotherapy as a treatment strategy for adolescents with major depression (March et al. 2007) A follow-up report on the cost-effectiveness of the three active treatments found that both fluoxetine and combination therapy are at least as cost-effective in the short term as other treatments commonly used in primary care, that fluoxetine is more cost-effective than combination therapy after 12 weeks of treatment, but also that combination therapy, while having the highest total costs, yielded the greatest improvements in Children's Depression Rating Scale—Revised. In addition, by 36 weeks the response to CBT had caught up to that of fluoxetine (81%) and was only slightly lower than that of combination therapy (86%) (Domino et al. 2008).

In a study of 58 adolescents with a bipolar spectrum disorder, patients were randomly assigned to 1) family-focused treatment and pharmacotherapy (including 21 sessions over 9 months of psychoeducation, communication training, and problem-solving skill training) or 2) enhanced care and pharmacotherapy (including 3 family sessions focused on relapse prevention). While the rates of recovery were the same in both groups, patients receiving the family-focused psychotherapy intervention recovered faster from their baseline depressive symptoms and spent fewer weeks in depressive episodes with a more favorable trajectory of depressive symptoms for 2 years (Miklowitz et al. 2008).

# Differential Effects of Psychotherapy

The foregoing studies have demonstrated relatively positive effects of psychotherapy. However, other studies have reported even more benefit that the meta-analytic survey, whereas some studies have shown no effect of psychotherapy at all. It may be worthwhile to look at these studies to ascertain which types of therapy seem to be most effective for which sort of youngsters.

Those studies reporting the best results (see Weisz and Weiss 1993 for a review) are those that are carried on in an academic setting with specially trained staff. The subjects are recruited (and not referred) for treatment of one particular symptom (e.g., academic problems, a specific phobia, obesity, shyness). One may then surmise that these children were doing well in other areas, because their parents had not sought help for grossly disturbed behavior, and the children and parents were motivated for treatment since they volunteered to be part of the study by answering some sort of advertisement or announcement. In contrast, those studies reporting poor results from psychotherapy have involved public or community clinics that serve lower socioeconomic families who may have difficulty keeping appointments or may be overwhelmed by difficulties (economic problems, issues of safety, medical illness) other than the problems of the identified patient. The patients treated have presented with extensive histories of oppositional behavior culminating in delinquency and often resulting in court-mandated therapy. For such children, therapy has not been shown to be particularly effective. Davidson et al. (W. S. Davidson, R. Gottschalk, L. Gensheimer, et al. "Interventions With Juvenile Delinquents, " unpublished manuscript, 1986; cited in Weisz and Weiss 1993) reviewed 91 intervention studies on delinquent youth and found no evidence of a positive effect. Similarly, a large intervention program for 2,800 violent and assaultive youth with serious emotional, neurological, or mental handicaps, which included a variety of treatments, recreational programs, and vocational training (North Carolina Department of Human Resources, "Report to the Governor and the General Assembly on the Willie M. Program," unpublished work, 1989), failed to reduce the arrest rate (29%) for youngsters who had been in the program for over 2 years versus those who had been in the program for only 1 month after the services had terminated (Weisz et al. 1990).

Some reasons for the failure of such programs may be proposed with some obvious uncertainty. These youngsters may have neurodevelopmental disorders (such as ADHD) that are not amenable to psychotherapy without concurrent medication; their immediate environment may encourage or reward deviant behavior while punishing or belittling more mainstream activities; and the families of such children may be so burdened by day-to-day difficulties as to be unavailable for therapeutic participation. Finally, the extent of prior trauma or deprivation experienced by these youngsters may render intervention at a later age so difficult as to require very long-term involvement before any change is observable. The point is that psychotherapy, as with any other form of treatment, has its indications and limitations. It should be applied judiciously and with appropriate caution. Psychotherapy may lead to excessive confidence when applied to relatively healthy children from highly motivated families who volunteer for a special project.

It may also lead to excessive pessimism when applied to undermotivated youths who may have comorbid neurological difficulties and are burdened by socioeconomic disadvantages, nonsupportive families, and a backlog of deprivation.

The studies abstracted above mainly describe the effects of psychotherapy for specialized groups. A more realistic appraisal of psychotherapy as it is practiced in the community for children with the full variety of problems who sought help can be found in several publications from the Anna Freud Center in London (Fonagy and Target 1994; Target and Fonagy 1994a, 1994b). These authors reviewed the charts of 763 children who had been treated and investigated the impact of intensive versus nonintensive psychotherapy on different disorders and on children in different stages of development. The therapy was provided by clinic staff experienced in principles of psychodynamic treatment. Effectiveness of treatment was measured by decrease in symptoms and by overall psychological functioning as determined by comparing pre- and posttreatment children's Global Assessment Scale scores. One study (Fonagy and Target 1994) looked at the result of treatment for children with disruptive disorders (those with externalizing symptoms). It was found that severely impaired children did better with intensive treatment (three to five sessions per week) than with nonintensive treatment (one to two sessions per week) whereas those with mild impairment did equally well in either treatment condition. A similar result was obtained when children with emotional disorders (internalizing symptoms) were considered (Target and Fonagy 1994a). The less severely impaired children did just as well with less frequent psychotherapy. The authors concluded that severely impaired children do not respond well to nonintensive therapy and should be seen in analysis, whereas mildly impaired children do not require intensive treatment and analysis is difficult to justify for this latter population.

Finally, the authors looked at effect of treatment on children of different ages. They reported that increased intensity of treatment is significantly related to improvement in children under age 12 but not for children over 12 who do equally well with either intensive or nonintensive treatment. However, duration of treatment was positively related to outcome for older children but not for younger children. The authors speculated that younger children may require more frequent sessions to be able to sustain a new relationship or to carry over learned beneficial behavior from one session to the next, but because their disorders were not as integrated into the personality, a shorter period of treatment could suffice. In contrast, older children are capable of maintaining a relationship with less frequent contact but have structuralized their disorders into their everyday personality function so that longer treatment is required before changes appear.

These studies are important, not only for demonstrating the effectiveness of psychotherapy but also because the therapy supplied, the patients treated, and the professionals providing care all are most representative of the way psychotherapy is practiced in the community. Therefore, studies like these may give a more valid picture of the effectiveness of psychotherapy than those reports from academic research departments or from public community clinics.

The appropriateness (and eventual effectiveness) of psychotherapy may be appreciated by the following case illustrations of two boys of similar age but with markedly different therapeutic needs.

# Case Vignettes

## Case 1

David was a 13-year-old boy who requested to see a therapist because of increasing feelings of sadness, a loss of interest in his usual activities, and a decrease in school performance. These symptoms began after his parents decided to separate and his father moved out of the family home. The separation was followed by frequent arguments between the estranged parents and by their exhibiting spiteful behavior toward each other in front of their children. For example, the father delayed paying household bills so that the family's television cable was disconnected and a cessation of power and telephone service was threatened. The mother, in retaliation, refused to let her husband enter their house and made it difficult for him to see his children. When the parents did encounter each other, a violent argument usually ensued with many recriminations and much mutual name calling. David witnessed these scenes and, in this context, became increasingly depressed.

In the first session, David was cooperative and open with his feelings, stating that he needed somebody he could "talk to." He openly described his symptoms and his current feeling of despair and disinterest. In time, he was able to express his anger at his parents for their behavior and his loss of his former respect for them. He found it difficult to comprehend how grown-ups, whom he had been taught to idealize, could act in such a spiteful and mean manner. These feelings of anger and disgust were in sharp conflict with his love for his parents who had always been kind to him in the past and, in fact, continued to treat him well despite the way they treated each other. David found himself devaluing his parents and then feeling guilty for his hostility toward them. However, his depression was the result of a greater psychic alteration than ambivalence toward his parents. David found himself forced to reevaluate his whole outlook regarding the world of adults. He could see little point in following social regulations or doing well in school if the adult world was so irrational and capricious. However, at the same time that he expressed disillusionment with adult society, David demonstrated relief at being in psychological contact with a mature and reliable adult in the therapeutic relationship.

David's symptoms improved rather rapidly as he was able to ventilate his anger in the safety of the therapeutic situation and to have his feelings understood and cared about by an adult who acted, temporarily, as a substitute parent. Interpretations could be kept at a minimum beyond the explanation that even adults can do foolish things in times of psychological stress but that, given his parents' rather sane behavior in the past, they would eventually settle down once this current upheaval had passed.

With David's permission, his parents were seen (individually), and the effect of their behavior was strongly communicated. As a result, they were able to reduce the frequency and magnitude of their arguments (at least in front of their children) and to leave their vindictive aspirations to their respective lawyers. They were able to formulate and abide by a separation agreement that prevented the excesses of behavior and dictated a fair division of responsibility and resources.

David responded to this amelioration in his environment favorably, but he was still distressed about his ambivalence toward his father. David sided with his mother but then felt guilty for blaming his father for his family's difficulties. He was very angry with his father but still wanted to love and respect him. These conflicting feelings were discussed in therapy, and David arrived at the conclusion that one could disagree with parents and even with their actions and still love them.

David's improvement allowed him to renew his former interest in friends, school, and age-appropriate activities and lessened his need for a confiding relationship with a neutral but empathic adult therapist. Therapy was gradually discontinued by mutual consent with the understanding that David could return at any time.

David responded well to therapy, which was largely effective in relieving his depression and other symptoms. A number of factors may be seen as contributing to a successful outcome: David had a history of excellent psychological functioning, free of organic problems, notable childhood traumas, or socioeconomic deprivation. His parents cared about him (despite their behavior toward each other) and participated in therapeutic efforts. David himself was highly motivated (he asked to see a therapist), very intelligent, and able to form a therapeutic relationship in a short time. In essence, this youngster had a healthy past and a healthy personality that reacted understandably to an unexpected psychological crisis.

## Case 2

Patrick was a 12-year-old boy mandated for therapy by the courts for recurrent substance abuse and minor brushes with the law (vandalism, shoplifting, chronic fighting in school). His repeated truancy, his disruption of classroom order, and his threatening teachers had resulted in his being placed in a special school for difficult children. Patrick often came to this setting seeming to be under the effects of smoking marijuana (which he denied). His behavior was highly inconsistent: at times Patrick could be cooperative and demonstrate impressive ability, while at other times he was sarcastic, hyperactive, hostile, and refused to participate in any regular activities. When confronted with his behavior during these times, Patrick loudly stated that he had to stand up for himself and show others his strength. He stated he saw no need to change and further that he liked others being afraid of him as this allowed him to get his own way and to feel respected and important.

Patrick's history revealed a host of familial and developmental problems. His natural father had begun taking drugs in the armed services and continued to do so after his return to civilian life. He abandoned Patrick and his mother when Patrick was still an infant, and his current whereabouts were unknown. Patrick's mother has been seen in numerous clinics for depression, but she repeatedly refused to follow through with treatment recommendations or to comply with taking medication. She remarried when Patrick was about age 5, and this marriage was very unstable with chronic arguing over economic difficulties.

Since attending a day care center at age 4, Patrick was found to display symptoms of ADHD (excessive hyperactivity, impulsivity, and distractibility). He had had numerous evaluations throughout his school years, all of which recommended treatment with stimulants. However, Patrick's mother refused to allow Patrick to take medication for fear he would become a "drug addict" like his father. At the same time, the mother complained that she could not control or discipline him and let him watch television for hours rather that provoke an angry confrontation by making him do chores or homework.

Patrick presented as a cheerful, friendly youngster. He was very talkative during the initial meeting, giving long, elaborate, and lively answers to questions often with more detail than necessary and diverging into unrelated topics. He tapped his foot or played with a paperclip throughout. Patrick saw no reason to be in therapy, stating he was satisfied with himself. He tended to blame his former difficulties on other people. He described rather shallow relationships that centered on joint activities rather than on the personal characteristics of others. He described himself as not needing to listen to others and as knowing how to take care of himself. He stated he knew all about therapists, who were either stupid or weird, and he was glad he had refused to see anyone when it had been recommended. While jovial and talkative, he could easily become angry if confronted. He said that he found school a waste of time and planned to quit when he could at age 16. However, he also said he wanted to become an electrician because they were "rich" and he wanted to make a lot of money. He had no idea of how one became an electrician or what the practice of this profession actually involved. Patrick did not attend his next two appointments. He was eventually arrested for selling drugs on the street.

Despite the attempt to meet Patrick on his own terms and to create a nonjudgmental, empathic treatment atmosphere, he declined to engage in any psychotherapeutic endeavor. Having grown up with a disorder that, when untreated, made schoolwork difficult and in a family plagued with economic concerns and parents preoccupied with their own difficulties, Patrick adopted the values of a peer subculture that rewarded his deviant behaviors. Therefore, Patrick denied any problems and did not consider himself in need of psychotherapy.

# Conclusion

The studies reviewed in this chapter may reveal a certain irony. Few, if any, represent the work of those practitioners who actually provide psychotherapy for most child patients. Clinicians who supply the bulk of psychotherapy rarely produce research reports or publish their results (beyond an interesting case report or a small, uncontrolled series), so that the test of effectiveness of therapy falls on individuals who do not practice it daily or for their livelihood. It remains an unsubstantiated hope that the positive effects reported by researchers, most of whom are not practitioners, reflect accurately the results obtained in private consulting offices. The initial reports from the Anna Freud Center (Fonagy and Target 1994; Target and Fonagy 1994a, 1994b) which closely approximate the typical professional's practice, appear to support the general conclusion that psychotherapy is effective, although more impaired children appear to require more intensive intervention. More studies such as these are needed to decide the appropriate allotment of resources in a most efficient manner.

# References

Abikoff H: Cognitive training in ADHD children: less to it than meets the eye. J Learn Disabil 24:205–209, 1991

Casey RJ, Berman JS: The outcome of psychotherapy with children. Psychol Bull 98:388–400, 1985

Domino M, Burns B, Silva S, et al: Cost-effectiveness of treatments for adolescent depression: results from TADS. Am J Psychiatry 165:588–596, 2008

Finney JW, Riley AW, Cataldo MF: Psychology in primary health care: effects of brief targeted therapy on children's medical care utilization. J Pediatr Psychol 16:447–461, 1991

Fonagy P, Target M: The efficacy of psychoanalysis for children with disruptive disorders. J Am Acad Child Adolesc Psychiatry 33:45–55, 1994

Freud A: Normality and Pathology in Childhood: Assessments of Development, The Writings of Anna Freud, Vol 6. New York, International Universities Press, 1965

Group for the Advancement of Psychiatry: Psychopathological Disorders in Childhood: Theoretical Considerations and a Proposed Classification (GAP Report 62). New York, Group for the Advancement of Psychiatry, 1966

Heinicke CM, Ramsey-Klee DM: Outcome of child psychotherapy as a function of frequency of session. J Am Acad Child Psychiatry 25:247–253, 1986

Henggeler SW, Schoenwald SK, Pickrel SG, et al: The contribution of treatment outcome research to the reform of children's mental health services: multisystemic therapy as an example. J Ment Health Adm 21:229–239, 1994

Jensen PS, Garcia JA, Glied S, et al: Cost-effectiveness of ADHD treatments: findings from the multimodal treatment study of children with ADHD. Am J Psychiatry 162:1628–1636, 2005

Johnson AM, Falstein EI, Szurek SA, et al: School phobia. Am J Orthopsychiatry 11:702–712, 1941

Kazdin AE, Bass D, Ayers WA, et al: Empirical and clinical focus of child and adolescent psychotherapy research. J Consult Clin Psychol 58:729–740, 1990

March J, Silva S, Petrycki S, et al: The treatment for adolescents with depression study (TADS). Arch Gen Psychiatry 64:1132–1144, 2007

Miklowitz D, Axelson D, Birmaher B, et al: Family focused treatment for adolescents with bipolar disorder: results of a 2-year randomized trial. Arch Gen Psychiatry 65:1053–1061, 2008

Moran G, Fonagy P, Kurtz A, et al: A controlled study of psychoanalytic treatment of brittle diabetes. J Am Acad Child Adolesc Psychiatry 30:926–935, 1991

Puig-Antich J, Lukens E, Davies M, et al: Psychosocial functioning in prepubertal major depressive disorders. I. Interpersonal relationships during the depressive episode. Arch Gen Psychiatry 42:500–507, 1985a

Puig-Antich J, Lukens E, Davies M, et al: Psychosocial functioning in prepubertal major depressive disorders. II. Interpersonal relationships after sustained recovery from affective episode. Arch Gen Psychiatry 42:511–517, 1985b

Satterfield JH, Satterfield BT, Schell AM: Therapeutic interventions to prevent delinquency in hyperactive boys. J Am Acad Child Adolesc Psychiatry 26:56–64, 1987

Target M, Fonagy P: Efficacy of psychoanalysis for children with emotional disorders. J Am Acad Child Adolesc Psychiatry 33:361–371, 1994a

Target M, Fonagy P: The efficacy of psychoanalysis for children: prediction of outcome in a developmental context. J Am Acad Child Adolesc Psychiatry 33:1134–1144, 1994b

Weiss G, Hechtman LT: Hyperactive Children Grown Up. New York, Guilford, 1986

Weisz JR, Weiss B: Effects of Psychotherapy With Children and Adolescents. New York, Sage, 1993

Weisz JR, Weiss B, Alicke MD, et al: Effectiveness of psychotherapy with children and adolescents: a meta-analysis for clinicians. J Consult Clin Psychol 55:542–549, 1987

Weisz JR, Walter BR, Weiss B, et al: Arrests among emotionally disturbed violent and assaultive individuals following minimal versus lengthy intervention through North Carolina's Willie M Program. J Consult Clin Psychol 58:720–728, 1990

## Summary of studies addressing effectiveness of psychotherapy for children and adolescents

| Article | Patient population | Treatment | Outcome |
|---|---|---|---|
| **Meta-analytic studies** | | | |
| Casey and Berman 1985 | Children, ages 3–12 years, from diverse sites (schools, hospitals, clinics). | Variety of verbal therapies, including cognitive, behavioral, and psychodynamic. | Surveyed 64 appropriate studies published between 1952 and 1983 with effect size of 0.71, indicating that average treated child improved more than 76% of untreated children. |
| Weisz et al. 1987 | Children, ages 4–18 years, from diverse sites (as above). Excluded subjects with retardation, physical disabilities, or seizures. | Variety of verbal therapies (as above) plus parent counseling. Excluded tutoring, bibliotherapy, and foster therapy. | Surveyed 105 appropriate studies published between 1958 and 1984 with effect size of 0.79, indicating that average treated child improved more than 79% of untreated children. |
| Kazdin et al. 1990 | Children, ages 4–18 years, from diverse sites including correctional facilities. | Varieties of verbal therapies. | Surveyed 105 appropriate studies published between 1970 and 1988 with effect size of 0.88, indicating that average treated child improved more than 81% of untreated children. |
| Weisz et al. 1993 | Children, ages 1.5–17.6 years, from diverse sites. | Variety of verbal therapies, including parent counseling. | Surveyed 110 appropriate studies published between 1967 and 1991 with effect size of 0.71, indicating that average treated child improved more than 76% of untreated children. |

**Summary of studies addressing effectiveness of psychotherapy for children and adolescents *(continued)***

| Article | Patient population | Treatment | Outcome |
|---|---|---|---|
| **Focused studies** | | | |
| Heinicke and Ramsey-Klee 1986 | Three matched groups of boys ages 7.8–10.1 years who had been receiving help for reading problems. | Three groups of psychoanalytically oriented outpatient therapy with different session frequency: once weekly, once weekly and then increased to four times weekly, or four times weekly. | All groups showed improved reading ability, self-esteem, and relationships, but greater session frequency correlated with greater improvement. |
| Finney et al. 1991 | Two groups of matched children whose parents were enrolled in a health maintenance organization (HMO). | Focused brief psychotherapy with parents for management of presenting problem. Children seen by Behavioral Pediatrics Service were matched with children not seen. Later follow-up by phone and tabulated HMO visits for medical reasons for each group. | Treatment group showed fewer visits to HMO for medical reasons. |
| Moran et al. 1991 | Children, ages 6–18 years, consecutively admitted for brittle diabetes. | Patients randomly assigned to standard treatment with or without psychoanalytically oriented therapy 3–5 times a week for average of 15 weeks. | Treated group showed better control of diabetes through measured blood sugars and better psychological functioning at later dates. |

## Summary of studies addressing effectiveness of psychotherapy for children and adolescents (continued)

| Article | Patient population | Treatment | Outcome |
|---|---|---|---|
| **Focused studies** (*continued*) | | | |
| Jensen et al. 2005 | 579 children with attention-deficit/hyperactivity disorder (ADHD) ages 7 to 9.9 years. | Patients were assigned to 14 months of medication management, behavioral treatment, both combined, or community care. Health care service costs were tallied throughout the study. | Costs varied fourfold, medication management being least expensive, followed by behavioral treatment, and then combined treatment. Community care was less intensive, had lower medication treatment costs, and was less effective. Medical management was more effective, more expensive than community care, less effective than combination treatment and behavioral treatment alone, but perhaps more cost-effective in routine treatment for children without comorbid disorders. For children with comorbid disorders, combination treatment may be more cost-effective due to its superior effectiveness. |
| March et al. 2007 | 327 patients with major depressive disorder ages 12–17 years. | Randomized controlled trial comparing fluoxetine and cognitive-behavioral therapy (CBT) (15 one-hour sessions during first 12 weeks). During first 12 weeks, partial responders given 6 additional weeks, and full responders given biweekly CBT for 6 weeks; after week 18, CBT every 6 weeks, and their combination (medication management plus CBT protocols). | Combination therapy is robustly superior to CBT and modestly and inconsistently superior to fluoxetine alone. Treatment with fluoxetine alone or in combination with CBT produces more rapid improvement in major depressive symptoms than CBT alone. CBT alone catches up to fluoxetine and to combination therapy toward end of treatment. Significant suicidal ideation persists in a minority of patients and is significantly more common in those given only medication than in those given combination therapy or CBT. Combined treatment appears superior to either monotherapy as treatment for major depression in adolescents. |

## Summary of studies addressing effectiveness of psychotherapy for children and adolescents *(continued)*

| Article | Patient population | Treatment | Outcome |
|---|---|---|---|
| **Focused studies** *(continued)* | | | |
| Domino et al. 2008 | 369 subjects who did not drop out and had evaluable outcome and cost data at 12 weeks. | Treatment as in March et al. 2007 study. | Both fluoxetine and combination therapy are at least as cost-effective in the short term as other treatments commonly used in primary care (using a threshold of $125,000 per quality-adjusted life year). Fluoxetine is more cost-effective than combination therapy after 12 weeks of treatment. Combination therapy had highest total costs but greatest improvements in Children's Depression Rating Scale. |
| Miklowitz et al. 2008 | 58 adolescents (mean age 14.5 years) with bipolar I or not otherwise specified disorder with a mood episode in the prior 3 months. | Patients randomly assigned to family-focused treatment for adolescents (FFT-A) and protocol pharmacotherapy or to enhanced care (EC) and protocol pharmacotherapy. FFT-A was 21 sessions over 9 months of psychoeducation, communication training, and problem-solving skills training. EC was three family sessions focused on relapse prevention. | Although no group differences in rates of recovery from index episode, patients in FFT-A recovered from baseline depression faster than patients in EC. Groups did not differ in time to recurrence of depression or mania, but patients given FFT-A spent less time in depressive episodes with more favorable trajectory of depressive symptoms for 2 years. FFT-A with pharmacotherapy is effective in stabilizing bipolar depressive symptoms for adolescents. |

**Summary of studies addressing effectiveness of psychotherapy for children and adolescents *(continued)***

| Article | Patient population | Treatment | Outcome |
|---|---|---|---|
| **Naturalistic studies** | | | |
| Fonagy and Target 1994 | 135 children with disruptive disorders were matched with 135 children with emotional disorders. | 67% of children received intensive therapy; the remainder received nonintensive therapy for up to 2 years. | Severely impaired children did best with intensive therapy; less impaired children did equally well with treatment. Effects of therapy determined by change in Global Assessment Scale scores, presence of symptoms, and general adaptation. |
| Target and Fonagy 1994a | 352 children with emotional disorders. | 72% of children received intensive therapy; the remainder nonintensive therapy for up to 2 years. | Same as above. |
| Target and Fonagy 1994b | Three matched groups of children ($n=127$ per group) compared according to age: less than 6, 6 to 12, older than 12. | Children seen in either intensive or nonintensive therapy for up to 2 years. | Younger children did best with intensive therapy even of shorter duration; older children did equally well with nonintensive therapy but did best with longer duration of treatment. |

# 10

# The Place of Long-Term and Intensive Psychotherapy

Allan Rosenblatt, M.D.

Previous chapters have set forth the cost-effectiveness of psychotherapy organized under various DSM-IV Axis I diagnostic categories (American Psychiatric Association 1994). In several categories (e.g., borderline personality disorder, schizophrenia, perfectionistic depressed patients, and more severely disturbed children), longer durations have been studied and reported (see Chapters 2, 3, 6, and 9 in this volume). More often, the studies cited have utilized psychotherapy of relatively brief duration and with frequencies of once weekly or less. The relative absence of longer term studies reflects the fact that research studies of psychotherapies lasting longer than 6 weeks or with frequencies higher than once-weekly sessions are markedly more complicated and expensive to conduct (see Doidge 1997; Gabbard 2000).

However, in clinical practice, the personality disorders of Axis II, whether encountered alone or in combination with Axis I disorders (a relatively common occurrence), are generally considered to require more extended therapy (see Gabbard 2000). Moreover, these conditions are often found to require a higher frequency of contact. In the National Institute of Mental Health (NIMH) Collaborative Study of Depression, 74% of the patients had diagnosable personality disorders, and they had significantly worse outcomes from the short-term treatments in the study than those patients without personality disorders (Shea et al. 1990). Blatt et al. (1995) analyzed data from this NIMH study and found that those self-critical "introjective" patients did poorly in brief treatment but were significantly more responsive to long-term intensive therapy. Similar findings occurred when Blatt (1992) analyzed the data from the Menninger Foundation Psychotherapy Research Project.

Personality disorders are considered to be one of the most important sources of chronic impairment in both treated and untreated psychiatric populations. Four studies from the United States, United Kingdom, and Germany all estimate their rate of prevalence to be between 10% and 13.5% (Casey and Tyrer 1986; Maier et al. 1992; Reich et al. 1988; Zimmerman and Coryell 1990). Those who suffer from these disorders are reported to be unemployed for longer periods, have more drug problems, are more prone to having interpersonal difficulties, and make more suicide attempts, all of which incur considerable costs (Gabbard 2000; Linehan and Heard 1999; Pilkonis et al. 1999; Reich et al. 1989).

# Search Methodology

A computer search of MEDLINE, from 1984 to 2007, was conducted using the key words "psychotherapy/economics"+"personality disorders" and "cost+psychotherapy." In addition, the recent online publication of An Open Door Review of Outcome Studies in Psychoanalysis, prepared by the Research Committee of the International Psychoanalytic Association, was used as a source, as well as the 1997 supplement of the journal *Psychoanalytic Inquiry*, titled "Extended Dynamic Psychotherapy," edited by Susan G. Lazar, M.D.

# Indications for Long-Term and Intensive Psychotherapy and Studies of Efficacy

The value of longer term psychotherapy was clearly demonstrated by Bannon et al. (1995) in their meta-analysis of three psychodynamic psychotherapy studies of patients with personality disorders that used stringent methodological criteria, including standardized diagnoses and operationalized outcome measures such as observer ratings and self-reports. The results show compelling evidence of the differential effectiveness of increasing frequency (and, therefore, intensity) of therapy. While patients in once-weekly treatment took over 8 years for remission of their disorder, this length of time was cut in half for patients in twice-weekly treatment.

Most of the more intensive forms of psychotherapy are based on psychodynamic principles, which in turn are derived from psychoanalytic theory. Psychoanalysis, as a modality of treatment, is a form of intensive psychotherapy, conducted three to five times a week over a period of several years. In addition, there are other modalities of intensive psychotherapy that are not psychodynamically based. Linehan's dialectical behavior therapy for borderline personality disorder is conducted twice weekly (using one individual and one group therapy session) over a period of a year (see Chapter 3). Therapy for schizophrenia either alone (see Chapter 2) or combined with Axis II disorders (see Hogg et al. 1990; Gabbard 1994) is often conducted more often than once weekly.

The literature on the effectiveness of psychoanalysis and intensive psychoanalytic psychotherapy is not usually reported according to DSM-IV categories, because the indications and suitability for such treatment cut across diagnostic headings. They are, instead, based on criteria that identify a kind of psychological organization that requires and is responsive to such intensive and insight-oriented therapy and that may be found in various constellations of symptoms.

Intensive therapy is generally considered to be indicated when psychopathology manifests itself in distorted, maladaptive, and often grossly self-destructive interpersonal relationships, in love relationships, and at work. There may be few or no specific symptoms (phobias, anxiety, etc.), as seen in DSM-IV Axis II categories of personality disorders, or there may be an admixture of characterological problems with Axis I symptoms.

In the latter case, Axis I symptoms either are embedded in a preexisting matrix of personality or character pathology or become encrusted with such additional pathology as a result of the social disruption occasioned by the primary illness. The resultant problems are not simple and are not usually susceptible to simple drug or brief therapy.

In the first instance, of symptoms embedded in a preexisting matrix, an analogy can be made to a streptococcal infection in an individual with preexisting illness, such as a compromised immune system, that makes it difficult to treat the infection easily and simply with a brief course of antibiotics. In the second instance, the analogy is to a streptococcal infection in a previously healthy patient that has led to the sequela of rheumatic heart disease or glomerulonephritis. Such chronic conditions are not usually treatable by short-term methods.

Character and personality problems that are thus associated with the specific DSM-IV Axis I disorders often need intensive psychotherapy and take time to treat. Indeed, it is likely that the cases of anxiety disorder that are resistant to simple drug therapy are just those that have associated character pathology or secondary problems arising from the primary illness. In an interesting physiological correlation with psychotherapy, Viinamaki et al. (1998) demonstrated normalization of serotonin metabolism, as assessed by SPECT (single-photon emission computed tomography), concomitant with clinical improvement in the psychotherapy of personality disorder, compared with no change in controls.

Several findings indicate that the length of psychotherapeutic treatment is correlated with its success, especially in personality disorders, including borderline personality disorder (see Dossmann et al. 1997; Fonagy 2002; Hoglend 1993; Howard et al. 1986; Kopta et al. 1994; Seligman 1995; von Rad et al. 1998). Therapy may require several years before significant improvement is noted (Howard et al. 1986).

Yet, there are formidable difficulties in devising appropriate outcome studies for extended psychotherapy, including problems of control groups, randomization of patients, varying and long duration of treatment, follow-up, statistical tests, and great expense (see Fonagy 2002). Consequently, there have been to date few controlled studies of effectiveness, although an increasing number of studies, particularly from Europe, present highly suggestive evidence of effectiveness. One such study with a naturalistic design examined 44 psychoanalytic patients and found a better outcome than for psychodynamically treated patients (Rudolf et al. 1994). A report from the Stockholm Outcome of Psychoanalysis and Psychotherapy Project (Sandell et al. 2000) found a moderate to large positive effect for psychotherapy and a very large positive effect for psychoanalysis. They also found long durations and high frequencies, in conjunction, to be associated with the most positive treatment outcomes. Another study compared two groups of patients with mixed diagnoses, one treated with psychoanalysis that was more intensive, had more sessions per week, and extended over a longer period of time, and the other with less intensive psychodynamic psychotherapy. At the end of treatment and at 1-year follow-up, the investigators found greater effectiveness for psychoanalysis (Grande et al. 2006).

In a meta-analysis of 23 studies of long-term psychodynamic psychotherapy, Leichsenring and Rabung (2008) examined its relative efficacy with regard to outcome and impact on functioning and symptoms compared with shorter treatments for complex mental disorders. These authors concluded that according to comparative analyses of controlled trials, long-term psychodynamic psychotherapy showed significantly better effectiveness and led to significantly greater improvement in target problems and personality functioning than briefer treatments for patients with complex mental disorders. In a subsequent publication, Leichsenring (2009) reviewed efficacy studies of both short- and long-term psychodynamic psychotherapy, reviewed and discussed process-outcome research that has corroborated central assumptions about the mechanisms of change of psychodynamic psychotherapy, discussed the applications of psychodynamic psychotherapy to specific disorders, and concluded that quasi-experimental studies have provided evidence that long-term psychodynamic psychotherapy lasting several years is effective. In another review of the empirical evidence for the efficacy of both short- and long-term psychodynamic psychotherapy, the effect sizes are as large as those reported for other therapies described as "empirically supported" and "evidence based." In addition, patients treated with psychodynamic psychotherapy maintain therapeutic gains and continue to improve after treatment ends (Shedler, in press).

With regard to designing cost-effectiveness studies for long-term psychotherapy, difficulty is added by the need for the measurement of both the cost of the illness and the outcome of treatment. For patients and their families, emotional illnesses have devastating effects of which the costs are not easy to measure. For example, both psychotic and nonpsychotic illnesses often disrupt marriages. Dysfunctional families have a damaging effect on children, leading to emotional disorders that then perpetuate the vicious circle of emotional illness.

Assessing symptom relief alone will not suffice to measure outcome, because the goal of intensive extended treatment necessarily goes beyond symptom relief to encompass behavioral changes. These changes enable greater social, marital, and vocational functioning, contributing to improvements that are not easily measurable in terms of cost savings. For example, a more stable family may save enormous costs associated with children who might otherwise have become seriously disturbed in a dysfunctional family setting. Similarly, a self-defeating individual who by virtue of an extended psychotherapy becomes able to resolve crippling conflicts may increase significantly his or her earning power.

# Studies Suggesting Cost-Effectiveness

Despite the above-noted obstacles, a number of studies suggest that intensive psychoanalytic therapy and psychoanalysis are cost-effective and, in some instances, afford a cost offset. Most are studies conducted in Europe, where the distinction between psychoanalysis and intensive psychoanalytic psychotherapy is somewhat blurred and these treatment approaches are seen as existing on a continuum. Some of the studies listed below combine results of psychoanalysis and intensive psychoanalytic psychotherapy but, even so, present significant implications for our review.

The patients in the studies discussed below represented a diagnostic mix, including personality disorders and affective disorders, and a number of patients had suffered symptoms for more than 10 years. Treatment settings included outpatient naturalistic studies, as well as hospital-based ones with severely impaired individuals. After several months to several years of treatment, substantial improvement was observed in most treated individuals. Sick leave and hospitalizations decreased, as did use of psychotropic drugs, and work capacity increased. It is notable that the longer the treatment, the better was the treatment success. On 4- to 6-year follow-ups, these gains were maintained and even increased. The quality of relationships had improved more at a 6-year follow-up than immediately after termination of treatment.

Duehrssen (1962) followed patients who had received psychoanalytic treatment (frequency of sessions varied) an average of 100 sessions under national health care in Germany. Out of the original population of 1,156 patients, independent assessors rated 55% as improved. At 5-year follow-up, 84% were available, and independent assessors rated 58% as still improved, having maintained their improvement. Sick leave was significantly reduced at termination of treatment, and a 5-year follow-up (Duehrssen and Jorswieck 1965) found that the mean number of days of hospitalization in a group of 125 treated patients was reduced 77%, from about 26 days to 6 days. An untreated group of 100 neurotic patients maintained about the same level of hospitalization of 24–25 days, whereas the general population of insured patients stayed about the same at 10–12 days. This study, despite some flaws (nonrandom assignment to groups), indicates not only that the substantial improvement was maintained over time but also that treated individuals displayed superior work capacity.

Heinzel et al. (1996) reported a German retrospective questionnaire study of 604 patients treated by 90 therapists with psychoanalytic psychotherapy at varied frequencies of one to four sessions per week, lasting over 3 years. Follow-up of up to 6 years showed a significant increase in self-rated well-being from "bad" to "good," the increase for physical health being most marked. The number of visits to the family doctor decreased by 40% and to medical specialists by 33%. Days of sickness absence decreased by 42%, and days of hospitalization decreased by 66%. It is notable that the quality of relationships had improved more at 6-year follow-up than immediately after termination of treatment. Again, this study demonstrates that gains from treatment were maintained, and even increased, over a period of years.

Savings in health care utilization were calculated, including allowances for reduced work loss. It was shown that, for the 2 years after termination, the monetary benefits alone of therapy were equal to about one-quarter of the costs of therapy. Since benefits were maintained after 6 years, extrapolation of savings indicates that after 8 years, a cost offset would begin to accrue, and after 20–30 years it would be substantial, aside from the secondary benefits to family members, especially children.

In another study of psychodynamic psychotherapy in Germany (Dossmann et al. 1997), 666 patients who had completed their therapy between January 1990 and December 1994 provided their self-assessment of physical, mental, social, and overall health on a 5-point rating scale and reported utilization of other health care, including medical visits, hospital days, medication, and frequency per year of lost work days at the beginning of therapy, at the end of therapy, and at the time when the questionnaire was filled out. The mean time since end of therapy was 2 years 3 months, and the range was 0–6 years. There was significant improvement on all reported measures. The savings in health cost per patient were $5,652 per individual patient and $9,553 for group patients, and lost work days declined by 41.6% demonstrating both cost offset and cost-effectiveness for long-term psychodynamic treatments. From the perspective of analyzing the impact of long-term treatment, for this study the most significant determinant of success was the positive effect of the duration of the analytic therapy.

A cost offset could also be inferred from the study of intensive treatment of children and adolescents with poorly controlled diabetes (Moran et al. 1991). Improved health and diabetic control were maintained at 1-year follow-up, as contrasted with a comparison group. The importance of this study is clear, in view of the known long-term complications of juvenile diabetes and the relatively poor outcome associated with other treatment methods (see Kent et al. 1994). Considering the expense associated with treatment of complications of this condition, this study clearly implies a cost-effectiveness of treatment.

Keller et al. (1998) reported a study on the effectiveness of psychoanalysis, so named, performed in a naturalistic setting in private practice. Thirty-five Jungian psychoanalysts in private practice in Berlin, Germany, participated in a questionnaire-based study of 259 patients who had terminated treatment, and 111 of those were followed up after a mean of 6 years. Psychoanalysis was conducted in 76% of the patients, the rest being treated with less intensive psychotherapy. A third of the patients had symptoms for more than 10 years. Personality disorder was diagnosed in 17% of the patients, and 46% were classified with affective disorders. The Schepank Impairment Severity Score, used to measure severity of illness, indicated that a substantial proportion of the sample was very severely handicapped, normally warranting full or partial hospitalization.

On 6-year follow-up, about 87% of patients reported their global well-being as moderate to very good, in contrast to 60% having reported their status at the start of treatment as very poor. The longer the treatment, the better was the treatment success at 6-year follow-up. Intake of psychotropic drugs was substantially reduced or eliminated. More that half of the patients reported a substantial reduction in the frequency of medical visits. Data from national insurers (available only in 47 of the 111 patients) revealed a 50% reduction in sickness absence and an 87.5% reduction in hospitalization days (in 58 patients). Despite limitations in design and methods, the study strongly suggests psychoanalysis can effect reduction of health care costs and has long-lasting therapeutic effects.

With regard to hospital and day hospital patients, Teufel and Volk (1988) studied the outcome, with a 3.9-year follow-up, of three to four times weekly inpatient psychoanalytic treatment with adjunctive group therapy of 147 patients at the Stuttgart Psychotherapeutic Hospital, a treatment facility that is exclusively psychoanalytically oriented. The average length of stay in the hospital was about 6 months. The patients were diagnosed as having severe personality disorder, neuroses, or psychosomatic conditions. Treatment outcome was measured along four dimensions: therapist's end-of-treatment rating of attainment of treatment goals set by the patient at the start of treatment; symptom reduction, measured by comparison of the patient's symptom questionnaire at start and at follow-up; the patient's report at follow-up of general well-being; and the patient's report of capacity for work at follow-up.

About 70% of the patients were rated as having moderate to good results in attainment of treatment goals, while about 60% rated themselves as having moderate to good symptom reduction. About 46% reported good or satisfying well-being, while another 34% reported moderate well-being, for a total of 80%. Two-thirds of the group reported being fully capable of work, with only 15% unable to hold any gainful employment. Only 18% of the sample failed to improve by any of the criteria.

The major limitations of this study are the lack of standardized measures and results, along with the absence of a comparison group. However, considering that these patients were sick enough to require hospitalization and that no psychotropic medication was given, the results appear significant, especially those with regard to work capacity. Again, because loss of employability is a major factor in assessing the social costs of illness, the cost-effectiveness of this inpatient psychoanalytic therapy seems clear-cut.

Several studies have reported on the use of a day treatment program for personality disorders, along with analytically oriented and cognitive-behavioral groups. Wilberg et al. (1998) studied 183 such low-functioning patients, most of whom were diagnosed with borderline personality disorders, in an 18-week program, with some receiving ancillary medication. There was moderately positive benefit, generally maintained at 1-year follow-up (Wilberg et al. 1999).

Bateman and Fonagy (1999) compared the effectiveness of a psychoanalytically oriented day care program for borderline personality disorders, which included individual and group therapy with standard psychiatric care, consisting of biweekly meetings with a psychiatrist but no formal psychotherapy. Outcome measures for the psychoanalytically treated group showed a significant decrease in frequency of suicide attempts, self-mutilation, depression, anxiety, interpersonal function, and social adjustment. The standard care group showed limited change, if not deterioration. Subsequent publications by these investigators studied 38 patients with borderline personality disorder treated with mentalization-based individual and group psychoanalytic psychotherapy in a partially hospitalized setting for up to 18 months versus the control treatment of standard psychiatric care. Patients were assigned in a randomized controlled design. Health care costs (psychiatric care, pharmacological treatment, and emergency room care) for the 6 months before treatment, the 18 months of treatment, and an 18-month follow-up period were measured, and no cost differences were found between the groups during pretreatment or treatment. The higher costs of care for patients treated with partial hospitalization were offset by less psychiatric inpatient care and reduced emergency room care for them during this period. During the 18-month treatment period, the annual costs were also significantly lower for both groups compared with their 6-month pretreatment costs. However, while the overall costs between the two groups were comparable during treatment, after discharge the average annual cost of health care for the partial hospitalization group was one-fifth of that for the general psychiatric care group. At follow-up, the mean annual cost savings associated with the study intervention were $12,000, thus recouping over 2 years the cost of the treatment and suggesting its cost-effectiveness for borderline patients (Bateman and Fonagy 2003). At 5-year follow-up after mentalization-based treatment, patients had some impaired social functioning but far superior clinical outcomes compared with treatment-as-usual patients with respect to suicidality (23% vs. 74%), diagnostic status (13% still diagnosable with borderline personality disorder vs. 87%), psychiatric outpatient service use (2 years vs. 3.5 years), use of medication (0.02 vs. 1.90 years using three or more medications), global function above 60 (45% vs. 10%), and vocational status (employed or in school 3.2 years vs. 1.2 years) (Bateman and Fonagy 2008).

Two studies of dialectical behavior psychotherapy administered to patients with borderline personality disorder also demonstrate cost-effectiveness. Linehan and colleagues (Linehan and Heard 1999; Linehan et al. 1991) showed that psychotherapy of 1 year or longer resulted in stays of only 8.46 hospital days, compared with 38.86 days in control subjects, as well as significantly less self-mutilation. It was calculated that regular psychotherapy saved $10,000 per patient per year (Heard 1994). Similarly, a study by Stevenson and Meares (1992) revealed that psychodynamic psychotherapy cut hospital use in half. They calculated that, for the 30 patients studied, in the year before therapy, hospital treatment alone cost up to $143,756 (in Australian dollars) per patient, with a total cost for all of $684,346. For the year after treatment, the cost per patient ranged up to $12,333 with a total cost of only $41,424 (Australian). The average cost of therapy per patient was $13,000, but the average decrease in hospital costs per patient was $21,431, representing a savings of $8,431 per patient. In addition, treated patients were significantly improved compared with patients receiving treatment as usual (Hall et al. 2001; Stevenson and Meares 1999; Meares et al. 1999).

In a study by Clarkin et al. (2001), 23 female patients (mean age 32.7 years) with borderline personality disorder reporting at least two incidents of self-injurious behavior in the last 5 years were recruited from inpatient, day hospital, and outpatient facilities. The patients served as their own controls (pre- vs. posttreatment). Patients were treated with a manualized transference-focused psychotherapy (TFP) twice weekly for 12 months. In this group, compared with the year prior to treatment, the number of patients who made suicide attempts decreased significantly (from 53% to 18%), as did the medical risk and severity of medical condition following self-injurious behavior. Comparing the year prior to treatment with the 12-month period of psychotherapy, the group had significantly fewer hospitalizations (a 67% reduction) as well as fewer inpatient days (an 89% reduction) during the year of treatment. The study sample was a relatively homogeneous group of severely disturbed borderline patients, none of whom abused psychoactive substances. The results strongly suggest that a twice-weekly treatment that focuses specifically on the relationship between patient and psychotherapist may be both clinically useful and cost-effective.

A later study by the same group (Clarkin et al. 2007) randomly assigned 90 patients with borderline personality disorder to 1 year of twice-weekly individual sessions of TFP, once-weekly supportive psychotherapy with additional sessions as needed, or weekly individual and group dialectical behavior therapy with available telephone consultation. Patients in all three treatment groups improved significantly in depression, anxiety, global functioning, and social adjustment, and both TFP and dialectical behavior therapy significantly improved suicidality. However, only TFP and supportive treatment improved impulsivity, and only TFP was significantly associated with improvement in irritability and verbal and direct assault. Although there were no reported cost data in this study, any treatment that is effective in severely ill patient populations will likely be cost-effective, at the very least by virtue of a decline in medical costs associated with suicidality.

For cocaine-dependent patients, Crits-Christoph et al. (1999) randomly assigned 487 patients to one of four treatments: individual drug counseling plus group drug counseling (GDC), cognitive therapy (CT) plus GDC, supportive-expressive (SE) therapy plus GDC, or to GDC alone. The treatments were intensive, including 36 possible individual sessions and 24 group sessions for 6 months. It was found that SE plus GDC and CT plus GDC retained patients better than the other treatment conditions. However, compared with the two psychotherapies with GDC and with GDC alone, individual drug counseling plus GDC led to superior reductions of overall drug use and cocaine use and a greater proportion of patients achieving abstinence. Although the results demonstrated the superiority of individual drug counseling to the psychotherapies in modifying cocaine use, a subsequent publication on the same study (Crits-Christoph et al. 2001) demonstrated that the superiority does not extend to other addiction-associated problems of psychiatric symptoms, employment, medical, legal, family, social, interpersonal, or alcohol use problems because, across treatments, all patients improved similarly from baseline.

For patients with pain disorders, Monsen and Monsen (2000) studied 40 pain patients, treating 20 with 33 sessions of psychodynamic body therapy (PBT) and 20 with treatment as usual or no treatment. From assessments of patients before therapy, at the end of therapy, and at 1-year follow-up, it was reported that patients treated with PBT had significantly greater improvement on levels of subjective experience of pain, general symptoms, interpersonal problems, personality characteristics, and affect consciousness. The improvements were durable, had increased at 1-year follow-up, and were consistent with the hypothesis that a psychodynamic approach would improve pain patients' capacity to recognize, distinguish, and tolerate distinctive affect states and acquire more differentiated expression of affects.

With regard to patients with eating disorders, Bachar et al. (1999) treated 25 patients with bulimia and 8 with anorexia with a psychoanalytic psychotherapy with its full components (as opposed to only some of its features as in interpersonal psychotherapy or expressive-supportive therapy) in comparison with CT. The bulimic patients were randomly assigned either to self-psychological treatment (SPT) or to control/nutritional counseling (C/NC), and the anorexic patients were randomly assigned either to SPT or to CT. SPT and CT were both delivered in an individual format of weekly sessions for a year and did not focus directly on the patient's eating attitudes or behavior. It was found that SPT led to significant improvement, CT to slight improvement, and C/NC to almost no changes. Sixty-four percent of SPT patients compared with 17% of CT patients and 14% of C/NC had remissions by the end of therapy in what were statistically significant differences.

Both SPT and CT had slight (not statistically significant) continued improvement during the year following termination of treatment.

# Conclusion

In Axis II disorders, psychopathology manifests itself in distorted, maladaptive, and often grossly self-destructive interpersonal relationships, in love relationships, and at work, even though specific symptoms such as phobias or anxiety may not be present. Axis I symptoms may be embedded in a preexisting matrix of personality or character pathology. Alternatively, they may become encrusted with such additional pathology as a result of the social disruption occasioned by the primary illness. In both instances the resultant problems are not simple and are not usually susceptible to simple drug or brief therapy. As a result, in such Axis II disorders, alone or in combination with Axis I disorders, intensive and extended psychotherapy is often required. There are daunting methodological problems inherent in outcome research calculating the cost-effectiveness for such intensive and extended psychotherapies. However, a number of studies indicate that such therapies can be cost-effective, although diagnostic categories are not identified.

# References

American Psychiatric Association: Diagnostic and Statistical Manual of Mental Disorders, 4th Edition. Washington, DC, American Psychiatric Association, 1994

Bachar E, Latzer Y, Kreitler S, et al: Empirical comparison of two psychological therapies: self psychology and cognitive orientation in the treatment of anorexia and bulimia. J Psychother Pract Res 8:115–128, 1999

Bannon E, Perry JC, Ianni F: The effectiveness of psychotherapy for personality disorders. Presentation at the International Society for the Study of Personality Disorders, Dublin, Ireland, 1995

Bateman A, Fonagy P: Effectiveness of partial hospitalization in the treatment of borderline personality disorder: a randomized controlled trial. Am J Psychiatry 156:1563–1569, 1999

Bateman A, Fonagy P: Health service utilization costs for borderline personality disorder patients treated with psychoanalytically oriented partial hospitalization versus general psychiatric care. Am J Psychiatry 160:169–171, 2003

Bateman A, Fonagy P: 8-Year follow-up of patients treated for borderline personality disorder: mentalization-based treatment versus treatment as usual. Am J Psychiatry 165:631–638, 2008

Blatt SJ: The differential effect of psychotherapy and psychoanalysis with anaclitic and introjective patients: the Menninger Psychotherapy Research Project revisited. J Am Psychoanal Assoc 40:691–724, 1992

Blatt SJ, Quinlan DM, Pilkonis PA, et al: Impact of perfectionism and need for approval on the brief treatment of depression: the National Institute of Mental Health Treatment of Depression Collaborative Research Program revisited. J Consult Clin Psychol 63:125–132, 1995

Casey PR, Tyrer PJ: Personality, functioning and symptomatology. J Psychiatr Res 20:363–374, 1986

Clarkin JF, Foelsch PA, Levy KN, et al: The development of a psychodynamic treatment for patients with borderline personality disorder: a preliminary study of behavioral change. J Pers Disord 15:487–495, 2001

Clarkin J, Levy K, Lenzenweger M, et al: Evaluating three treatments for borderline personality disorder: a multiwave study. Am J Psychiatry 164:922–928, 2007

Crits-Christoph P, Siqueland L, Blaine J, et al: Psychosocial treatments for cocaine dependence: National Institute on Drug Abuse collaborative cocaine treatment study. Arch Gen Psychiatry 56:493–502, 1999

Crits-Christoph P, Siqueland L, McCalmont E, et al: Impact of psychosocial treatments on associated problems of cocaine-dependent patients. J Consult Clin Psychol 69:825–830, 2001

Doidge N: Empirical evidence for the efficacy of psychoanalytic psychotherapies and psychoanalysis: an overview. Psychoanalytic Inquiry 17 (suppl 1, ed. Lazar SG):102–150, 1997

Dossmann R, Kutter P, Heinzel R, et al: The long-term benefits of intensive psychotherapy: a view from Germany. Psychoanalytic Inquiry 17 (suppl 1, ed. Lazar SG):74–86, 1997

Duehrssen A: [Catamnestic results with 1004 patients following analytic psychotherapy.] Z Psychosom Med 8:94–113, 1962

Duehrssen A, Jorswiek E: [An empirical and statistical inquiry into the therapeutic potential of psychoanalytic treatment.] Nervenarzt 36:166–169, 1965

Fonagy P: Open Door Review of Outcome Studies in Psychoanalysis, 2nd Edition. London, International Psychoanalytical Association, 2002

Gabbard GO (ed.): Psychodynamic Psychiatry in Clinical Practice. Washington, DC, American Psychiatric Press, 1994, pp 156–163

Gabbard GO: Psychotherapy of personality disorders. J Psychother Pract Res 9:1–6, 2000

Grande T, Dilg R, Jakobsen T, et al: Differential effects of two forms of psychoanalytic therapy: results of the Heidelberg-Berlin study. Psychother Res 16:470–485, 2006

Hall J, Caleo S, Stevenson J, et al: An economic analysis of psychotherapy for borderline personality disorder patients. J Ment Health Policy Econ 4:3–8, 2001

Heard H: Behavior therapies for borderline patients. Paper presented at the 147th annual meeting of the American Psychiatric Association. Philadelphia, PA, May 21–26, 1994

Heinzel R, Breyer F, Klein T: Ambulante psychoanalyse in Deutschland: Eine katamnestische evaluation studie. Fakultat fur Wirtschaftswissenschaften und Statistik, Diskussionbeitrage, Universitat Konstanz 1:281, 1996

Hogg B, Jackson HJ, Rudd RP, et al: Diagnosing personality disorders in recent-onset schizophrenia. J Nerv Ment Dis 178:194–199, 1990

Hoglend P: Personality disorders and long-term outcome after brief dynamic psychotherapy. J Pers Disord 7:168–181, 1993

Howard KI, Kopta SM, Krause MS, et al: The dose-effect relationship in psychotherapy. Am Psychol 41:159–164, 1986

Keller W, Westhoff G, Dilg R, et al: Studt and the study group on empirical psychotherapy research in analytical psychology. Berlin, Benjamin Franklin Free University of Berlin, Department of Psychosomatic Medicine and Psychotherapy, 1998

Kent LA, Gill GV, Williams G: Mortality and outcome of patients with brittle diabetes and recurrent ketoacidosis. Lancet 344:778–781, 1994

Kopta SM, Howard KI, Lowry JL, et al: Patterns of symptomatic recovery in psychotherapy. J Consult Clin Psychol 62:1009–1016, 1994

Leichsenring F: Applications of psychodynamic psychotherapy to specific disorders, in Textbook of Psychotherapeutic Treatments. Edited by Gabbard GO, APPI, 2009, pp 97–132

Leichsenring F, Rabung S: Effectiveness of long-term psychodyamic psychotherapy: a meta-analysis. JAMA 300:1551–1587, 2008

Linehan MM, Heard HI: Borderline personality disorder, in Cost Effectiveness of Psychotherapy. Edited by Miller NE, Magruder KM. New York, Oxford University Press, 1999, pp 291–305

Linehan MM, Armstrong HE, Suarez A, et al: Cognitive-behavioral treatment of chronically parasuicidal borderline patients. Arch Gen Psychiatry 48:1060–1064, 1991

Maier W, Lichtermann D, Klingler T, et al: Prevalences of personality disorder (DSM-III-R) in the community. J Pers Disord 6:187–196, 1992

Meares R, Stevenson J, Comerford A: Psychotherapy with borderline patients: I. A comparison between treated and untreated cohorts. Aust N Z J Psychiatry 33:467–472; discussion 478–481, 1999

Monsen K, Monsen J: Chronic pain and psychodynamic body therapy: a controlled outcome study. Psychotherapy 37:257–269, 2000

Moran G, Fonagy P, Kurtz A, et al: A controlled study of psychoanalytic treatment of brittle diabetes. J Am Acad Child Adolesc Psychiatry 30:926–935, 1991

Pilkonis PA, Neighbors BD, Corbitt EM: Personality disorders: treatments and cost, in Cost-Effectiveness of Psychotherapy: A Guide for Practitioners, Researchers, and Policymakers. Edited by Miller NE, Magruder KM. New York, Oxford University Press, 1999, pp 279–290

Reich J, Nduaguba M, Yates W: Age and sex distribution of DSM-III personality cluster traits in a community population. Compr Psychiatry 29:298–303, 1988

Reich J, Yates W, Nduaguba M: Prevalence of DSM-III personality disorders in the community. Soc Psychiatry Psychiatr Epidemiol 24:12–16, 1989

Rudolf G, Manz R, Ori C: [Outcome of psychoanalytic therapy]. Z Psychosom Med Psychother 40:25–40, 1994

Sandell R, Blomberg J, Lazar A, et al: Varieties of long-term outcome among patients in psychoanalysis and long-term psychotherapy: a review of findings in the Stockholm outcome of psychoanalysis and psychotherapy project (STOPPP). Int J Psychoanal 81:921–942, 2000

Seligman ME: The effectiveness of psychotherapy. The Consumer Reports study. Am Psychol 50:965–974, 1995

Shea MT, Pilkonis PA, Beckham E, et al: Personality disorders and treatment outcome in the NIMH Treatment of Depression Collaborative Research Program. Am J Psychiatry 147:711–718, 1990

Shedler J: The efficacy of psychodynamic psychotherapy. Am Psychol (in press)

Stevenson J, Meares R: An outcome study of psychotherapy for patients with borderline personality disorder. Am J Psychiatry 149:358–362, 1992

Stevenson J, Meares R: Psychotherapy with borderline patients: II. A preliminary cost benefit study. Aust N Z J Psychiatry 33:473–477; discussion 478–481, 1999

Teufel R, Volk W: Erfolg und Indikation stationarer psychotherapeutischer Langzeittherapie, in Biopsycho-soziale Medizin. Edited by Ehlers W, Traue H, Czogalik D. Berlin, Springer-PSZ Drucke, 1988, pp 331–346

Viinamäki H, Kuikka J, Tiihonen J, et al: Change in monoamine transporter density related to clinical recovery: a case-control study. Nor J Psychiatry 52:39–44, 1998

von Rad M, Senf W, Brautigam W: [Psychotherapy and psychoanalysis in patient management: results of the Heidelberg Catamnesis Project]. Psychother Psychosom Med Psychol 48:88–100, 1998

Wilberg T, Karterud S, Urnes O, et al: Outcomes of poorly functioning patients with personality disorders in a day treatment program. Psychiatr Serv 49:1462–1467, 1998

Wilberg T, Urnes O, Friis S, et al: One-year follow-up of day treatment for poorly functioning patients with personality disorders. Psychiatr Serv 50:1326–1330, 1999

Zimmerman M, Coryell WH: Diagnosing personality disorders in the community. A comparison of self-report and interview measures. Arch Gen Psychiatry 47:527–531, 1990

## Summary of studies addressing cost-effectiveness of long-term and intensive psychotherapy

| Article | Patients | Treatment | Outcome |
| --- | --- | --- | --- |
| Duehrssen 1962 | 1,156 analytic psychotherapy patients; 845 available for follow-up. | Analytic psychotherapy; average 100 sessions, frequency varied. | 55% satisfactorily improved or better. 58% still improved at 5 years. Follow-up: sick leave significantly reduced. |
| Duehrssen and Jorswiek 1965 | 5-year follow-up of 100 of above group, compared with untreated neurotic patients and with general population of insured patients. | Analytic psychotherapy. | Days in hospital originally higher for neurotic group but reduced 77% (from 26 days to 6 days); days in hospital for untreated group (24–25) and general population (10–12) remained about the same. Data from insurance company regarding hospital days. Treated patients had superior work capacity. |
| Teufel and Volk 1988 | 147 patients with severe personality disorder, neuroses, or psychosomatic conditions. | Inpatient psychotherapy (three to four times per week) with adjunctive group therapy. | 70% moderate to good results in attainment of treatment goals as measured by therapists' ratings at end of treatment. 60% moderate to good symptom reduction assessed by questionnaire at start and at follow-up. 80% moderate to good well-being assessed by patient report. 65% fully capable of work assessed by patient report. |
| Moran et al. 1991 | 22 children and adolescents with brittle diabetes. | Relatively brief psychoanalytic therapy (three to four times per week). Focus on developmental conflicts. | Significant improvement in diabetic control, measured by hospitalizations, hemoglobin A1c levels, and growth in height. Maintained at 1-year follow-up. Comparison group with only medical intervention had less improvement, which was not maintained. Outcome suggestive of cost-effectiveness. |

## Summary of studies addressing cost-effectiveness of long-term and intensive psychotherapy *(continued)*

| Article | Patients | Treatment | Outcome |
|---|---|---|---|
| 1. Stevenson and Meares 1999 | 30 severely dysfunctional borderline personality disorder (BPD) patients referred from community. | Individual psychodynamic psychotherapy: Outpatient individual psychotherapy (two times per week) for 12 months, follow-up 12 months after termination. Patients served as own controls (pre– vs. posttreatment), along with a waiting-list comparison group. | Significant reduction in impulsivity, anger, suicidal behavior. Medical visits cut to one-seventh of pretreatment rates. Work absenteeism, hospital admissions, and inpatient days decreased significantly after treatment. |
| 2. Meares et al. 1999 | | | Significant decrease in BPD symptoms compared with waiting-list group. |
| 3. Hall et al. 2001 | | | Substantial savings in health care usage comparing 12 months pre- and posttreatment. |
| Heinzel et al. 1996 | 604 psychoanalysis and psychoanalytic psychotherapy patients. | Psychoanalytic psychotherapy one to four times per week for 3 or more years. | Follow-up of 6 years and use of retrospective questionnaire. Substantial improvement in self-rated total well-being, most marked regarding physical health, both maintained at follow-up. Visits to family medical doctor down by 40%; visits to specialists down by 33%. Days of sickness absence down by 42%; days of hospitalization down by 66%. Savings in health care utilization for the 2 years after termination equaled one-fourth of costs, suggestive of cost offset. |

## Summary of studies addressing cost-effectiveness of long-term and intensive psychotherapy *(continued)*

| Article | Patients | Treatment | Outcome |
|---|---|---|---|
| Dossmann et al. 1997 | 666 patients of psychodynamic psychotherapy who had completed their therapy between January 1990 and December 1994. | Psychodynamic and psychoanalytic psychotherapeutic treatments in Germany for the time period. | Patients were asked for their self-assessment of physical, mental, social, and overall health on a 5-point rating scale and to report utilization of other health care, including medical visits, hospital days, medication, and frequency per year of lost work days for three points in time: beginning of therapy, at end of therapy, and the time when questionnaire was filled out. Mean time since end of therapy was 2 years 3 months, and the range was 0–6 years. There was significant improvement on all reported measures; the most significant determinant of success was the positive effect of the duration of the analytic therapy. The savings in health cost per patient were $5,652 per individual patient and $9,553 for group patients, and lost work days declined by 41.6%, demonstrating both cost offset and cost-effectiveness for long-term psychodynamic treatments. |

## Summary of studies addressing cost-effectiveness of long-term and intensive psychotherapy *(continued)*

| Article | Patients | Treatment | Outcome |
|---|---|---|---|
| Keller et al. 1998 | 111 psychoanalytic patients, many considered severe enough to warrant hospitalization. | Jungian psychoanalysis (76%) or psychotherapy. | Patients followed for mean of 6 years. Retrospective questionnaire with rating scale for impairment; objective data regarding health care utilization. Rating of global well-being by 60% as poor at start vs. 87% as moderate to very good at follow-up. Reduced intake of psychotropics; reduction in frequency of medical visits; reduced hospitalization; reduced sickness and work absence. Data suggestive of effective treatment of severely ill and reduction of health care costs. |
| Bachar et al. 1999 | 33 patients with eating disorder: 25 with bulimia, 8 with anorexia. | Bulimic patients randomly assigned either to self-psychological treatment (SPT) or to control/nutritional counseling (C/NC). Anorexic patients randomly assigned either to SPT or to cognitive therapy (CT). SPT and CT both delivered in an individual format of weekly sessions for a year and did not focus directly on the patient's eating attitudes or behavior. | SPT led to significant improvement, CT to slight improvement, C/NC to almost no changes. 64% of SPT patient compared with 17% of CT patients and 14% of C/NC had remissions by the end of therapy (statistically significant differences). Both SPT and CT had slight (not statistically significant) continued improvement during the year following termination of treatment. |

## Summary of studies addressing cost-effectiveness of long-term and intensive psychotherapy *(continued)*

| Article | Patients | Treatment | Outcome |
|---|---|---|---|
| 1. Bateman and Fonagy 1999<br><br>2. Bateman and Fonagy 2003 | 38 patients with BPD. | Psychoanalytic psychotherapy, individual and group, in a partially hospitalized setting for up to 18 months vs. the control treatment of standard psychiatric care. Patients assigned in a randomized controlled design. | Health care utilization costs were compared for the two groups of patients before treatment, during treatment, and at 18-month follow-up. Costs were the same for both groups before and during treatment, with the greater cost of treatment for the study treatment offset by lower inpatient and emergency room costs. At 18-month follow-up, however, annual health care costs for patients in the partial hospitalization group were only one-fifth of those in the psychiatric general care control group. |
| Bateman and Fonagy 2008 | As above. | As above. | At 5-year follow-up after mentalization-based treatment, patients had some impaired social functioning, but far superior clinical outcomes compared with treatment-as-usual patients with respect to suicidality (23% vs. 74%), diagnostic status (13% still diagnosable with BPD compared with 87%), psychiatric outpatient service use (2 years vs. 3.5 years), use of medication (0.02 vs. 1.90 years using three or more medications), global function above 60 (45% vs. 10%), and vocational status (employed or in school 3.2 years vs. 1.2 years). |

## Summary of studies addressing cost-effectiveness of long-term and intensive psychotherapy *(continued)*

| Article | Patients | Treatment | Outcome |
|---|---|---|---|
| 1. Crits-Christoph et al. 1999<br><br>2. Crits-Christoph et al. 2001 | 487 patients with cocaine dependency. | Patients were randomly assigned to one of four treatments: individual drug counseling plus group drug counseling (GDC), CT plus GDC, supportive-expressive (SE) therapy plus GDC, or GDC alone.<br>Treatment was intensive, including 36 possible individual sessions and 24 group sessions for 6 months. | SE plus GDC and CT plus GDC retained patients better than the other treatment conditions.<br>However, compared with the two psychotherapies with GDC and with GDC alone, individual drug counseling plus GDC led to superior reductions of overall drug use and cocaine use and a greater proportion of patients achieving abstinence.<br>Although the study demonstrated the superiority of individual drug counseling to psychotherapies in modifying cocaine use, that superiority does not extend to other addiction-associated problems of psychiatric symptoms, employment, medical, legal, family, social, interpersonal, or alcohol use problems because, across treatments, all patients improved similarly from baseline. |
| Monsen and Monsen 2000 | 40 patients with pain disorders. | 20 patients were treated with 33 sessions of psychodynamic body therapy (PBT).<br>20 received treatment as usual or no treatment. | Patients were assessed before therapy, at the end of therapy, and at 1-year follow-up.<br>Patients treated with PBT had significantly greater improvement on levels of subjective experience of pain, general symptoms, interpersonal problems, personality characteristics, and affect consciousness.<br>Improvements were durable and had increased at 1-year follow-up. |

**Summary of studies addressing cost-effectiveness of long-term and intensive psychotherapy *(continued)***

| Article | Patients | Treatment | Outcome |
| --- | --- | --- | --- |
| Clarkin et al. 2001 | 23 female patients with BPD and at least two incidents of self-injurious behavior in the last 5 years, no substance abuse, mean age 32.7 years. | Outpatient psychotherapy two times a week for 12 months, using manualized transference-focused psychotherapy (TFP). Patients served as own controls (pre- vs. post- treatment). 17 of 23 patients completed treatment. No separate control group. | Comparing 12 months prior to treatment with 12 months of treatment: decreased self-destructive acts, decreased number and severity of suicide attempts, decreased medical and psychiatric hospitalizations and number of hospital days. |
| Clarkin et al. 2007 | 90 patients with BPD. | Patients randomly assigned to 1 year of twice-weekly individual sessions of TFP, once-weekly supportive psychotherapy with additional sessions as needed, or weekly individual and group dialectical behavior therapy (DBT) with available telephone consultation. | Patients in all three treatment groups improved significantly in depression, anxiety, global functioning, and social adjustment. Both TFP and DBT significantly improved suicidality. Only TFP and supportive treatment improved impulsivity. Only TFP was significantly associated with change in irritability and verbal and direct assault. |

# 11 | Epilogue

William H. Sledge, M.D.
Susan G. Lazar, M.D.
Robert J. Waldinger, M.D.

For many years within psychiatry, biology and psychopharmacology have been major foci of interest while there has been a significant decline in the awareness of the importance of psychotherapy. In addition, psychiatrists are being trained with much less emphasis on learning to do psychotherapy. To our minds, these trends represent a distorted view of the value of psychiatric treatments. There is no question that psychotherapy is effective, as has been amply demonstrated by a large body of research (Spiegel 1999). Nevertheless, in this era of medicine dominated by cost considerations, practitioners are increasingly asked to demonstrate the cost-effectiveness of the services they provide. More than many treatments, both within and outside of psychiatry, psychotherapy in particular has been required to demonstrate its usefulness in cost terms.

This volume on the cost-effectiveness of psychotherapy is meant for policy makers in public and private settings, clinicians, teachers of psychotherapists who design curricula to teach effective treatments, and interested parties to whom support for psychotherapy is important. This book examines the research literature addressing the cost-effectiveness of various psychotherapeutic approaches for a number of the most important psychiatric conditions. The authors believe that the preponderance of the literature reviewed attests in a general way to the cost-effectiveness of the psychotherapies for the conditions examined.

The concept of cost-effectiveness is a contemporary and sophisticated standard. Previously, psychiatric treatments, especially psychotherapy, were held to the stringent standard of cost offset, in order to lobby effectively for its inclusion within the benefit packages of some insurance programs. Cost offset indicates the savings in other medical costs when a specific treatment is provided. Clearly, a treatment that is justified only by virtue of its leading to cost offset or savings in other medical costs is not automatically accepted as necessary and is being held to a standard different from that of other, presumably more obviously necessary, medical care. Another problem with the older concept of cost offset as it has been applied to psychotherapy is that it is restricted to measuring costs saved only in other kinds of medical and surgical care. Newer studies of the outcomes of psychotherapy also measure the cost savings associated with fewer psychiatric hospitalizations, reduced disability, increased work productivity, and even the financial aspects of a life saved from the threat of suicide.

Cost-effectiveness is a broader standard altogether than that of cost offset in that it attempts to describe the value in effectiveness per unit of cost. Thus a treatment that is held to be cost-effective may be effective but not necessarily inexpensive to provide. In addition, data on cost-effectiveness of psychotherapy are often not available for many illnesses. Nonetheless, a conclusion about its likely cost-effectiveness can often be made indirectly by comparing the high costs of untreated illness with the known efficacy of specific psychotherapeutic approaches. The chapters in this volume on psychotherapy of anxiety disorders, posttraumatic stress disorder, and substance abuse take this approach.

There are many different kinds of psychotherapy and many different studies of their value for different illnesses. Consequently, many conclusions have been asserted; for example, a variety of cognitive-behavioral treatment, dialectical behavior therapy, is very helpful for borderline personality disorder (Linehan et al. 1991, 1993, 1994) as is a psychodynamic approach (Bateman and Fonagy 1999, 2003, 2008; Stevenson and Meares 1992, 1995). A psychodynamic approach is less helpful for schizophrenia (Gunderson et al. 1984) than family therapy (Tarrier et al. 1989). The value of different treatments can be assessed in different ways using a variety of standards. The gold standard for research demonstrating efficacy is the prospective, double-blind randomized control study in which treatments are compared with each other and/or with a nontreatment control. Other variables besides the differing treatment approaches are controlled as strictly as possible. Therefore, in an efficacy study investigators prefer to use patients who are as similar as possible. It is important to question whether this rigorous approach to establishing efficacy, often used in drug trials to assess medications, can be similarly meaningful in the much less easily controlled situation of psychotherapy. The establishment of effectiveness, as opposed to efficacy, is measured in more realistic clinical situations with the more usual, heterogeneous patient populations in the real world. Effectiveness studies are meant to inform the average practitioner about the potential benefits from providing a particular kind of treatment.

With the emphasis on the commercialization of medicine, costs have become much more of a consideration determining policy. And as cost considerations began increasingly to drive policy decisions, the authors of this volume undertook the task of assessing the cost-effectiveness of psychotherapy to determine if the case could be made according to these standards. Measuring monetarily the cost of providing care is much easier than measuring monetarily its outcome, especially in its more intangible components such as the relief of suffering and pain. Thus it would be a great loss clinically if we were limited to making medical decisions only by virtue of the most obvious cost considerations. It is also important to remember that psychotherapy is a very personal enterprise. A decision that a given treatment is more valuable on the basis only of cost-effectiveness standards (such as the costs of providing group vs. individual treatment) may completely overlook all of the less readily measurable personal values that are not captured by financial calculations.

Even though psychotherapy has been held to a higher standard than other medical treatments, the authors of this volume conclude that in addition to its effectiveness, a good case can be made for the cost-effectiveness of psychotherapy. The establishment of cost-effectiveness provides a powerful statement about a treatment modality. Nonetheless, while cost-effectiveness is an important concept, these authors feel that there would be much lost if it is used as the sole criterion for making a treatment available. Therefore, when evidence of the cost-effectiveness of a given treatment is not present, the conclusion about its value may still be far from clear. Rather, the decision to support a particular treatment should be made based on a delicate balance of considering both the scientific evidence that supports it and the values of the society in which it is offered.

# References

Bateman A, Fonagy P: Effectiveness of partial hospitalization in the treatment of borderline personality disorder: a randomized controlled trial. Am J Psychiatry 156:1563–1569, 1999

Bateman A, Fonagy P: Health service utilization costs for borderline personality disorder patients treated with psychoanalytically oriented partial hospitalization versus general psychiatric care. Am J Psychiatry 160:169–171, 2003

Bateman A, Fonagy P: Eight-year follow-up of patients treated for borderline personality disorder: mentalization-based treatment versus treatment as usual. Am J Psychiatry 165:631–638, 2008

Gunderson JG, Frank AF, Katz HM, et al: Effects of psychotherapy in schizophrenia: II. Comparative outcome of two forms of treatment. Schizophr Bull 10:564–598, 1984

Linehan MM, Armstrong HE, Suarez A, et al: Cognitive-behavioral treatment of chronically parasuicidal borderline patients. Arch Gen Psychiatry 48:1060–1064, 1991

Linehan MM, Heard HL, Armstrong HE: Naturalistic follow-up of a behavioral treatment for chronically parasuicidal borderline patients. Arch Gen Psychiatry 50:971–974, 1993

Linehan MM, Tutek DA, Heard HL, et al: Interpersonal outcome of cognitive behavioral treatment for chronically suicidal borderline patients. Am J Psychiatry 151:1771–1776, 1994

Spiegel D (ed): Efficacy and Cost-Effectiveness of Psychotherapy. Washington DC, American Psychiatric Press, 1999

Stevenson J, Meares R: An outcome study of psychotherapy for patients with borderline personality disorder. Am J Psychiatry 149:358–362, 1992

Stevenson J, Meares R: Borderline patients at five-year follow up. Paper presented at the Annual Congress of the Royal Australia and New Zealand College of Psychiatrists, Cairns, Australia, 1995

Tarrier N, Barrowclough C, Vaughn C, et al: Community management of schizophrenia. A two-year follow-up of a behavioural intervention with families. Br J Psychiatry 154:625–628, 1989

# Subject Index

*Page numbers printed in* **boldface** *type refer to tables or figures.*

AA (Alcoholics Anonymous), 185, 187, 198
ABCT (alcohol behavioral couples therapy), 187–188
Abdominal pain
in irritable bowel syndrome, 247
recurrent pediatric, 246
Abend et al. (1983), 63
Abramowitz et al. (2003), 110
Abuse victims. *See also* Sexual abuse/assault
posttraumatic stress disorder among, 4, 23, 87, 94–95
Acamprosate, for alcoholism, 190
ACRA (adolescent community reinforcement approach), for marijuana use disorders, 196
Acupuncture, for alcoholism, 185
Addiction disorders. *See* Substance abuse/dependence
ADHD. *See* Attention-deficit/hyperactivity disorder
Adolescent community reinforcement approach (ACRA), for marijuana use disorders, 196
Affective disorders
alcoholism and, 178
in children and adolescents, 3, 268, 275–276, 279–280
costs of, 3, 104, 135–137, 139–141
depression, 24, 135–157, **162–173**
disability due to, 2, 135–136, 137, 138, 139–140
epidemiology of, 3, 136
substance abuse and, 176, 198

Afghanistan war veterans, 4, 90
AFM (applied family management), for schizophrenia, 36, **56, 57**
Agoraphobia
classification of, 111–112
cost-effectiveness of psychotherapy for, 112
epidemiology of, 111
panic disorder with or without, 105, 111–112
cognitive-behavioral therapy for, 108, 109
Alcohol abuse/dependence, 184–192. *See also* Substance abuse/dependence
alcohol behavioral couples therapy for, 187–188
behavioral broad spectrum treatment of, 190
cognitive-behavioral therapy for, 185–186, 188
computer/Internet-based approaches to, 190
considerations in treatment of, 184–185
contingency management approach to, 189
contracting intervention for, 191
costs of, 177–178
culture and, 179
effectiveness and cost-effectiveness of treatments for, 175, 186, 189–192, **213–219**
epidemiology of, 177–178

Alcohol abuse/dependence *(continued)*
  health risks of, 178
  motivational enhancement therapy
      for, 185, 186, 187, 190
  outcome measures for treatment of,
      185
  in pregnancy, 179
  psychiatric comorbidity with, 176,
      178
  psychotherapy combined with
      medication for, 190
  residential treatment of, 185, 187,
      189, 191
  screening and brief intervention for,
      188–189, 191–192
  treatment in adolescents, 189
  treatment matching for, 185–186
  treatment modalities for, 185
      comparing costs of, 186
  twelve-step programs for, 185, 186,
      187, 189
Alcohol behavioral couples therapy
      (ABCT), 187–188
Alcoholics Anonymous (AA), 185, 187,
      198
Alessi et al. (2007), 189
Alterman et al. (2001), 182, **210**
Alzheimer's disease, caregivers for
      patients with
  psychotherapy for, 233
  social support and cardiac changes
      in, 239
American Board of Psychiatry and
      Neurology, 10
American Psychiatric Association, 5, 6,
      105
Amir et al. (1998), 92, **100**
Amitriptyline, for depression, 146, **162**
Andersen (1992), 236
Andrews (1989), 18
Anger, myocardial infarction and,
      239
Angina, 240–241, **260–261**
Anglin and Hser (1990), 200
Anorexia, 299–300, **307**

Antidepressants
  for depression, 135, 136, 141,
      **162–164, 166–171**
    in adolescents, 276, **286**
    combined with psychotherapy,
        142, 143, 144, 146–147,
        151, 156
    combined with psychotherapy in
        diabetes, 242–243
  for generalized anxiety disorder,
      107, 114, **132**
  for panic disorder, 109, 114, **126,
      132**
    combined with cognitive-
        behavioral therapy, 105,
        107, 109, **124, 128, 132**
Antipsychotics, for schizophrenia, 33,
      37–38, 40
  akathisia induced by, 40
  compliance with, 41
  cost-effectiveness of, 42, **60**
  psychosocial treatment and, 38
Antisocial personality disorder, 4, 176,
      178, 198
Anxiety disorders, 23, 103–116. *See also
      specific anxiety disorders*
  borderline personality disorder and,
      62, 75
  case vignette of, 115–116
  in children and adolescents, 3,
      113
  costs of, 3, 23, 103–104, 140
  depression and, 108
  disability due to, 2
  epidemiology of, 3, 103–104
  generalized anxiety disorder,
      113–115, **132–134**
  medical illness and, 233
    diabetes, 241
  obsessive-compulsive disorder,
      110–111, **129**
  panic disorder, 104–110, **122–128**
  phobic disorder, 111–113, **130–131**
  posttraumatic stress disorder, 23,
      87–95, **98–102**

psychotherapy for
combined with
pharmacotherapy, 103
effect on years lived with
disability, 94, 107–108,
112–113, 114
search methodology for studies
of, 104
substance abuse and, 176, 198
alcoholism, 178
undertreatment of, 116
Applied family management (AFM),
for schizophrenia, 36, **56, 57**
Arathuzik (1994), 246
Arnow and Constantino (2003), 144
Aronson (1989), 64
Arthritis, 246
Attention-deficit/hyperactivity
disorder (ADHD), 277
medical costs of children with, 275
pharmacotherapy for, 275
parental objection to, 269, 281
psychotherapy for, 268, 274–275,
**286**
Avants et al. (1998), 193
Avants et al. (2004), 196
Aversion therapies, for alcoholism, 185

Babor et al. (2007), 192, **218**
Bachar et al. (1999), 299–300, **307**
Baines et al. (2004), 248, **264**
Ball et al. (1996), 110
Bannon et al. (1995), 290–991
Barlow et al. (1984), 113
Barlow et al. (2000), 105, **124**
Barrett et al. (2006), 191, **217**
Bassler and Hoffmann (1994), 112,
113, **132**
Bateman and Fonagy (1999), 74, 76,
**85**, 297, **308**, 312
Bateman and Fonagy (2000), 75, 77
Bateman and Fonagy (2003), 76, **85**,
297, **308**, 312
Bateman and Fonagy (2008), 76, **86**,
297, **308**, 312

Beck Depression Inventory, 67, 70,
145, **162**, 248
Beck et al. (1992), 105
Beecham et al. (2006), 17
Behavioral contracting, for alcoholism,
185, 191
Behavioral family therapy (BFT), for
schizophrenia, 36, 39, 41, **57**
Bell South pilot project (1991–1993),
15
Bellack et al. (2000), 36, 41, **56**
Benzodiazepines
for generalized anxiety disorder,
114
for panic disorder, **123**
Berglund et al. (2003), 36, 41, **57**
Bernbaum et al. (1989), 242
BFT (behavioral family therapy), for
schizophrenia, 36, 39, 41, **57**
Bipolar disorder
costs of, 137
epidemiology of, 136
psychotherapy for, 144
combined with
pharmacotherapy for
adolescents, 276, **287**
cost-effectiveness of, 15, 135,
145–146, 149
Bischof et al. (2008), 188
Blatt (1992), 144, 290
Blatt et al. (1995), 144, 290
Blumenthal and Wei (1993), 239
Board certification, 10
Bolton et al. (2003), 144
Borderline personality disorder (BPD),
4, 15, 23, 61–77
case vignette of, 62–63
clinical features of, 62
comorbidity with, 62, 75
diagnostic criteria for, 64
emergency room visits due to, 61,
62, 63
parenting deficits due to, 62–63
pharmacotherapy for, 63
prevalence of, 62

Borderline personality disorder (BPD)
(*continued*)
  psychotherapy for, 63–77, **81–86,
    305, 308, 310**
    cognitive analytic therapy, 67, 74
    common elements of effective
      therapies, 77
    comorbidity and, 75
    control groups in studies of, 68,
      74–75
    cost-effectiveness of, 64–65,
      66–67, 69, 75–77, 297–298
    day treatment programs,
      296–297
    defining and standardizing
      treatment for, 64, 73–74
    dialectical behavior therapy, 64,
      70–72, 74, **84–85,** 291, 312
    economic variables and, 75–76
    future research on, 73–76
    group psychotherapy, 69–70,
      **84**
    individual psychotherapy,
      65–69, **81–83**
    long-term psychotherapy, 68,
      74, 76, 289, 292
    manual-assisted cognitive-
      behavior therapy, 68–69, 74
    methodological problems in
      studies of, 64, 73–76
    partial hospitalization with
      individual and group
      psychoanalytic
      psychotherapy, 72–73,
      **85–86**
    premature termination of, 63,
      64, 67
    psychodynamic psychotherapy,
      65–66
    randomization for studies of, 75
    search methodology for studies
      of, 61
    transference-focused
      psychotherapy, 67–68, 298
  suicide and, 62–63, 67

treatment utilization in, 62
underdiagnosis and undertreatment
  of, 62
Borderline Personality Disorder Study
  of Cognitive Therapy
  (BOSCOT), 69
Bosmans et al. (2007), 145, 153–154,
  156, **172**
Bower and Rowland (2006), 16
Bower et al. (2000), 145, 148, **165**
BPD. *See* Borderline personality
  disorder
Brandon (2001), 182
Brazier et al. (2006), 76
Breast cancer, 6, 236, 237, 238, 246,
  **258**
Breastfeeding, depression management
  during, 142–143, 155
Brief dynamic psychotherapy, for panic
  disorder, 103, 107, **123**
Brief motivational counseling, for
  alcoholism, 185
Brom et al. (1989), 91, **98**
Brooker et al. (1994), 35, **52**
Brooner et al. (2007), 195
Brown and Schulberg (1995), 141
Brown et al. (1972), 35
Browne et al. (2002), 145, 149–150,
  **167**
Buie and Adler (1982), 63
Bulimia, 299–300, **307**
Bupropion
  for depression, 151, **169**
  for tobacco cessation, 183
Burden of mental illness, 2
Burke et al. (2002), 201
Butler et al. (1987), 113, **132**

Cain et al. (1986), 238
California Drug and Alcohol
  Treatment Assessment
  (CALDATA) study, 182, 199–200
Cancer, 235–238
  alcohol use and, 178
  case vignette of, 231–232

psychiatric comorbidity with, 235
psychotherapy for patients with, 6,
    232, 236–238, **256–259**
    impact on health care costs,
        237–238
    impact on quality of life, 237,
        238
    for pain management, 236, 246
smoking and, 177, 182
Cannabis use. *See* Marijuana use
    disorders
"Cardiac cripple," 239
Cardiac defibrillator, 241, **261**
Cardiac disease, 5–6, 239–241
    psychosocial interventions for
        patients with, 239–241,
        **260–261**
        cost-effectiveness of, 240
        effect on quality of life, 239–240
    type A personality and, 239
Caregivers of Alzheimer's disease
    patients
    psychotherapy for, 233
    social support and cardiac changes
        in, 239
Carpal tunnel syndrome, 244–245
Carroll and Rounsaville (1992), 198,
    201
Carroll and Rounsaville (1995), 189
Carroll et al. (1994), 194–195, 201,
    202
Carroll et al. (1998), 201
Carroll et al. (2001), 194
Casey and Berman (1985), 272, 273,
    **284**
CAT (cognitive analytic therapy)
    for borderline personality disorder,
        67, 74
    in diabetes, 242
CBT. *See* Cognitive-behavioral therapy
CHAMPUS system, 18
Chen et al. (2006), 199, **224**
Cheung et al. (2003), 237, **257**
Chiesa et al. (2002), 16–17
Child PTSD Reaction Index, 92

Children and adolescents, 24, 267–282
    adolescent community
        reinforcement approach for
        marijuana use disorders in, 196
    affective disorders in, 3, 268,
        275–276, 279–280
    anxiety disorders in, 3, 113
        cognitive-behavioral therapy
            combined with
            pharmacotherapy for
            obsessive-compulsive
            disorder, 110–111
        psychotherapy for posttraumatic
            stress disorder, 92, 93, **99**
    case vignettes of psychotherapy
        with, 279–281
    cognitive-behavioral family
        intervention for recurrent
        abdominal pain in, 246
    cost-effectiveness of psychotherapy
        with, 267–268, 275–276,
        **284–288**
    costs of mental illness in, 268
    differential effects of psychotherapy
        with, 276–279
        related to environmental and
            family factors, 277–278
        related to intensity of treatment,
            278
        related to patient age, 278
        related to treatment setting, 277
    factors affecting efficacy of
        psychotherapy with, 269–271
        adult dependency and treatment
            decisions, 269–270
        developmental level, 269
        family factors, 270
        goal of treatment, 271
        socioeconomic status, 270
        therapist skill and training,
            270–271
    focused studies on efficacy of
        psychotherapy with, 273–276
        for adolescents with depression,
            275–276

Children and adolescents *(continued)*
  focused studies on efficacy of
      psychotherapy with *(continued)*
    for children with attention-
        deficit/hyperactivity
        disorder, 268, 274–275
    for children with diabetes,
        241–242, 273–274
    for children with learning
        disorders, 274
    medical service utilization and,
        274
  long-term psychotherapy with,
      289
  mental health care parity for, 21
  meta-analytic studies of
      psychotherapy with, 272–273
  search methodology for studies of,
      268
  trauma and abuse of, 4
  treatment settings for, 268
  types of psychotherapy outcome
      studies for, 271–276
Children's Depression Rating Scale—
    Revised, 276
Children's Global Assessment Scale,
    278
Chisholm (2005), 37, **59**, 145,
    150–151, **168**
CHOICE Project, 37, **59**, 151, **168**
Chronic fatigue syndrome/myalgic
    encephalopathy, 248, **266**
Cisler et al. (1998), 186, **214**
Clark et al. (1994), 105
Clark et al. (1999), 107, **124**
Clarkin et al. (2001), 67–68, 74, **82**,
    298, **310**
Clarkin et al. (2007), 298, **310**
Classification of mental disorders,
    6–7
Clinical case management, 230
Clozapine, for schizophrenia, 40, 42
CM. *See* Contingency management
    approaches

Cocaine use/addiction. *See also*
    Substance abuse/dependence
  contingency-based programs for
      methadone-maintained
      patients with, 195–196
  cost-effectiveness of treatment for,
      175, 299
  effectiveness of treatment for, 200
  meta-analysis of treatment outcome
      studies for, 192–193
  predictors of treatment seeking for,
      192
  in pregnancy, 179
  psychiatric comorbidity with, 176
  psychotherapy for, 194–195, 299,
      **309**
Cognitive analytic therapy (CAT)
  for borderline personality disorder,
      67, 74
  in diabetes, 242
Cognitive therapy (CT)
  for cocaine dependence, 299
  for eating disorders, 299–300, **307**
  for posttraumatic stress disorder,
      94
Cognitive-behavioral therapy (CBT),
    9, 10
  for borderline personality disorder,
      65, 69, **83**
    cognitive-behavior therapy, 69
    manual-assisted cognitive-
        behavior therapy, 68–69
  in cardiovascular disease, 239,
      240–241
  in chronic fatigue syndrome, 248
  for depression, 141, 142, 146, 147,
      148–149, 151, 152, 153, 154,
      **162–165, 169–172**
    in adolescents, 276, **286**
  for generalized anxiety disorder,
      107, 113–114
  immunological effects of, 230
  in irritable bowel syndrome, 247
  in musculoskeletal disease, 244–245

for obsessive-compulsive disorder, combined with pharmacotherapy, 110–111

for pain, 244–245, 246

for panic disorder, combined with pharmacotherapy, 103, 105–110

for posttraumatic stress disorder, 93, 95, **100**

for schizophrenia, 38

for social phobia, 112

for substance abuse, 180, 201

alcoholism, 185–186, 188

cocaine, 194–195

marijuana, 196–197

nicotine, 182–183

Cohen et al. (1997), 233

Collaborative Study of Depression, 289–290

Colorectal cancer, 236–237, **259**

COMBINE trial, 190

Commercialization of medicine, 313

Community reinforcement approach

for adolescent marijuana use disorders, 196

for alcoholism, 185

Computer-based approaches to alcoholism, 189

Concepts of mental illness, 5–7

Confidentiality, 8

Confrontational interventions for alcoholism, 185, 186–187

Consultation-liaison psychiatry, 230, 244–245

Contingency management (CM) approaches

for alcoholism, 189

for cocaine addiction, 195–196

for dually diagnosed patients, 199

for marijuana use disorders, 197

for opiate dependence, 194

Coronary heart disease. *See* Cardiac disease

Cost-benefit analysis, 13, 14

Cost-effectiveness of psychotherapy, 1, 8, 13–15, 22, 311–313

for anxiety disorders, 116, **133–134**

generalized anxiety disorder, 114

obsessive-compulsive disorder, 111

panic disorder, 105–110, 114

phobic disorder, 112–113

posttraumatic stress disorder, 91, 92, 93, 94, 95, **98–102**

for borderline personality disorder, 64–65, 66–67, 69, 75–77, **81–86,** 297–298

for children and adolescents, 267–268, 275–276, **284–288**

vs. cost offset, 13–14, 311–312

for depression, 144–157, **161–173,** 231

long-term psychotherapy, 293–300, **304–310**

for medically ill patients, 231–249, **256–266**

meta-analyses of studies of, 8, 16

for schizophrenia, 15, 39, 42, **47–60**

for specific diagnostic groups, 15–17, 22

for substance abuse, 175–176, 199–200, **210–226**

Costs of medical care, 233

Costs of mental illness, 2–3

affective disorders, 3, 104, 135–137, 139–141, 144, 155

anxiety disorders, 3, 23, 103–104, 110, 111, 140

in children and adolescents, 268

attention-deficit/hyperactivity disorder, 275

schizophrenia, 31–32, 104

substance abuse/dependence, 176, 177–180

Costs of psychotherapy, 11–13

accountant perspective of, 12

dimensions of, 11–13

Costs of psychotherapy *(continued)*
  economist or societal perspective of, 12
  management perspective of, 11–12
  methodology for determination of, 11–12
  production characteristics and, 12
  service units and, 12
Cost-utility analysis, 14
  of depression management, 150
Cottraux et al. (2000), 112, **131**
Counseling
  for alcoholism, 185, 188
  for depression
    individual counseling by social worker, 146
    nondirective counseling, 147–149
    via telephone, 148, **165, 172**
  nutritional, for eating disorders, 299
Couples therapy
  for alcoholism, 185, 187–188
  for depression, 149, **166**
Crack cocaine, 179. *See also* Cocaine use/addiction
Creed et al. (2003), 247–248
Criminal activity
  posttraumatic stress disorder among victims of, 4, 90–91, 92
  substance abuse and, 176, 180
    effect of treatment interventions on, 199, 200
Crits-Christoph and Siqueland (1996), 192–193
Crits-Christoph et al. (1999), 299, **309**
Crits-Christoph et al. (2001), 299, **309**
CT. *See* Cognitive therapy
Culture
  and definitions of mental illness, 5
  substance abuse/dependence and, 179–180, 202

DALYs (disability-adjusted life years), 14, 107, 114, 137
Davidson et al. (1986), 277

Davidson et al. (2007), 190, 240, **260**
Day treatment programs, for borderline personality disorder, 72–73, 76, 296–297
DBT. *See* Dialectical behavior therapy for borderline personality disorder
Delinquent youth, 277, 280–281
Delusions, 32
Dennis et al. (2004), 196, **220**
Depression, 24, 135–157
  anxiety disorders and, 108
  borderline personality disorder and, 62, 75
  case vignette of, 155
  in children and adolescents, 3, 268, 275–276, 279–280
  chronic pelvic pain and, 245
  costs of, 3, 135–137, 139–141, 144, 155
  disability due to, 2, 24, 135–136, 137, 138, 139–140
  effects compared with chronic medical illness, 138–139
  epidemiology of, 3, 135–136
  functional impairment due to, 3, 138
  health care utilization/costs and, 139, 140–141
  medical expenditures and, 233
  medical illness and, 229, 233
    diabetes, 241, 242–243
  psychotherapy for, 141–157, **162–173**
    for adolescents, 275–276, **286**
    for chronic depression, 144
    cognitive-behavioral therapy, 141, 142, 146, 147, 148–149, 151, 152, 153, 154
    combined with pharmacotherapy, 142, 143, 144, 146–147, 151, 156
    with comorbid panic disorder, **122**

cost-effectiveness of, 135, 136, 144–157, 231
couples therapy, 149
duration of, 141, 289
effect of perfectionism on outcome of, 144
effects on quality of life, 150
efficacy of, 135, 141–144
group interpersonal psychotherapy, 144
individual counseling by social worker, 146
interpersonal psychotherapy, 141, 142–143, 145, 147, 153–154
for low-income minority women, 151
maintenance treatment, 141, 143
for medical inpatients, 145
mindfulness-based cognitive therapy, 143
nondirective counseling, 147–149
for postpartum depression, 142–143, 152–153, 155
in primary care settings, 146–148, 150, 151–152, 153
problem-solving treatment, 142, 146, **163**
QI-Meds and QI-Therapy, 152, **170**
search methodology for studies of, 136
self-management therapy, 154
for subthreshold depression, 154–155, 156
telephone counseling, 148
severity of, 136
sexual victimization and, 90
smoking cessation and, 183
somatic symptoms of, 229
suicide and, 136, 137, 155
in transplant recipients, 248
Treatment of Adolescents With Depression Study, 275–276

treatment-resistant, 137
undertreatment of, 136
in U.S. workforce, 140
in war veterans, 4, 90
Desipramine, for cocaine addiction, 194
Diabetes mellitus, 241–244
family expressed emotion and, 35, 241
psychiatric comorbidity with, 241
psychotherapy for patients with, 241–244, **262**
children and adolescents, 241–242, 273–274, **285**, 295, **304**
cost-effectiveness of, 242–243
depression treatment and, 242–244
*Diagnostic and Statistical Manual of Mental Disorders* (DSM), 5, 6
borderline personality disorder in, 64
generalized anxiety disorder in, 113
posttraumatic stress disorder in, 88
schizophrenia in, 32
Diagnostic Interview for Borderlines, 69, 70
Dialectical behavior therapy (DBT) for borderline personality disorder, 64, 70–72, **84–85**, 312
with comorbid substance use disorders, 71–72
cost-effectiveness of, 71, 76, 297–298
frequency and duration of, 74, 291
Difede et al. (2007), 93, **101**
Disability due to mental illness, 1–2, 5
depression, 2, 24, 135–136, 137, 138, 139–140
Disability-adjusted life years (DALYs), 14, 107, 114, 137
Disruptive behavior disorders, psychotherapy for youth with, 278, **286**
Dissociative disorders, 4

Disulfiram, for alcoholism, 187
Doggrell (2006), 190
Doidge et al. (1994), 18
Domino et al. (2008), 276, **287**
Donovan and Wells (2007), 197
Doran et al. (2004), 189, **214**
Dossmann et al. (1997), 17, 292, 295,
   **306**
Drummond (1993), 110
Drummond (1997), 188
Druss et al. (2000), 233
DSM. *See Diagnostic and Statistical
   Manual of Mental Disorders*
Dually diagnosed patients, 176, 185,
   197–199, 202. *See also* Substance
   abuse/dependence
   contingency management for, 199
   cost-effectiveness of interventions
      for, 198
   outcome related to intensity of
      services for, 198, 199
   prognosis for, 198
   residential treatment for, 198
Duehrssen (1962), 294, **304**
Duehrssen and Jorswiek (1965), 8, 294,
   **304**
Dunn et al. (2007), 93–94, **101**, 145,
   154, **173**
Duration of treatment, 17–19. *See also*
   Long-term and intensive
   psychotherapy
Durham et al. (2005), 93, 95, **100, 108,**
   114, **134**
Dysthymia
   cost-effectiveness of therapy for,
      149–150
   costs of, 137
   epidemiology of, 136
   sertraline vs. psychotherapy for,
      142, **167**

EAP (employee assistance program),
   15, 16
Earthquake survivors, 92
Eating disorders, 299–300, **307**

ECA (Epidemiologic Catchment Area)
   surveys, 104, 110, 111, 113, 137
Eckman et al. (1992), 37, **58**
ECT (experiential-cognitive therapy),
   for panic disorder, **126**
Edgell et al. (2000), 145, 149, **166**
EE (expressed emotion), 35, 41
Effectiveness studies, 312–313
Elderly persons
   generalized anxiety disorder in, 113
   hip fractures in, 244
Electromyography feedback, for
   generalized anxiety disorder, 113
EMDR (eye movement desensitization
   and reprocessing), 88
Employee assistance program (EAP),
   15, 16
Epidemiological Catchment Area
   (ECA) surveys, 104, 110, 111, 113,
   137
Epidemiology, 1–5
   of anxiety disorders, 3, 103–104
      generalized anxiety disorder, 113
      obsessive-compulsive disorder,
         110
      panic disorder, 104–105
      phobic disorder, 111
      posttraumatic stress disorder, 4,
         87, 88–89
   of bipolar disorder, 136
   of borderline personality disorder,
      62
   of depression, 3, 135, 136
   of personality disorders, 290
   of schizophrenia, 4, 31
   of substance abuse, 4, 177–179
Epstein and McCrady (1998), 187–188
Esophageal cancer, 236, **259**
Experiential-cognitive therapy (ECT),
   for panic disorder, **126**
Exposure therapy
   for panic disorder, **123**
   for posttraumatic stress disorder,
      91–93, 94, 95
   for social phobia, 112, **130, 131**

Expressed emotion (EE), 35, 41
Eye movement desensitization and
    reprocessing (EMDR), 88

Falloon et al. (1987), 34, 39, **48**
Family interventions (FIs)
    for affective disorders, **162, 166**
        adolescent bipolar disorder, 276,
            **287**
        cost-effectiveness of, 145–146
        integrated family and individual
            therapy for bipolar
            disorder, 144
    for caregivers of Alzheimer's disease
        patients, 233
    for marijuana use disorders, 196
    for pediatric recurrent abdominal
        pain, 246
    for schizophrenia, 23, 33, 34, 312
        case vignette of, 39–40
        clinical effectiveness of, 34–38,
            41–42
        cost-effectiveness of, 39, 43
        discrepancy in outcomes of, 41
        summary of studies on, **47–57**
Fava et al. (1994), 142
Fava et al. (1996), 142
Fava et al. (1998), 142
Fawzy et al. (1990), 236
Fawzy et al. (1993), 236
Feuerstein et al. (1999), 244
Finney et al. (1991), 274, **285**
First Chicago Corporation study, 139
FIs. *See* Family interventions
Fluoxetine, for adolescent depression,
    276, **286**
Foa (1997), 92, **99**
Foa et al. (1991), 91, **98**
Foa et al. (2003), 94, **102**
Follette and Cummings (1970), 8
Fonagy (2002), 292
Fonagy and Target (1994), 278, 282,
    **288**
Forester et al. (1985), 238
Fosbury et al. (1997), 242

Frank et al. (1990), 141
Freeborn et al. (2000), 187
French et al. (2008), 189, **219**
Frequency of treatment, 18, 289. *See
    also* Long-term and intensive
    psychotherapy
Friedli et al. (2000), 145, 147–148, 156,
    **164**
Fromm-Reichmann (1950), 33
Frueh et al. (1996), 91–92, **98**
Functional status
    depression and, 3, 138
    personality disorders and, 290
        borderline personality disorder,
            62
    posttraumatic stress disorder and,
        87, 89, 95

Gabbard (2000), 289
Gabbard et al. (1997), 15, 33, 63, 65, 77
GAD. *See* Generalized anxiety disorder
Gastrointestinal cancers, 236–237, **259**
Gastrointestinal disorders, 246–248
Gava et al. (2007), 111, **129**
Gavard et al. (1993), 233
GDC (group drug counseling), for
    cocaine dependence, 299
Gellert et al. (1993), 236
General medical providers of mental
    health care, 2
Generalized anxiety disorder (GAD),
    23, 113–115
    case vignette of, 115–116
    comorbidity with, 113, 114
    epidemiology of, 113
    psychotherapy for, 113–114,
        **132–134**
        cognitive-behavioral therapy,
            107, 113–114
        combined with
            pharmacotherapy, 107
        cost-effectiveness of, 114
        endurance of effects of, 114
        inpatient treatment with, 113
Gerstein et al. (1994), 192, **226**

Glick et al. (1990), 34, **49**
Glick et al. (1993), 34, **49**
Goenjian et al. (1997), 92, **99**
Gordon et al. (2007), 184, **213**
Gould et al. (1995), 240
Grande et al. (2006), 292
Greenberg et al. (1999), 107
Greist (1998), 110
Gross et al. (2006), 195
Group drug counseling (GDC), for
    cocaine dependence, 299
Group psychotherapy
    for alcoholism, 185, 187
    for bipolar disorder, 149
    for borderline personality disorder,
        69–70, **84–86**
        dialectical behavior therapy
            with, 70–72
        partial hospitalization with,
            72–73
    cost-effectiveness of, 8
    for depression, 144
    for dysthymia, 142
    effects on immune functioning, 230
    for medically ill patients, 6
        with cancer, 6, 236–238, 246
        with cardiac disease, 240
        transplant recipients, 248
    for methadone-maintained patients,
        193, 195
    for panic disorder, **125**
    for personality disorders, 16
    for phobic disorder, 112
    for posttraumatic stress disorder,
        92–94
    for smoking cessation, 184
    for social phobia, 112, **131**
Gunderson et al. (1984), 33, 312
Guthrie et al. (1993), 246–247
Gutierrez-Recacha et al. (2006), 38,
    **60**
Gynecological cancers, 238

Haas et al. (1988), 34, **49**
Haddock et al. (1997), 245

Halfway house, for schizophrenic
    patients, 40
Hall et al. (1998), 183
Hall et al. (2001), 66, 75, 76, **81**, 298,
    **305**
Hallucinations, 32, 33
    cultural views of, 5
Hallucinogen abuse, 175. *See also*
    Substance abuse/dependence
Haloperidol, for schizophrenia, 38, 40
Halpin et al. (2006), 183–184, **212**
Hamblen et al. (2009), 91
Hampson et al. (2001), 242, **262**
Harvard Center for Risk Analysis
    Cost-Effectiveness Registry, 150,
    **168**
Harvey and Rapee (1995), 114
Hay Huggins (1990), 19
Health care expenditures, 233
Health maintenance organizations
    (HMOs), 11, 20, 90, 140, 143, 268,
    274
Heard (1994), 71, 75, 298
Heart disease, 5–6, 239–241
    psychosocial interventions for
        patients with, 239–241,
        **260–261**
        cost-effectiveness of, 240
        effect on quality of life, 239–240
    type A personality and, 239
Heimberg (1993), 112
Heimberg et al. (1990), 112
Heimberg et al. (1998), 112, **131**
Heinicke and Ramsey-Klee (1986),
    274, **285**
Heinzel et al. (1996), 294, **305**
Hellman et al. (1990), 233
Hengeveld et al. (1988), 145, **162**
Heroin dependence. *See* Opiate
    dependence
Hester and Miller (2006), 190
Heuzenroeder et al. (2004), 107, 114,
    **132**
Hip fracture, 244
HIV-positive patients, 245

HMOs (health maintenance organizations), 11, 20, 90, 140, 143, 268, 274
Hofmann (2004), 112, **131**
Hogarty (2002), 37
Hogarty et al. (1986), 34–35, 37, **47**
Hogarty et al. (1991), 34–35, 37, **47**
Hogarty et al. (1995), 37
Hogarty et al. (1997), 37
Hoglend (1993), 292
Hoke (1989), 68, 73, **81**
Holder et al. (1991), 185, 187, 188, 189, **213**
Hooley et al. (1986), 35
Hopkins Symptom Checklist–90, 70, 92
Hopkins Symptom Checklist–90—Revised, 67
Howard (1993), 188
Howard et al. (1986), 74, 292
Huxley et al. (2000), 145, 149, **166**
Hypnosis, for alcoholism, 185
Hypochondriasis, 115

IBS (irritable bowel syndrome), 246–248
IES (Impact of Event Scale), 92
IFIT (integrated family and individual therapy), for bipolar disorder, 144
IGP (interpersonal group psychotherapy), for borderline personality disorder, 69–70
Imipramine
    for depression, 141, **162, 168**
    for panic disorder, 109, **124, 128**
Immunological effects of psychological stress, 229–230
IMPACT intervention, in diabetes, 242–243
Impact of Event Scale (IES), 92
Implantable cardioverter-defibrillator, 241, **261**
Income and mental illness, 5
Inhalant abuse, 175. *See also* Substance abuse/dependence
    culture and, 179–180

Inpatient psychiatric care. *See also* Partial hospitalization
    for borderline personality disorder, 62–63
        dialectical behavior therapy for reduction of, 70–72
    effectiveness of long-term psychotherapy during, 296
    insurance coverage for, 20
    psychoanalytically oriented psychotherapy for severe anxiety disorders, 112, 113, **132**
Insurance coverage for mental health care, 7, 17–22
    for inpatient psychiatric care, 20
    managed care and patterns of, 19–21
    parity of, 7, 20, 21–22
    utilization related to, 17–19
Integrated family and individual therapy (IFIT), for bipolar disorder, 144
Intensive psychotherapy. *See* Long-term and intensive psychotherapy
Internet-based approaches to alcoholism, 189
Interpersonal group psychotherapy (IGP), for borderline personality disorder, 69–70
Interpersonal psychotherapy (IPT)
    for depression, 141, **162, 172**
        cost-effectiveness of, 145, 147, 153–154
        group therapy, 144
        in postpartum period, 142–143
    for dysthymia, 149–150, **167**
Iraq war veterans, 4, 90
Irritable bowel syndrome (IBS), 246–248
Irwin et al. (1999), 202
Israel et al. (1996), 188
Issakidis et al. (2004), 94, **102**, 107–108, 112–113, 114, **133**

Jacobsen et al. (2002), 238, **256**
Jacobson (1996), 233
Jarrett et al. (2001), 143
Jenike (1993), 110, **129**
Jensen et al. (2005), 275, **286**
Johannesson et al. (1995), 240
Johnson et al. (1941), 271
Johnson et al. (2007), 244, **263**
Johnson-Masotti et al. (2000), 245
Jones and Vischi (1979), 8
Joyce et al. (1999), 69
Juvenile delinquency, 277, 280–281

Kadden et al. (1989), 198
Kamlet et al. (1992), 144, 145, **162**
Kashner et al. (1995), 233, 234
Katon (1987), 233
Katon et al. (2002), 106, **125**
Katon et al. (2006), 109, **127,** 242–243
Kazdin et al. (1990), 273, **284**
Keefe and Caldwell (1997), 246
Keller et al. (1998), 295–296, **307**
Kennedy et al. (2003), 107, **126**
Kent et al. (1004), 295
Kernberg (1975), 63
Kessler et al. (1982), 8, 235
Kessler et al. (2001), 192
Kessler et al. (2006), 105
Kessler et al. (2008), 5
Kidney transplant recipients, 248,
    **264**
King et al. (2000), 145, 148, **165**
Kissane et al. (2007), 237, **258**
Klarreich et al. (1998), 16
Klesges et al. (1999), 183
Klosko et al. (1990), 105
Koenigsberg and Handley (1986), 35
Koenigsberg et al. (1993), 35
Koerner and Linehan (2000), 72
Koons et al. (1998), 71, 74, **84**
Kopta et al. (1994), 292
Kosten et al. (1989), 198, **223**
Kraemer (2007), 191, **218**
Kraft et al. (1997), 194, **219**
Krizay (1990), 19

Kuchler et al. (2007), 236–237, **259**
Kunz et al. (2004), 191, **215**

Laberge et al. (1993), 105, **1122**
Landon and Barlow (2004), 108, **126**
Landry (1996), 189
Lash et al. (2005), 191, **215**
Lave et al. (1998), 145, 147, 153–154,
    **164**
Law and Tang (1995), 181–182
Learning disorders, 274
Leff et al. (1989), 34, 35, **50**
Leff et al. (1990), 34, **50**
Leff et al. (2000), 145, 149, **166**
Lehtinen (1993), 39, **52**
Leichsenring (2009), 292–293
Leichsenring and Rabung (2008), 292
Lemieux et al. (2006), 6, 237
Leukemia, 236
Levenson et al. (1990), 233
Levini et al. (2002), 112
Levitan and Kornfeld (1981), 244
Levy (2008), 72
Lewin et al. (2009), 241, **261**
Liberman et al. (1986), 37, **58**
Liberman et al. (1987), 39, **48**
Lichtenstein et al. (1996), 181
Lincoln et al. (2003), 112
Linden et al. (1996), 239–240
Linehan (1987), 70
Linehan (1993), 70
Linehan and Heard (1999), 297
Linehan et al. (1991), 64, 70–71, 73, 74,
    76, **84,** 297, 312
Linehan et al. (1993), 312
Linehan et al. (1994), 312
Linehan et al. (1999), 71–72, 73, 74, 75, **85**
Linn and Linn (1981), 238
Linn et al. (1982), 236
Linton (1994), 246
Liver cancer, 236–237, 259
Long-term and intensive
    psychotherapy, 18–19, 24,
    289–300, **304–310**
    cost-effectiveness of, 293–300

dialectical behavior therapy, 74, 291
indications for and efficacy of,
    290–293
methodological problems in
    devising studies of, 292
for personality disorders, 289–291,
    292
    borderline personality disorder,
        68, 74, 76, 289, 292
    psychodynamic psychotherapy,
        290–291
    search methodology for studies of,
        290
Loscalzo (1996), 246
Lost productivity, 2–3, 15
    due to anxiety disorders, 3, 104
        panic disorder, 106
    due to depression, 3, 135, 137, 140, 155
    due to schizophrenia, 31–32
    in workplace, 4–5, 16
Low back pain, 244, 246, **263**
Lubin et al. (1998), 93, **100**
Luborsky et al. (1993), 198, **224**
Luborsky et al. (2004), 235, **265**
Lung cancer, 236
Lymphoma, 236

MACT (manual-assisted cognitive-
    behavior therapy), for borderline
    personality disorder, 68–69, 74,
    76, **82**
Malingering, 9
Managed care, 10–11, 17, 19–21. *See
    also* Insurance coverage for mental
    health care
Manning et al. (1986), 19
Manual-assisted cognitive-behavior
    therapy (MACT), for borderline
    personality disorder, 68–69, 74,
    76, **82**
Manualized approach to psychother-
    apy, 9
March (1995), 111, **129**
March et al. (1994), 111, **129**
March et al. (1998), 93, **100**

March et al. (2007), 276, **286**
Marcotte and Wilcox-Gok (2001), 5
Marijuana use disorders, 175, 178.
    *See also* Substance abuse/
    dependence
    contingency management approach
        to, 197
    efficacy and cost-effectiveness of
        psychotherapy for, 196–197,
        **220, 222**
    meta-analysis of treatment outcome
        studies for, 192–193
    motivational enhancement therapy/
        cognitive-behavioral therapy
        for, 196–197
Marital therapy. *See* Couples therapy
Marks (1988), 110
Marks et al. (1993), 105
Mason and Kocsis (1991), 198
Mattson (2002), 185
May (1968), 33
Maynard et al. (1999), 198
Mayou et al. (1997), 239
McCrady and Langenbucher (1996),
    187, 189
McFarlane et al. (1995), 34, 39, **54**
McHugh et al. (2007), 109–110, **128**
McLellan et al. (1983), 198
MDFT (multidimensional family
    therapy), for marijuana use
    disorders, 196
Mead (1956), 179
Meares et al. (1999), 66, **82**, 298, **305**
Mecca (1997), 199–200
Medical illness, 6, 24, 227–249. *See also
    specific illnesses*
    case vignette of, 231–232
    disability and costs of depression
        compared with, 138–140
    emotional disorders in patients
        with, 228–229
    emotional distress, psychopathol-
        ogy and, 229–230
        effect on medical expenditures,
            233

Medical illness *(continued)*
  psychological interventions in,
    230–231, **256–266**
    cost-effectiveness of, 231
    for patients with cancer,
      235–238, **256–259**
    for patients with cardiovascular
      disease, 239–241,
      **260–261**
    for patients with chronic fatigue
      syndrome/myalgic
      encephalopathy, 248, **266**
    for patients with diabetes,
      241–244, **262**
    for patients with gastrointestinal
      disorders, 246–248
    for patients with HIV, 245
    for patients with musculoskeletal
      disease, 244–245, **263**
    for patients with pain, 245–246
    for patients with somatization
      disorder, 234
    role of, 231–232
    search methodology for studies
      of, 232–233
    for transplant recipients, 248,
      **264**
  substance-related, 201
    alcohol, 178
    nicotine, 177, 182
MEDLINE searches, 33–34, 61,
  87–88, 136, 176–177, 232, 268,
  290
Melanoma, 236
Menninger Foundation Psychotherapy
  Research Project, 290
Mental health care providers, 2,
  10–11
  psychotherapists, 10–11
  training of, 9, 10, 311
Mental Health Parity Act of 1996, 21
Mental health services
  inadequacy of, 7
  insurance coverage for, 7, 17–22
  utilization of, 7, 8, 9

Mental illness. *See also specific disorders*
  among American workers, 4–5
  burden of, 2
  concepts of, 5–7
  culture and, 5
  diagnostic categories of, 6–7
  disability due to, 1–2, 5
  economic costs of, 2–3
  epidemiology of, 1–5
  impact on income, 5
  misconceptions and prejudices
    about, 7–8, 9
  perceptions of medical illness
    compared with, 6, 7–8
  prevalence of, 2
  stigma of, 6, 7–8
  undertreatment of, 2
Mersch (1995), 112, **130**
Mescaline, 179
MET (motivational enhancement
  therapy)
  for alcoholism, 185, 186, 187
  for marijuana use disorders,
    196–197
Methadone-maintained patients
  contingency management for
    cocaine dependence among,
    195–196
  cost-effectiveness data for, 200
  harm reduction counseling for, 196
  interventions for stimulant abuse
    among, 197
  psychosocial treatments for,
    193–194, 195
  treatment matching for, 193
Methamphetamine addiction, 197
Meyer et al. (1981), 233, 234–235
MFGs (multiple family groups), for
  schizophrenia, 39
MI (myocardial infarction), 239–240
Miklowitz et al. (2003), 144
Miklowitz et al. (2008), 276, **287**
Miller et al. (1995), 186
Miller et al. (1998), 192, **226**
Miller et al. (2003), 150, **168**

Milrod et al. (2007), 110, **128**
Mind-body relationship, 228–229
Mindfulness-based cognitive therapy,
    for depression, 143
Mohrer et al. (2005), 184, **211**
Monsen and Monsen (2000), 299, **309**
Montero et al. (2001), 36, **57**
Moore et al. (2007), 195, **221**, 240–241,
    **261**
Moran et al. (1991), 241–242, 273–274,
    **285**, 295, **304**
Mortimer and Segal (2005), 190, **216**
Mosher (1999), 36
Motivational enhancement therapy
    (MET)
    for alcoholism, 185, 186, 187, 190
    for marijuana use disorders,
        196–197
Mueser et al. (2001), 36, 41, **57**
Multicenter Comparative Treatment
    Study of Panic Disorder, 109, **128**
Multidimensional family therapy
    (MDFT), for marijuana use
    disorders, 196
Multimodal Treatment Study of
    Children With ADHD, 275
Multiple family groups (MFGs), for
    schizophrenia, 39
Mumford et al. (1982), 234
Mumford et al. (1984), 8, 23
Mundt (2006), 190, **218**
Munroe-Blum and Marziali (1995), 64,
    69–70, 73, **84**
Murgraff et al. (2007), 188
Musculoskeletal disease, 245–246, **263**
Mynors-Wallis (1996), 145, 146, **163**
Mynors-Wallis et al. (1997), 16
Mynors-Wallis et al. (2000), 142, 156
Myocardial infarction (MI), 239–240,
    **260**

Naltrexone
    for alcoholism, 190
    for opiate dependence, 194
National Cancer Institute, 182

National Comorbidity Survey, 2, 104,
    110, 111, 113, 177, 178
National Comorbidity Survey
    Replication, 2, 3, 5, 88, 105, 110,
    111, 113, 136, 138
National Institute of Mental Health
    (NIMH)
    Collaborative Study of Depression,
        289–290
    Epidemiologic Catchment Area
        (ECA) surveys, 104, 110, 111,
        113, 137
    Multimodal Treatment Study of
        Children With ADHD, 275
    Treatment of Depression
        Collaborative Research
        Program, 141, 144
National Institute on Alcohol Abuse
    and Alcoholism, 185
National Vietnam Veterans
    Readjustment Study, 89
Nicotine. *See* Smoking/tobacco
    addiction
Nicotine replacement therapy (NRT),
    181–182, 183, 184
NIMH. *See* National Institute of
    Mental Health
North Carolina Department of
    Human Resources (1989), 277
Nortriptyline
    for depression, 147, **164**
    for smoking cessation, 183
NRT (nicotine replacement therapy),
    181–182, 183, 184
Nunes et al. (1991), 198
Nurses, 10
Nutritional counseling, for eating
    disorders, 299

Obsessive-compulsive disorder
    (OCD), 23, 110–111, 116, 229
    cognitive-behavioral therapy for,
        110–111, **129**
        for children and adolescents,
            110–111

Obsessive-compulsive disorder (OCD)
   (*continued*)
   cognitive-behavioral therapy for
      (*continued*)
      combined with
         pharmacotherapy, 23, 110
      cost-effectiveness of, 111
   costs of, 23, 110, 111
   epidemiology of, 110
O'Dowd et al. (2006), 248, **266**
Oehrberg et al. (1995), 105, **122**
O'Hara et al. (2000), 143
Olanzapine, for schizophrenia, 42
Olfson and Pincus (1994), 18
Olfson et al. (2002), 19
Olivier et al. (2007), 183
Olmstead et al. (2007), 197, **222**
Onken and Blaine (1990), 189
Opiate dependence. *See also* Substance
   abuse/dependence
   cost-effectiveness of treatments for,
      175, 195, **219, 221**
   culture and, 179
   meta-analysis of treatment outcome
      studies for, 192–193
   methadone-maintained patients
      with
      contingency management for
         cocaine dependence
         among, 195–196
      cost-effectiveness data for,
         200
      harm reduction counseling for,
         196
      interventions for stimulant abuse
         among, 197
      psychosocial treatments for,
         193–194, 195
      treatment matching for, 193
   predictors of treatment seeking for,
      192
   psychiatric comorbidity with, 176
Ornish (1990), 6
Osteoarthritis, 246
Otto et al. (2000), 106, **125**

Padgett et al. (1988), 242
Pain disorders, 245–246
   cancer-related, 236, 246
   chronic pelvic pain, 245
   cognitive-behavioral therapy for,
      244–245, 246
   depression and, 138
   low back pain, 244, 246, **263**
   psychodynamic body therapy for,
      299, **309**
Palmer et al. (2006), 69, 74, 76, 77, **83**
Pampallona et al. (2004), 156
Pancreatic cancer, 236–237, **259**
Panic attacks, 105
Panic disorder, 23, 104–110
   with or without agoraphobia, 105,
      108, 109, 111–112
   cognitive-behavioral therapy for,
      105–110, **122–128**
      combined with
         pharmacotherapy, 103,
         105–107, 109, 114
      cost-effectiveness of, 105–110,
         114
      effectiveness of, 105, 108
      guidelines for, 105
      impact on health care utilization,
         109
      long-term follow-up of, 108
      modifications of, 107
   comorbidity with, 105
   epidemiology of, 104–105
   physical symptoms of, 229
   psychodynamic psychotherapy for,
      110
   social morbidity of, 104
Paroxetine
   for depression, 151, **169**
   in irritable bowel syndrome,
      247–248
   for panic disorder, 105, 109, **122,
      128**
Partial hospitalization, for borderline
   personality disorder, 72–73, 76,
   296–297

Paul Wellstone and Pete Domenici
    Mental Health and Addiction
    Equity Act, 22
PBT (psychodynamic body therapy),
    for pain disorders, 299, **309**
Peirce et al. (2006), 197
Pelvic pain, chronic, 245
Perphenazine, for schizophrenia, 40
Perry et al. (1999), 64
Personal therapy, for schizophrenia,
    37, 42
Personality
    problems associated with Axis I
        disorders, 291, 300
    type A, 239
Personality disorders. *See also specific*
    *personality disorders*
    borderline personality disorder, 4,
        15, 23, 61–77, **81–86**
    cost-effectiveness of psychotherapy
        for, 16–17
    day treatment programs for,
        296–297
    functional impairment due to, 290
    long-term and intensive
        psychotherapy for, 289–291,
        292
    normalization of serotonin
        metabolism after
        psychotherapy for, 292
    prevalence of, 290
    substance abuse and, 176, 198
    suicide and, 290
Peters et al. (2000), 245–246
Petrou et al. (2006), 145, 152–153, **171**
Petry et al. (2005), 196
Pharmacotherapy, 10–11, 18. *See also*
    *specific drugs and classes*
    for alcoholism, 185, 187
        combined with psychotherapy,
        190
    for anxiety disorders, combined
        with psychotherapy, 103
        generalized anxiety disorder,
        107, 114

        obsessive-compulsive disorder,
        110–111, **129**
        panic disorder, 105–107, 109,
        114, **122–128**
    for attention-deficit/hyperactivity
        disorder, 269, 275, 281
    for borderline personality disorder,
        63
    for depression, 135, 136, 141, **162**
        combined with psychotherapy,
        142, 143, 144, 146–147,
        151, 156
        combined with psychotherapy
        for adolescents, 276
    for dysthymia, combined with
        interpersonal psychotherapy,
        149–150
    methadone maintenance for opiate
        dependence, 193–194
    for schizophrenia, 33, 37–38
        compliance with, 41
        cost-effectiveness of, 42, **60**
        psychosocial treatment and, 38
Phenelzine, for social phobia, 112, **131**
Phobic disorders, 23, 111–113. *See also*
    Agoraphobia; Social phobia
    case vignette of, 115–116
    epidemiology of, 111
    psychotherapy for, 112–113,
        **130–131**
Pirraglia et al. (2004), 150, **168**
PMRT (progressive muscle relaxation
    training), for cancer patients, 237,
    **257**
Postpartum depression, 142–143,
    152–153, 155, **171**
Posttraumatic stress disorder (PTSD),
    23, 87–95
    clinical features of, 88
    epidemiology of, 4, 87, 88–89
    eye movement desensitization and
        reprocessing for, 88
    functional impairment due to, 87,
        89, 95
    gender distribution of, 88

Posttraumatic stress disorder (PTSD)
(*continued*)
health care utilization and, 90–91
health problems and, 87, 89
morbidity of trauma and rape in
women, 4, 90–91
psychotherapy for, 87–95, **98–102**
case vignette of, 94–95
for children and adolescents, 92,
93
cognitive-behavioral therapy,
93, 95
cost-effectiveness of, 91, 92, 93,
94, 95, **102**
efficacy of, 91–94
exposure therapies, 91–93, 94,
95
for rape and crime victims, 92
review articles of, 94
search methodology for studies
of, 87–88
self-management therapy,
93–94, 154
stress inoculation training, 91
for survivors of terrorist attacks,
92, 93
trauma management therapy for
combat veterans, 91–92
risk factors for, 88
substance abuse and, 4, 88–89
among war veterans, 4, 87, 89–90
Powell et al. (1985), 187
Pregnancy
interventions for postpartum
depression, 142–143, 152–153,
155, **171**
substance abuse in, 179
Problem-solving treatment (PST) for
depression, 142, 146, **163**
in diabetes, 242, 243
Progressive muscle relaxation training
(PMRT), for cancer patients, 237,
**257**
Project MATCH, 185

PST (problem-solving treatment) for
depression, 142, 146, **163**
in diabetes, 242, 243
Psychiatrists, 2, 10–11
Psychoanalysis and psychoanalytic
psychotherapy, 9, 18, 291
for borderline personality disorder,
**85–86**
with children and adolescents, 271,
273–274
cost-effectiveness of, 293–297,
**304–305, 307**
for eating disorders, 299–300
effectiveness of, 292
Psychodynamic body therapy (PBT),
for pain disorders, 299, **309**
Psychodynamic psychotherapy, 9, 10,
17
for borderline personality disorder,
65–66, 312
compared with interpersonal
group psychotherapy, 69–
70
cost-effectiveness of, 295, 298,
**306**
effectiveness of long-term
treatment with, 292–293
for obsessive-compulsive disorder,
110
for panic disorder, 110, **128**
for personality disorders, 290–291
for posttraumatic stress disorder,
91, 95
for substance abuse, 180
Psychoeducation, 230
Psychological stress, 229–230
cardiovascular effects of, 239
immunological effects of, 229–230
Psychologists, 10
Psychotherapists, 8, 10–11
Psychotherapy, 8–9. *See also specific types
of psychotherapy*
for anxiety disorders, 23, 103–116,
**122–134**

for borderline personality disorder, 23, 61–77, **81–86**

for children and adolescents, 24, 267–282, **284–288**

cost-effectiveness of, 1, 8, 13–17, 22, 311–313

costs of, 11–13

definition of, 8–9, 230

for depression, 24, 135–157, **162–173**

insurance coverage for, 7, 17–22

lack of public knowledge about, 8–9

long-term and intensive, 18–19, 24, 289–300, **304–310**

manualized approach to, 9

for medically ill patients, 6, 24, 227–249, **256–266**

for posttraumatic stress disorder, 23, 87–95, **99–102**

reimbursement for, 10–11

for schizophrenia, 23, 31–43, **47–60**

for substance abuse, 24, 175–202, **210–226**

theoretical approaches to, 9, 10

utilization of, 17–19

PsycLIT searches, 34, 61

PTSD. *See* Posttraumatic stress disorder

Public knowledge about psychotherapy, 8–9

Puig-Antich (1985), 275

QI-Meds and QI-Therapy, for depression, 152, **170**

Quality-adjusted life years (QALYs), 14, 150, 157, 184, 185, 190

Quality-of-life effects of psychotherapy
in cancer, 237, 238
in cardiovascular disease, 239–240, 241
in irritable bowel syndrome, 247
in pain disorders, 246

RAND Corporation studies, 19, 21, 138

Rape. *See* Sexual abuse/assault

Rational-emotive therapy, for social phobia, 112, **130**

Ravindran et al. (1999), 142

Rayburn and Otto (2003), 105

Rees et al. (1998), 107

Regier et al. (1993), **225**

Reimbursement for psychotherapy, 10–11

Relaxation training
for cancer patients, 237, **257**
for generalized anxiety disorder, 113
for low back pain, 246
for panic disorder, 110, **128**

Residential treatment for substance abuse
alcoholism, 185, 187, 189, 191
cost-effectiveness of, 200
dually diagnosed patients, 198

Retzer et al. (1991), 145, **162**

Revicki et al. (2005), 151, **169**

Rheumatoid arthritis, 246

Richardson et al. (1990), 236

Rigotti and Pasternak (1996), 182

Risperidone, for schizophrenia, 38, 42, **60**

Roberge et al. (2005), 108, 109, **127**

Rosenheck et al. (1999), 233

Rosset and Andreoli (1995), 145, 146, **163**

Rounsaville et al. (1986), 198

Rudolf et al. (1994), 292

Rund et al. (1994), 34, 39, **53**

Ryle (1997), 67

Ryle and Golynkina (2000), 67, 74, **82**

Saeman (1994), 15

Saitz (2007), 192

Salvador-Carulla et al. (1995), 105–106, **123**

Sandell et al. (2000), 292

Sanders et al. (1994), 246

Satterfield et al. (1987), 274–275

SBI (screening and brief intervention) for alcoholism, 188–189, 191–192

Schepank Impairment Severity Score, 295

Schildhaus et al. (1998), 200

Schizoaffective disorder, 135, 145

Schizophrenia, 23, 31–43
  antipsychotics for, 33
    compliance with, 41
    cost-effectiveness of, 42, **60**
    psychosocial treatment and, 38
  brain pathology in, 33
  costs of, 31–32, 104
  definition of, 32
  diagnostic criteria for, 32
  disability due to, 2
  family expressed emotion and, 35, 41
  prevalence of, 4, 31
  psychosocial interventions for, 31–43, **47–60**
    case vignette of, 39–40
    cost-effectiveness of, 15, 39, 42, **59–60**
    discrepancy between outcomes of, 40–41
    effectiveness of, 34–38, 41–42, 312
    family interventions, 34–38, 312
    literature on, 34
    long-term psychotherapy, 289
    personal therapy, 37, 42
    pharmacotherapy and, 38
    search methodology for studies of, 33–34
    social skills training, 34–38
  substance abuse and, 198, 199
  subtypes of, 32

Schoenbaum et al. (2005), 145, 151–152, **170**

School phobia, 271

Schooler et al. (1997), 36, 41, **55**

Schulberg et al. (2002), 150, **167**

Schweikert et al. (2006), 244–245, **263**

Scott and Freeman (1992), 146, 156, **162**

Screening and brief intervention (SBI) for alcoholism, 188–189, 191–192

Searles (1965), 33

SEGT (supportive-expressive group therapy), for breast cancer patients, 237

Selective serotonin reuptake inhibitors (SSRIs)
  for depression, 151, **169**
    in adolescents, 276, **286**
  in irritable bowel syndrome, 247–248
  for panic disorder, 107, 114, **132**

Self-control, 7–8, 9

Self-control training, for alcoholism, 185

Self-destructive behaviors, in borderline personality disorder, 62

Self-help groups, 231

Self-management therapy, for comorbid posttraumatic stress disorder and depression, 93–94, 154, **173**

Self-psychological treatment (SPT), for eating disorders, 299–300, **307**

Seligman (1995), 292

Serotonin-norepinephrine reuptake inhibitors (SNRIs), for generalized anxiety disorder, 107, 114, **132**

Sertraline, for dysthymia, 142, 149, **167**

Services Research Outcomes Study (SROS), 200

Sexual abuse/assault, 4, 23
  borderline personality disorder and, 62
  chronic pelvic pain and, 245
  gastrointestinal disorders and, 246
  long-term effects of, 90
  posttraumatic stress disorder and, 4, 90–91, 95
    psychotherapy for, 92, 94–95, **98–99**

SFM (supportive family management), for schizophrenia, 36, **56, 57**

SFT (single family therapy), for schizophrenia, 39

Shaffer et al. (1997), 193

Sharp et al. (1997), 105

Shea et al. (1990), 290

Shea et al. (1992), 141

Shedler (in press), 293

Sick role, 7

Sigmon and Stitzer (2005), 195

Simon et al. (2007), 243–244

Simple phobia, 111. *See also* Phobic disorders

Single family therapy (SFT), for schizophrenia, 39

SIT (stress inoculation training), for posttraumatic stress disorder, 91, 94

Smit et al. (2006), 145, 153, **172**

Smith et al. (1986), 233, 234

Smith et al. (1995), 233, 234

Smoking cessation, 181–184, **210–213**
  cognitive-behavioral therapy for, 182–183
  cost-effectiveness of interventions for, 175, 182, 183, 184
  guidelines for health professionals, 181, 182
  nicotine replacement therapy for, 181–182, 183, 184
  outcomes related to intensity of treatment for, 182–184
  physician advice and encouragement for, 181, 182
  for preoperative patients, 183
  psychotherapy for, 181
  success rates for, 181, 183
  workplace interventions for, 184

Smoking/tobacco addiction, 181–184
  costs of, 177
  culture and, 179
  epidemiology of, 177, 178
  health risks of, 177, 182

SNRIs (serotonin-norepinephrine reuptake inhibitors), for generalized anxiety disorder, 107, 114, **132**

Social Adjustment Scale, 70

Social effectiveness therapy, for social phobia, 112, **130**

Social isolation, 229

Social phobia, 111
  psychotherapy for, 112, **130–131**

Social skills training (SST)
  for alcoholism, 185
  for combat-related posttraumatic stress disorder, 92
  for schizophrenia, 23, 33, 34
    case vignette of, 39–40
    clinical effectiveness of, 34–38, 41–42
    cost-effectiveness of, 39, 43
    summary of studies on, **58**
  for social phobia, 112, **130, 131**

Social workers, 10
  depression counseling by, 146

Solomon et al. (1992), 94, **102**

Somatization disorder, 234

Spiegel (1994), 238

Spiegel (1995), 238

Spiegel (1996), 233, 235

Spiegel (1999), 311

Spiegel and Bloom (1983), 246

Spiegel and Bruce (1997), 105, **123**

Spiegel and Wissler (1987), 34, **48**

Spiegel et al. (1981), 238

Spiegel et al. (1989), 6, 236

SPT (self-psychological treatment), for eating disorders, 299–300, **307**

SROS (Services Research Outcomes Study), 200

SSRIs (selective serotonin reuptake inhibitors), for panic disorder, 107, 114, **132**

SST. *See* Social skills training

State-Trait Anxiety Inventory, 237

Stead and Lancaster (2005), 184, **212**

Stevenson and Meares (1992), 65–66, 68, 74, 75, 76, **81**, 298, 312
Stevenson and Meares (1995), 312
Stevenson and Meares (1999), 298, **305**
Stigma, 6, 7–8
Stimulant abuse, 175, 197. *See also* Substance abuse/dependence
Stockholm Outcome of Psychoanalysis and Psychotherapy Project, 292
Stomach cancer, 236–237, **259**
Stone (1990), 74
Strain et al. (1991), 244
Stress, 229–230
    cardiovascular effects of, 239
    immunological effects of, 229–230
Stress inoculation training (SIT), for posttraumatic stress disorder, 91, 94
Stress management training
    for alcoholism, 185
    for cancer patients, 238
Strong Kinnaman et al. (2007), 199
Stuart et al. (2000), 105
Sturm (1997), 21
Substance abuse/dependence, 24, 175–202, **210–226**. *See also specific substances of abuse*
    age and, 179
    alcohol addiction, 184–192
    borderline personality disorder and, 75
        dialectical behavior therapy for, 71–72
    brief interventions for, 176
    case vignette of, 180–181
    cost-effectiveness of interventions for, 175–176, 199–200, 299
    costs of, 176, 177–180
    criminal activity and, 176, 180
    culture and, 179–180, 202
    disability due to, 1, 2
    epidemiology of, 4, 177–179
    genetic factors and, 180
    health risks of, 201
    marijuana, cocaine, and opiate dependence, 192–197, 299

multimodal treatment for, 176
posttraumatic stress disorder and, 4, 88–89
predictors of treatment seeking for, 192
in pregnancy, 179
psychiatric comorbidity with, 176, 185, 197–199 (*See also* Dually diagnosed patients)
quitting without formal treatment for, 175–176
search methodology for studies of, 176–177
sexual victimization and, 90
survey studies of treatments for, 199–200, 202
therapeutic effect of treatments for, 199–200
time between onset and treatment seeking for, 192
tobacco addiction, 181–184
treatment matching for, 185–186, 193, 202
Suicide, 15
    adolescent, 3
    anxiety disorders and, 104
    depression and, 136, 137, 155
    incidence of, 137
    personality disorders and, 290
        borderline personality disorder, 62–63, 67
    sexual victimization and, 4
Support groups, 231
Supportive family management (SFM), for schizophrenia, 36, **56, 57**
Supportive listening, in irritable bowel syndrome, 246–247
Supportive psychotherapy, 9
    for borderline personality disorder, 298
    for posttraumatic stress disorder, 91
    for social phobia, 112, **131**
Supportive-expressive group therapy (SEGT), for breast cancer patients, 237

TADS (Treatment of Adolescents With Depression Study, 275–276, **286, 287**

Target and Fonagy (1994), 18, 278, 282, **288**

Tarrier et al. (1989), 34, 39, **51,** 312

Tarrier et al. (1991), 34, 39, **51**

Tarrier et al. (1994), 34, 35–36, 39, **51**

Taylor (1996), 112, **130**

Teasdale et al. (2000), 143

Telch and Lucas (1994), 105

Telephone counseling, for depression, 148, **165, 172**

Terrorist attack survivors, 92, 93, **100, 101**

Teufel and Volk (1988), 296, **304**

TFP (transference-focused psychotherapy), for borderline personality disorder, 67–68, 298

Time-limited psychotherapy, for borderline personality disorder, 67, 69–70

Tobacco use. *See* Smoking/tobacco addiction

Tracy et al. (2007), 199

Training in psychotherapy, 9, 10, 311

Transference-focused psychotherapy (TFP), for borderline personality disorder, 67–68, 298

Transplant recipients, 248, **264**

Trauma
  alcohol-related, 178
  posttraumatic stress disorder among victims of, 4, 23, 87, 88, 91–95

Trauma and grief-focused brief psychotherapy, 92, **99**

Trauma management therapy, 91–92

TrEAT (Trial for Early Alcohol Treatment), 190

Treatment of Adolescents With Depression Study (TADS), 275–276, **286, 287**

Treatment of Depression Collaborative Research Program, 141, 144

Treatment Strategies in Schizophrenia Study, 36

Trial for Early Alcohol Treatment (TrEAT), 190

Trijsburg et al. (1992), 238

Turner and Jensen (1993), 246

Turner et al. (1995), 112, **130**

Tutty et al. (2000), 145, 148, **165**

Twelve-step programs, 180
  for alcohol abuse, 185, 186, 187, 189
  for methamphetamine addiction, 197

Type A personality, 239

Tyrer et al. (2004), 68–69, 74, 76, 77, **82**

UKATT Research Team (2005), 190, **216**

UKATT Research Team (2008), 190

United Behavioral Health, 21

U.S. Department of Health and Human Services (1996), 181

Utilization of mental health services, 7, 8, 9
  insurance coverage and, 7, 17–19

van Balkom et al. (1998), 110

Van Dulmen et al. (1996), 247

Vandrey et al. (2007), 195–196

Vaughn et al. (1982), 35

Verbosky et al. (1993), 145, 146, **163,** 233

Victimization of women, 4, 90–91

Videotaped self-confrontation, for alcoholism, 185, 186–187

Vietnam War veterans, 4, 89

Viinamaki et al. (1998), 292

Vincelli et al. (2003), 107, **126**

Violence
  alcohol-related, 179
  posttraumatic stress disorder and, 4, 87–91

Vocational rehabilitation, for schizophrenia, 40

Von Korff et al. (1998), 145, 146–147, **164**

von Rad et al. (1998), 292
Vos et al. (2005), 38, **59**, 152, **171**

Wade et al. (1998), 105
Waldinger (1987), 63
Waldinger and Frank (1989), 63
Waldinger and Gunderson (1984), 63,
    64
Waldinger and Gunderson (1987), 63
Walker et al. (2000), 143
Walker et al. (2003), 90
War veterans, posttraumatic stress
    disorder among, 4, 87, 89–90, 95
    psychotherapy for, 91–94, **98, 101**
Weiss and Hechtman (1986), 274
Weissman (1993), 142
Weisz and Weiss (1993), 272, 273, 277,
    **284**
Weisz et al. (1987), 272–273, **284**
Weisz et al. (1990), 277
Weisz et al. (1992), 273
Wells and Sturm (1995), 231
Wells et al. (2007), 154–155, 156, **173**
West et al. (2000), 182, 183
Westmaas et al. (2000), 182
White et al. (2006), 188
Wiborg and Dahl (1996), 107, **123**
Wilberg et al. (1998), 296
Wilberg et al. (1999), 296

Wolfenden et al. (2005), 183
Wolff et al. (1997), 231
Woody et al. (1983), 198
Woody et al. (1985), 198
Woody et al. (1995), 193–194, 198
Workplace mental illness, 4–5
    alcohol abuse, 178
    cost-effectiveness of psychotherapy
        for, 15–16
    depression, 140, 155
World Health Organization, 1, 137,
    150–151
    CHOICE Project, 37, **59**, 151, **168**
    Technical Report Series 873, 192
World Health Organization (1998),
    192
World Trade Center attacks, 93, **101**
Wu et al. (2005), 32
Wyatt et al. (1995), 31

Years lived with disability (YLDs), 14,
    94, 107–108, 112–113, 114
Yoga therapy, for methadone-
    maintained patients, 193

Zarkin et al. (2005), 190, **217**
Zhang et al. (1994), 35, **54**
Zhang et al. (1998), 35, **56**
Zients (1993), 18

# Index of Treatment Studies

*Page numbers printed in* **boldface** *type refer to tables or figures.*

Agoraphobia treatment
  Bassler and Hoffmann (1994), 112,
    **132**
  Landon and Barlow (2004), 108,
    **126**
  Roberge et al. (2005), 108, **127**
  Williams and Falbo (1996), 114
Alcoholism treatment, **213–219**
  Alessi et al. (2007), 189
  Babor et al. (2007), 192, **218**
  Barrett et al. (2006), 191, **217**
  Bischof et al. (2008), 188
  Carroll and Rounsaville (1995), 189
  Cisler et al. (1998), 186, **214**
  Davidson et al. (2007), 190
  Doggrell (2006), 190
  Doran et al. (2004), 189, **214**
  Drummond (1997), 188
  Epstein and McCrady (1998),
    187–188
  Freeborn et al. (2000), 187
  French et al. (2008), 189, **219**
  Hester and Miller (2006), 190
  Holder et al. (1991), 185, 187, 188,
    189, **213**
  Howard (1993), 188
  Israel et al. (1996), 188
  Kraemer (2007), 191, **218**
  Kunz et al. (2004), 191, **215**
  Landry (1996), 189
  Lash et al. (2005), 191, **215**

Mattson (2002), 185
McCrady and Langenbucher
    (1996), 187, 189
Miller et al. (1995), 186
Mortimer and Segal (2005), 190,
    **216**
Mundt (2006), 190, **218**
Murgraff et al. (2007), 188
Onken and Blaine (1990), 189
Powell et al. (1985), 187
Saitz (2007), 192
UKATT Research Team (2005),
    190, **216**
UKATT Research Team (2008),
    190
White et al. (2006), 188
Zarkin et al. (2005), 190, **217**
Anxiety disorders treatment, **98–102,**
    **122–134**
  Abramowitz et al. (2003), 110
  Amir et al. (1998), 92, **100**
  Ball et al. (1996), 110
  Barlow et al. (1984), 113
  Barlow et al. (2000), 105, **124**
  Bassler and Hoffmann (1994), 112,
    **132**
  Beck et al. (1992), 105
  Brom et al. (1989), 91, **98**
  Butler et al. (1987), 113, **132**
  Clark et al. (1994), 105
  Clark et al. (1999), 107, **124**

Anxiety disorders treatment *(continued)*
    Cottraux et al. (2000), 112, **131**
    Difede et al. (2007), 93, **101**
    Drummond (1993), 110
    Dunn et al. (2007), 93–94, **101**
    Durham et al. (2005), 108, 114, **134**
    Durham et al. (2005), 93, 95, **100**
    Foa (1997), 92, **99**
    Foa et al. (1991), 91, **98**
    Foa et al. (2003), 94, **102**
    Frueh et al. (1996), 91–92, **98**
    Gava et al. (2007), 111, **129**
    Goenjian et al. (1997), 92, **99**
    Greenberg et al. (1999), 107
    Greist (1998), 110
    Hamblen et al. (2009), 91
    Harvey and Rapee (1995), 114
    Heimberg (1993), 112
    Heimberg et al. (1990), 112
    Heimberg et al. (1998), 112, **131**
    Heuzenroeder et al. (2004), 107,
        114, **132**
    Hofmann (2004), 112, **131**
    Issakidis et al. (2004), 94, **102**, 107–
        108, 112–113, 114, **133**
    Jenike (1993), 110, **129**
    Katon et al. (2002), 106, **125**
    Katon et al. (2006), 109, **127**
    Kennedy et al. (2003), 107, **126**
    Kessler et al. (2006), 105
    Klosko et al. (1990), 105
    Laberge et al. (1993), 105, **1122**
    Landon and Barlow (2004), 108,
        **126**
    Levini et al. (2002), 112
    Lincoln et al. (2003), 112
    Lubin et al. (1998), 93, **100**
    March (1995), 111, **129**
    March et al. (1994), 111, **129**
    March et al. (1998), 93, **100**
    Marks (1988), 110
    Marks et al. (1993), 105
    McHugh et al. (2007), 109–110,
        **128**
    Mersch (1995), 112, **130**

    Milrod et al. (2007), 110, **128**
    Oehrberg et al. (1995), 105, **122**
    Otto et al. (2000), 106, **125**
    Rayburn and Otto (2003), 105
    Rees et al. (1998), 107
    Roberge et al. (2005), 108, **127**
    Salvador-Carulla et al. (1995), 105–
        106, **123**
    Sharp et al. (1997), 105
    Solomon et al. (1992), 94, **102**
    Spiegel and Bruce (1997), 105, **123**
    Stuart et al. (2000), 105
    Taylor (1996), 112, **130**
    Telch and Lucas (1994), 105
    Turner et al. (1995), 112, **130**
    van Balkom et al. (1998), 110
    Vincelli et al. (2003), 107, **126**
    Wade et al. (1998), 105
    Wiborg and Dahl (1996), 107, **123**
    Williams and Falbo (1996), 114
Attention-deficit/hyperactivity
    disorder treatment
    Abikoff (1991), 269
    Jensen et al. (2005), 275, **286**
    Puig-Antich (1985), 275
    Satterfield et al. (1987), 274–275
    Weiss and Hechtman (1986), 274

Bipolar disorder treatment
    Huxley et al. (2000), 149, **166**
    Miklowitz et al. (2003), 144
    Miklowitz et al. (2008), 276, **287**
    Retzer et al. (1991), 145–146, **162**
Borderline personality disorder
    treatment, **81–86, 305, 308, 310**
    Abend et al. (1983), 63
    Aronson (1989), 64
    Bateman and Fonagy (1999), 74, 76,
        **85**, 297, **308**, 312
    Bateman and Fonagy (2000), 75, 77
    Bateman and Fonagy (2003), 76, **85**,
        297, **308**, 312
    Bateman and Fonagy (2008), 76, **86**,
        297, **308**, 312
    Brazier et al. (2006), 76

Buie and Adler (1982), 63
Clarkin et al. (2001), 67–68, 74, **82,** 298, **310**
Clarkin et al. (2007), 298, **310**
Gabbard et al. (1997), 63, 65, 77
Hall et al. (2001), 66, 75, 76, **81**
Heard (1994), 71, 75, 298
Hoke (1989), 68, 73, **81**
Howard et al. (1986), 74
Joyce et al. (1999), 69
Kernberg (1975), 63
Koerner and Linehan (2000), 72
Koons et al. (1998), 71, 74, **84**
Levy (2008), 72
Linehan (1987), 70
Linehan (1993), 70
Linehan and Heard (1999), 70, 297
Linehan et al. (1991), 64, 70–71, 73, 74, 76, **84,** 297, 312
Linehan et al. (1993), 312
Linehan et al. (1994), 312
Linehan et al. (1999), 71–72, 73, 74, 75, **85**
Meares et al. (1999), 66, **81,** 298, **305**
Munroe-Blum and Marziali (1995), 64, 69–70, 73, **84**
Palmer et al. (2006), 69, 74, 76, 77, **83**
Perry et al. (1999), 64
Ryle (1997), 67
Ryle and Golynkina (2000), 67, 74, **82**
Stevenson and Meares (1992), 65–66, 68, 74, 75, 76, **81,** 298, 312
Stevenson and Meares (1995), 312
Stevenson and Meares (1999), 298, **305**
Stone (1990), 74
Tyrer et al. (2004), 68–69, 74, 76, 77, **82**
Waldinger (1987), 63
Waldinger and Frank (1989), 63
Waldinger and Gunderson (1984), 63, 64
Waldinger and Gunderson (1987), 63
Wilberg et al. (1998), 296
Wilberg et al. (1999), 296

Cancer treatment, **256–259**
Andersen (1992), 236
Arathuzik (1994), 246
Cain et al. (1986), 238
Cheung et al. (2003), 237, **257**
Fawzy et al. (1990), 236
Fawzy et al. (1993), 236
Forester et al. (1985), 238
Gellert et al. (1993), 236
Jacobsen et al. (2002), 238, **256**
Kissane et al. (2007), 237, **258**
Kuchler et al. (2007), 236–237, **259**
Lemieux et al. (2006), 6, 237
Linn and Linn (1981), 238
Linn et al. (1982), 236
Loscalzo (1996), 246
Richardson et al. (1990), 236
Spiegel (1994), 238
Spiegel (1995), 238
Spiegel (1996), 235
Spiegel and Bloom (1983), 246
Spiegel et al. (1981), 238
Spiegel et al. (1989), 6, 236
Trijsburg et al. (1992), 238
Cardiac disease treatment, **260–261**
Blumenthal and Wei (1993), 239
Davidson et al. (2007), 240, **260**
Gould et al. (1995), 240
Johannesson et al. (1995), 240
Lewin et al. (2009), 241, **261**
Linden et al. (1996), 239–240
Mayou et al. (1997), 239
Moore et al. (2007), 240–241, **261**
Child and adolescent treatment, **284–288**
Abikoff (1991), 269
Casey and Berman (1985), 272, 273, **284**
Davidson et al. (1986), 277
Domino et al. (2008), 276, **287**

Child and adolescent treatment
  (*continued*)
  Finney et al. (1991), 274, **285**
  Fonagy and Target (1994), 278, 282,
    **288**
  Heinicke and Ramsey-Klee (1986),
    274, **285**
  Jensen et al. (2005), 275, **286**
  Johnson et al. (1941), 271
  Kazdin et al. (1990), 273, **284**
  March et al. (2007), 276, **286**
  Miklowitz et al. (2008), 276, **287**
  Moran et al. (1991), 241–242,
    273–274, **285, 295, 304**
  North Carolina Department of
    Human Resources (1989), 277
  Puig-Antich (1985), 275
  Sattfield et al. (1987), 274–275
  Target and Fonagy (1994), 278, 282,
    **288**
  Weiss and Hechtman (1986), 274
  Weisz and Weiss (1993), 272, 273,
    277, **284**
  Weisz et al. (1987), 272–273, **284**
  Weisz et al. (1992), 273
Cocaine abuse treatment
  Avants et al. (2004), 196
  Crits-Christoph and Siqueland
    (1996), 192–193
  Crits-Christoph et al. (1999), 299,
    **309**
  Crits-Christoph et al. (2001), 299,
    **309**
  Petry et al. (2005), 196
  Sigmon and Stitzer (2005), 195
  Vandrey et al. (2007), 195–196
Cost-effectiveness of psychotherapy
  Duehrssen and Jorswiek (1965), 8,
    294, **304**
  Follette and Cummings (1970), 8
  Gabbard et al. (1997), 15, 33
  Jones and Vischi (1979), 8
  Kessler et al. (1982), 8
  Klarreich et al. (1998), 16
  Mumford et al. (1984), 8, 23

Mynors-Wallis et al. (1997), 16
Saeman (1994), 15
Spiegel (1999), 311
Wells and Sturm (1995), 231
Wolff et al. (1997), 231

Depression treatment, **162–173**
  Arnow and Constantino (2003), 144
  Blatt (1992), 144, 290
  Blatt et al. (1995), 144, 290
  Bolton et al. (2003), 144
  Bosmans et al. (2007), 145,
    153–154, 156, **172**
  Bower et al. (2000), 145, 148, **165**
  Brown and Schulberg (1995), 141
  Browne et al. (2002), 145, 149–150,
    **167**
  Chisholm (2005), 145, 150–151,
    **168**
  Domino et al. (2008), 276, **287**
  Dunn et al. (2007), 145, 154, **173**
  Edgell et al. (2000), 145, 149, **166**
  Fava et al. (1994), 142
  Fava et al. (1996), 142
  Fava et al. (1998), 142
  Frank et al. (1990), 141
  Friedli et al. (2000), 145, 147–148,
    156, **164**
  Hengeveld et al. (1988), 145, **162**
  Huxley et al. (2000), 145, 149, **166**
  Jarrett et al. (2001), 143
  Kamlet et al. (1992), 144, 145, **162**
  King et al. (2000), 145, 148, **165**
  Lave et al. (1998), 145, 147,
    153–154, **164**
  Leff et al. (2000), 145, 149, **166**
  March et al. (2007), 276, **286**
  Miller et al. (2003), 150, **168**
  Mynors-Wallis (1996), 145, 146, **163**
  Mynors-Wallis et al. (2000), 142,
    156
  O'Hara et al. (2000), 143
  Pampallona et al. (2004), 156
  Petrou et al. (2006), 145, 152–153,
    **171**

Pirraglia et al. (2004), 150, **168**
Ravindran et al. (1999), 142
Retzer et al. (1991), 145, **162**
Revicki et al. (2005), 151, **169**
Rosset and Andreoli (1995), 145, 146, **163**
Schoenbaum et al. (2005), 145, 151–152, **170**
Schulberg et al. (2002), 150, **167**
Scott and Freeman (1992), 146, 156, **162**
Shea et al. (1992), 141
Smit et al. (2006), 145, 153, **172**
Teasdale et al. (2000), 143
Tutty et al. (2000), 145, 148, **165**
Verbosky et al. (1993), 145, 146, **163**, 233
Von Korff et al. (1998), 145, 146–147, **164**
Vos et al. (2005), 152, **171**
Walker et al. (2000), 143
Weissman (1993), 142
Wells and Sturm (1995), 231
Wells et al. (2007), 154–155, 156, **173**
Diabetes treatment
    Bernbaum et al. (1989), 242
    Fosbury et al. (1997), 242
    Hampson et al. (2001), 242, **262**
    Katon et al. (2006), 242–243
    Kent et al. (1994), 295
    Moran et al. (1991), 241–242, 273–274, **285**, 295, **304**
    Padgett et al. (1988), 242
    Simon et al. (2007), 243–244
Dialectical behavior therapy, **84–85**
    Heard (1994), 298
    Koerner and LInehan (2000), 72
    Koons et al. (1998), 71, 74, **84**
    Levy (2008), 72
    Linehan (1987), 70
    Linehan (1993), 70
    Linehan and Heard (1999), 297
    Linehan et al. (1991), 64, 70–71, 73, 74, 76, **84**, 297, 312

Linehan et al. (1993), 312
Linehan et al. (1994), 312
Linehan et al. (1999), 71–72, 73, 74, 75, **85**
Dual diagnosis treatment
    Carroll and Rounsaville (1992), 198
    Chen et al. (2006), 199, **224**
    Kadden et al. (1989), 198
    Kosten et al. (1989), 198, **223**
    Luborsky et al. (1993), 198, **224**
    Mason and Kocsis (1991), 198
    Maynard et al. (1999), 198
    McLellan et al. (1983), 198
    Nunes et al. (1991), 198
    Rounsaville et al. (1986), 198
    Strong Kinnaman et al. (2007), 199
    Tracy et al. (2007), 199
    Woody et al. (1983), 198
    Woody et al. (1985), 198
    Woody et al. (1995), 198

Eating disorders treatment
    Bachar et al. (1999), 299–300, **307**
Expressed emotion and mental disorders
    Brown et al. (1972), 35
    Hooley et al. (1986), 35
    Koenigsberg and Handley (1986), 35
    Koenigsberg et al. (1993), 35
    Vaughn et al. (1982), 35

Gastrointestinal disease treatment
    Creed et al. (2003), 247–248
Generalized anxiety disorder treatment, **132–134**
    Barlow et al. (1984), 113
    Bassler and Hoffmann (1994), 113, **132**
    Butler et al. (1987), 113, **132**
    Durham et al. (2005), 114, **134**
    Harvey and Rapee (1995), 114
    Heuzenroeder et al. (2004), 114, **132**
    Issakidis et al. (2004), 114, **133**

HIV disease treatment
  Johnson-Masotti et al. (2000), 245

Insurance coverage and treatment
    utilization
  Andrews (1989), 18
  Doidge et al. (1994), 18
  Dossmann et al. (1997), 17
  Hay Huggins (1990), 19
  Krizay (1990), 19
  Manning et al. (1986), 19
  Olfson and Pincus (1994), 18
  Olfson et al. (2002), 19
  Target and Fonagy (1994), 18
  Zients (1993), 18
Irritable bowel syndrome treatment
  Creed et al. (2003), 247–248
  Guthrie et al. (1993), 246–247
  Van Dulmen et al. (1996), 247

Long-term and intensive
    psychotherapy, **304–310**
  Bachar et al. (1999), 299–300, **307**
  Bannon et al. (1995), 290–991
  Bateman and Fonagy (1999), 74, 76,
    **85**, 297, **308**, 312
  Bateman and Fonagy (2003), 76, **85**,
    297, **308**, 312
  Bateman and Fonagy (2008), 76, **86**,
    297, **308**, 312
  Blatt (1992), 144, 290
  Blatt et al. (1995), 144, 290
  Clarkin et al. (2001), 67–68, 74, **82**,
    298, **310**
  Clarkin et al. (2007), 298, **310**
  Crits-Christoph et al. (1999), 299,
    **309**
  Crits-Christoph et al. (2001), 299,
    **309**
  Dossmann et al. (1997), 292, 295,
    **306**
  Duehrssen (1962), 294, **304**
  Duehrssen and Jorswiek (1965), 8,
    294, **304**
  Fonagy (2002), 292

Gabbard (2000), 289
Grande et al. (2006), 292
Hall et al. (2001), 298, **305**
Heard (1994), 298
Heinzel et al. (1996), 294, **305**
Hoglend (1993), 292
Howard et al. (1986), 292
Keller et al. (1998), 295–296, **307**
Kopta et al. (1994), 292
Leichsenring (2009), 292–293
Leichsenring and Rabung (2008),
    292
Linehan and Heard (1999), 297
Linehan et al. (1991), 297
Meares et al. (1999), 66, **81**, 298,
    **305**
Monsen and Monsen (2000), 299,
    **309**
Moran et al. (1991), 241–242,
    273–274, **285**, 295, **304**
Rudolf et al. (1994), 292
Sandell et al. (2000), 292
Seligman (1995), 292
Shea et al. (1990), 290
Shedler (in press), 293
Stevenson and Meares (1992),
    65–66, 68, 74, 75, 76, **81**, 298,
    312
Stevenson and Meares (1999), 298,
    **305**
Teufel and Volk (1988), 296, **304**
von Rad et al. (1998), 292
Wilberg et al. (1998), 296
Wilberg et al. (1999), 296

Marijuana abuse treatment
  Crits-Christoph and Siqueland
    (1996), 192–193
  Dennis et al. (2004), 196, **220**
  Olmstead et al. (2007), 197, **222**
Medical illness and psychosocial
    interventions, **256–266**
  Andersen (1992), 236
  Arathuzik (1994), 246
  Baines et al. (2004), 248, **264**

Bernbaum et al. (1989), 242
Blumenthal and Wei (1993), 239
Cain et al. (1986), 238
Cheung et al. (2003), 237, **257**
Cohen et al. (1997), 233
Creed et al. (2003), 247–248
Davidson et al. (2007), 240, **260**
Druss et al. (2000), 233
Fawzy et al. (1990), 236
Fawzy et al. (1993), 236
Feuerstein et al. (1999), 244
Forester et al. (1985), 238
Fosbury et al. (1997), 242
Gavard et al. (1993), 233
Gellert et al. (1993), 236
Gould et al. (1995), 240
Guthrie et al. (1993), 246–247
Haddock et al. (1997), 245
Hampson et al. (2001), 242, **262**
Hellman et al. (1990), 233
Jacobsen et al. (2002), 238, **256**
Jacobson (1996), 233
Johannesson et al. (1995), 240
Johnson et al. (2007), 244, **263**
Johnson-Masotti et al. (2000), 245
Kashner et al. (1995), 233, 234
Katon (1987), 233
Katon et al. (2006), 242–243
Keefe and Caldwell (1997), 246
Kessler et al. (1982), 235
Kissane et al. (2007), 237, **258**
Kuchler et al. (2007), 236–237, **259**
Lemieux et al. (2006), 6, 237
Levenson et al. (1990), 233
Levitan and Kornfeld (1981), 244
Lewin et al. (2009), 241, **261**
Linden et al. (1996), 239–240
Linn and Linn (1981), 238
Linn et al. (1982), 236
Linton (1994), 246
Loscalzo (1996), 246
Luborsky et al. (2004), 235, **265**
Mayou et al. (1997), 239
Meyer et al. (1981), 233, 234–235
Moore et al. (2007), 240–241, **261**

Moran et al. (1991), 241–242,
273–274, **285**, 295, **304**
Mumford et al. (1982), 234
O'Dowd et al. (2006), 248, **266**
Padgett et al. (1988), 242
Peters et al. (2000), 245–246
Richardson et al. (1990), 236
Rosenheck et al. (1999), 233
Sanders et al. (1994), 246
Schweikert et al. (2006), 244–245,
**263**
Simon et al. (2007), 243–244
Smith et al. (1986), 233, 234
Smith et al. (1995), 233, 234
Spiegel (1994), 238
Spiegel (1995), 238
Spiegel (1996), 233, 235
Spiegel and Bloom (1983), 246
Spiegel et al. (1981), 238
Spiegel et al. (1989), 6, 236
Strain et al. (1991), 244
Trijsburg et al. (1992), 238
Turner and Jensen (1993), 246
Van Dulmen et al. (1996), 247
Verbosky et al. (1993), 233
Musculoskeletal disease treatment, **263**
Feuerstein et al. (1999), 244
Johnson et al. (2007), 244, **263**
Levitan and Kornfeld (1981), 244
Schweikert et al. (2006), 244–245,
**263**
Strain et al. (1991), 244

Obsessive-compulsive disorder
treatment, **129**
Abramowitz et al. (2003), 110
Ball et al. (1996), 110
Drummond (1993), 110
Gava et al. (2007), 111, **129**
Greist (1998), 110
Jenike (1993), 110, **129**
March (1995), 111, **129**
March et al. (1994), 111, **129**
Marks (1988), 110
van Balkom et al. (1998), 110

Opiate dependence treatment,
193–194
Avants et al. (1998), 193
Brooner et al. (2007), 195
Carroll et al. (1994), 194–195
Carroll et al. (2001), 194
Crits-Christoph and Siqueland
(1996), 192–193
Gross et al. (2006), 195
Kraft et al. (1997), 194, **219**
Moore et al. (2007), 195, **221**
Shaffer et al. (1997), 193
Woody et al. (1995), 193–194

Pain disorders treatment
Arathuzik (1994), 246
Haddock et al. (1997), 245
Keefe and Caldwell (1997), 246
Linton (1994), 246
Loscalzo (1996), 246
Monsen and Monsen (2000), 299,
**309**
Peters et al. (2000), 245–246
Sanders et al. (1994), 246
Spiegel and Bloom (1983), 246
Turner and Jensen (1993), 246
Panic disorder treatment, **122–128**
Barlow et al. (2000), 105, **124**
Beck et al. (1992), 105
Clark et al. (1994), 105
Clark et al. (1999), 107, **124**
Durham et al. (2005), 108, **134**
Greenberg et al. (1999), 107
Heuzenroeder et al. (2004), 107,
**132**
Issakidis et al. (2004), 107–108, **133**
Katon et al. (2002), 106, **125**
Katon et al. (2006), 109, **127**
Kennedy et al. (2003), 107, **126**
Kessler et al. (2006), 105
Klosko et al. (1990), 105
Laberge et al. (1993), 105, **1122**
Landon and Barlow (2004), 108,
**126**
Marks et al. (1993), 105

McHugh et al. (2007), 109–110,
**128**
Milrod et al. (2007), 110, **128**
Oehrberg et al. (1995), 105, **122**
Otto et al. (2000), 106, **125**
Rayburn and Otto (2003), 105
Rees et al. (1998), 107
Roberge et al. (2005), 109, **127**
Salvador-Carulla et al. (1995),
105–106, **123**
Sharp et al. (1997), 105
Spiegel and Bruce (1997), 105, **123**
Stuart et al. (2000), 105
Telch and Lucas (1994), 105
Vincelli et al. (2003), 107, **126**
Wade et al. (1998), 105
Wiborg and Dahl (1996), 107, **123**
Williams and Falbo (1996), 114
Personality disorders treatment,
**81–86, 305, 308, 310**
Abend et al. (1983), 63
Aronson (1989), 64
Bateman and Fonagy (1999), 74, 76,
**85, 297, 308,** 312
Bateman and Fonagy (2000), 75, 77
Bateman and Fonagy (2003), 76, **85,**
297, **308,** 312
Bateman and Fonagy (2008), 76, **86,**
297, **308,** 312
Beecham et al. (2006), 17
Brazier et al. (2006), 76
Buie and Adler (1982), 63
Chiesa et al. (2002), 16–17
Clarkin et al. (2001), 67–68, 74, **82,**
298, **310**
Clarkin et al. (2007), 298, **310**
Gabbard (2000), 289
Gabbard et al. (1997), 63, 65, 77
Hall et al. (2001), 66, 75, 76, **81**
Heard (1994), 71, 75, 298
Hoke (1989), 68, 73, **81**
Howard et al. (1986), 74
Joyce et al. (1999), 69
Kernberg (1975), 63
Koerner and Linehan (2000), 72

Koons et al. (1998), 71, 74, **84**
Levy (2008), 72
Linehan (1987), 70
Linehan (1993), 70
Linehan and Heard (1999), 297
Linehan et al. (1991), 64, 70–71, 73,
    74, 76, **84,** 297, 312
Linehan et al. (1993), 312
Linehan et al. (1994), 312
Linehan et al. (1999), 71–72, 73, 74,
    75, **85**
Meares et al. (1999), 66, **81,** 298,
    **305**
Munroe-Blum and Marziali (1995),
    64, 69–70, 73, **84**
Palmer et al. (2006), 69, 74, 76, 77,
    **83**
Perry et al. (1999), 64
Ryle (1997), 67
Ryle and Golynkina (2000), 67, 74,
    **82**
Shea et al. (1990), 289
Stevenson and Meares (1992),
    65–66, 68, 74, 75, 76, **81,** 298
Stevenson and Meares (1995), 312
Stevenson and Meares (1999), 298,
    **305**
Stone (1990), 74
Tyrer et al. (2004), 68–69, 74, 76,
    77, **82**
Viinamaki et al. (1998), 292
Waldinger (1987), 63
Waldinger and Frank (1989), 63
Waldinger and Gunderson (1984),
    63, 64
Waldinger and Gunderson (1987),
    63
Wilberg et al. (1998), 296
Wilberg et al. (1999), 296
Phobic disorders treatment, **130–131**
Bassler and Hoffmann (1994), 112,
    **132**
Cottraux et al. (2000), 112, **131**
Heimberg (1993), 112
Heimberg et al. (1990), 112
Heimberg et al. (1998), 112, **131**
Hofmann (2004), 112, **131**
Issakidis et al. (2004), 112–113, **133**
Landon and Barlow (2004), 108,
    **126**
Levini et al. (2002), 112
Lincoln et al. (2003), 112
Mersch (1995), 112, **130**
Roberge et al. (2005), 108, **127**
Taylor (1996), 112, **130**
Turner et al. (1995), 112, **130**
Posttraumatic stress disorder
    treatment, **98–102**
Amir et al. (1998), 92, **100**
Brom et al. (1989), 91, **98**
Difede et al. (2007), 93, **101**
Dunn et al. (2007), 93–94, **101**
Durham et al. (2005), 93, 95, **100**
Foa (1997), 92, **99**
Foa et al. (1991), 91, **98**
Foa et al. (2003), 94, **102**
Frueh et al. (1996), 91–92, **98**
Goenjian et al. (1997), 92, **99**
Hamblen et al. (2009), 91
Issakidis et al. (2004), 94, **102**
Lubin et al. (1998), 93, **100**
March et al. (1998), 93, **100**
Solomon et al. (1992), 94, **102**
Primary care counseling
Bower and Rowland (2006), 16

Schizophrenia treatment, **47–60**
Bellack et al. (2000), 36, 41, **56**
Berglund et al. (2003), 36, 41, **57**
Brooker et al. (1994), 35, **52**
Chisholm (2005), 37, **59**
Eckman et al. (1992), 37, **58**
Falloon et al. (1987), 34, 39, **48**
Fromm-Reichmann (1950), 33
Glick et al. (1990), 34, **49**
Glick et al. (1993), 34, **49**
Gunderson et al. (1984), 33, 312
Gutierrez-Recacha et al. (2006), 38,
    **60**
Haas et al. (1988), 34, **49**

Schizophrenia treatment *(continued)*
 Hogarty (2002), 37
 Hogarty et al. (1986), 34–35, 37, **47**
 Hogarty et al. (1991), 34–35, 37, **47**
 Hogarty et al. (1995), 37
 Hogarty et al. (1997), 37
 Leff et al. (1989), 34, 35, **50**
 Leff et al. (1990), 34, **50**
 Lehtinen (1993), 39, **52**
 Liberman et al. (1986), 37, **58**
 Liberman et al. (1987), 39, **48**
 May (1968), 33
 McFarlane et al. (1995), 34, 39, **54**
 Mosher (1999), 36
 Mueser et al. (2001), 36, 41, **57**
 Rund et al. (1994), 34, 39, **53**
 Schooler et al. (1997), 36, 41, **55**
 Searles (1965), 33
 Spiegel and Wissler (1987), 34, **48**
 Tarrier et al. (1989), 34, 39, **51**, 312
 Tarrier et al. (1991), 34, 39, **51**
 Tarrier et al. (1994), 34, 35–36, 39, **51**
 Vos et al. (2005), 38, **59**
 Wu et al. (2005), 32
 Wyatt et al. (1995), 31
 Zhang et al. (1994), 35, **54**
 Zhang et al. (1998), 35, **56**
Smoking cessation, **210–213**
 Alterman et al. (2001), 182, **210**
 Brandon (2001), 182
 Centers for Disease Control and Prevention (1993), **210**
 Centers for Disease Control and Prevention (1994), **210**
 Gordon et al. (2007), 184, **213**
 Hall et al. (1998), 183
 Halpin et al. (2006), 183–184, **212**
 Klesges et al. (1999), 183
 Law and Tang (1995), 181–182
 Lichtenstein et al. (1996), 181
 Mohrer et al. (2005), 184, **211**
 Olivier et al. (2007), 183
 Rigotti and Pasternak (1996), 182
 Stead and Lancaster (2005), 184, **212**

U.S. Department of Health and Human Services (1996), 181
 West et al. (2000), 182, 183
 Westmaas et al. (2000), 182
 Wolfenden et al. (2005), 183
Social phobia treatment, **130–131**
 Cottraux et al. (2000), 112, **131**
 Heimberg (1993), 112
 Heimberg et al. (1990), 112
 Heimberg et al. (1998), 112, **131**
 Hofmann (2004), 112, **131**
 Mersch (1995), 112, **130**
 Taylor (1996), 112, **130**
 Turner et al. (1995), 112, **130**
Stimulant abuse treatment
 Donovan and Wells (2007), 197
 Peirce et al. (2006), 197
Substance abuse treatment, **210–226**
 Alessi et al. (2007), 189
 Alterman et al. (2001), 182, **210**
 Anglin and Hser (1990), 200
 Avants et al. (1998), 193
 Avants et al. (2004), 196
 Babor et al. (2007), 192, **218**
 Barrett et al. (2006), 191, **217**
 Bischof et al. (2008), 188
 Brandon (2001), 182
 Brooner et al. (2007), 195
 Burke et al. (2002), 201
 Carroll and Rounsaville (1992), 198, 201
 Carroll and Rounsaville (1995), 189
 Carroll et al. (1994), 194–195, 201, 202
 Carroll et al. (1998), 201
 Carroll et al. (2001), 194
 Chen et al. (2006), 199, **224**
 Cisler et al. (1998), 186, **214**
 Crits-Cristoph and Siqueland (1996), 192–193
 Crits-Cristoph et al. (1999), 299, **309**
 Crits-Cristoph et al. (2001), 299, **309**
 Davidson et al. (2007), 190
 Dennis et al. (2004), 196, **220**

Doggrell (2006), 190
Donovan and Wells (2007), 197
Doran et al. (2004), 189, **214**
Drummond (1997), 188
Epstein and McCrady (1998), 187–188
Freeborn et al. (2000), 187
French et al. (2008), 189, **219**
Gerstein et al. (1994), 192, **226**
Gordon et al. (2007), 184, **213**
Gross et al. (2006), 195
Hall et al. (1998), 183
Halpin et al. (2006), 183–184, **212**
Hester and Miller (2006), 190
Holder et al. (1991), 185, 187, 188, 189, **213**
Howard (1993), 188
Irwin et al. (1999), 202
Israel et al. (1996), 188
Kadden et al. (1989), 198
Kessler et al. (2001), 192
Klesges et al. (1999), 183
Kosten et al. (1989), 198, **223**
Kraemer (2007), 191, **218**
Kraft et al. (1997), 194, **219**
Kunz et al. (2004), 191, **215**
Landry (1996), 189
Lash et al. (2005), 191, **215**
Law and Tang (1995), 181–182
Lichtenstein et al. (1996), 181
Luborsky et al. (1993), 198, **224**
Mason and Kocsis (1991), 198
Mattson (2002), 185
Maynard et al. (1999), 198
McCrady and Langenbucher (1996), 187, 189
McLellan et al. (1983), 198
Mecca (1997), 199–200
Miller et al. (1995), 186
Miller et al. (1998), 192, **226**
Mohrer et al. (2005), 184, **211**
Moore et al. (2007), 195, **221**

Mortimer and Segal (2005), 190, **216**
Mundt (2006), 190, **218**
Murgraff et al. (2007), 188
Nunes et al. (1991), 198
Olivier et al. (2007), 183
Olmstead et al. (2007), 197, **222**
Onken and Blaine (1990), 189
Peirce et al. (2006), 197
Petry et al. (2005), 196
Powell et al. (1985), 187
Regier et al. (1993), **225**
Rigotti and Pasternak (1996), 182
Rounsaville et al. (1986), 198
Saitz (2007), 192
Schildhaus et al. (1998), 200
Shaffer et al. (1997), 193
Sigmon and Stitzer (2005), 195
Stead and Lancaster (2005), 184, **212**
Strong Kinnaman et al. (2007), 199
Tracy et al. (2007), 199
UKATT Research Team (2005), 190, **216**
UKATT Research Team (2008), 190
U.S. Department of Health and Human Services (1996), 181
Vandrey et al. (2007), 195–196
West et al. (2000), 182, 183
Westmaas et al. (2000), 182
White et al. (2006), 188
Wolfenden et al. (2005), 183
Woody et al. (1983), 198
Woody et al. (1985), 198
Woody et al. (1995), 193–194, 198
World Health Organization (1998), 192
Zarkin et al. (2005), 190, **217**

Transplantation and psychotherapy
Baines et al. (2004), 248, **264**